Watkins' Manual of Foot and Ankle Medicine and Surgery

FIFTH EDITION

Watkins' Manual of Foot and Ankle Medicine and Surgery

FIFTH EDITION

Leon Watkins, DPM, FACFAS, CWS
Gulf South Medical Group
Metairie, Louisiana

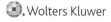

Wolters Kluwer

Philadelphia · Baltimore · New York · London
Buenos Aires · Hong Kong · Sydney · Tokyo

Acquisitions Editor: Tulie McKay
Senior Development Editor: Stacey Sebring
Editorial Coordinator: Sunmerrilika Baskar
Marketing Manager: Kirsten Watrud
Production Project Manager: Bridgett Dougherty
Manager, Graphic Arts & Design: Stephen Druding
Manufacturing Coordinator: Beth Welsh
Prepress Vendor: S4Carlisle Publishing Services

5th edition

9 8 7 6 5 4 3 2 1

Printed in Singapore

Library of Congress Cataloging-in-Publication Data

ISBN-13: 978-1-9751-7552-8

ISBN-10: 1-975175-52-2

Cataloging in Publication data available on request from publisher.

MKO722

Dedicated to my wife, Maria, and my children,
Maxwell and Oliver

CONTENTS

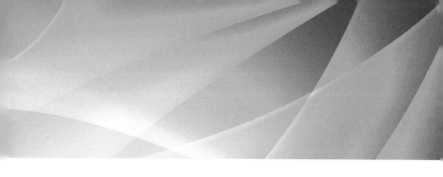

Watkins' Manual of Foot and Ankle Medicine and Surgery

FIFTH EDITION

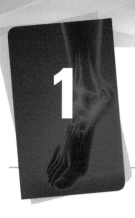

1 ANATOMY

CRANIAL NERVES

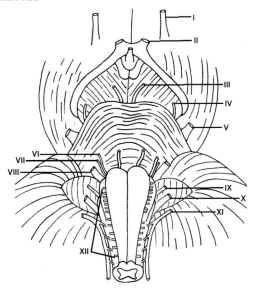

Nerve	Name[a]	Function	Type
I	Olfactory	Smell	Sensory
II	Optic	Vision	Sensory
III	Oculomotor	Eye muscles, accommodation	Motor
IV	Trochlear	One eye muscle	Motor
V	Trigeminal	Sensation to face/oral, muscles of mastication	Both
VI	Abducens	One eye muscle	Motor
VII	Facial	Taste, muscles of facial expression, secretions of lacrimal, mucosal, and some salivary glands	Both
VIII	Vestibulocochlear (or Auditory)	Hearing, sense of equilibrium	Sensory
IX	Glossopharyngeal	Sensation from pharynx, taste, one pharyngeal muscle, secretion of one salivary gland	Both
X	Vagus	Sensation from pharynx and larynx, taste, muscles of palate, pharynx, larynx, and one tongue muscle, parasympathetic to thorax and upper abdomen	Both
XI	Accessory	Two neck muscles	Motor
XII	Hypoglossal	Tongue muscles	Motor

[a]Mnemonic for names of cranial nerves: *O*n *O*ld *O*lympus *T*owering *T*op *A* *F*in *A*nd *G*erman *V*iewed *A* *H*op.

BLOOD SUPPLY TO THE TALUS

Posterior tubercle: The medial calcaneal artery anastomoses with a branch from the peroneal artery to supply this area.

Body: Supplied by the artery of the sinus tarsi and the artery of the tarsal canal; both anastomose

with each other as well as with the deltoid branches.

Head/neck: Supplied by direct branches off the dorsalis pedis artery or anterior tibial artery and the anastomoses that the dorsalis pedis makes with the deltoid branches and the artery of the sinus tarsi

Anterior Tibial Artery/Dorsalis Pedis
Supplies 36.2% of talus
Supplies most of the head and neck of talus (dorsal medial 2/3rds)
Lateral tarsal branch contributes to the tarsal canal artery
Medial tarsal branch contributes to the artery of the tarsal canal

Lateral tarsal artery

Artery of the tarsal sinus

Perforating Peroneal Artery
Supplies 16.9% of talus
Contributes to the artery of the tarsal sinus
Supplies the lateral process, lateral 1/3 of the body, and lateral plantar portion of the talar head
Calcaneal branches of the peroneal artery contribute to posterior process

Medial tarsal artery

Medial and lateral plantar arteries

Artery of the tarsal canal

Deltoid artery

Interosseus membrane

Posterior Tibial Artery
Supplies 47% of talux *(most important)*
BRANCHES: Deltoid artery (supplies medial body)
             Artery of the tarsal canal (supplies most of the body)
             Calaneal branch (supplies the posterior process)

Peroneal artery

NERVES TO THE LOWER EXTREMITY

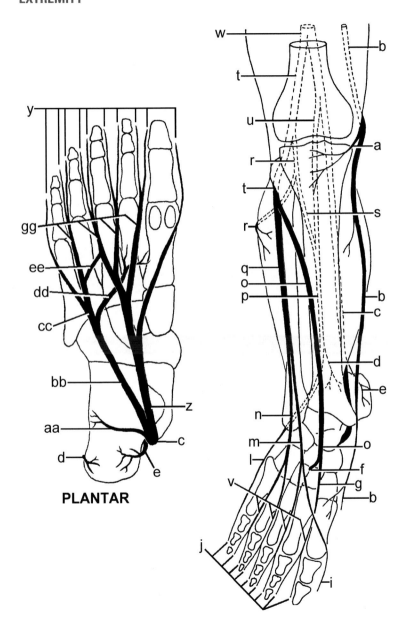

PLANTAR

a. Infrapatellar branch of the saphenous nerve

b. Saphenous nerve (L3, L4)

c. Tibial nerve

d. Lateral calcaneal nerve

e. Medial calcaneal nerve

f. Lateral branch of deep peroneal nerve

g. Medial branch of deep peroneal nerve

i. 1st dorsal digital proper nerve

j. 2nd to 10th dorsal digital proper nerve

l. Lateral dorsal cutaneous nerve

m. Medial dorsal cutaneous nerve

n. Intermediate dorsal cutaneous nerve

o. Deep peroneal nerve

p. Sural nerve

q. Superficial peroneal nerve

r. Lateral sural cutaneous nerve

s. Peroneal communicating branch

t. Common peroneal nerve

u. Medial sural cutaneous nerve

v. 1st to 4th common dorsal digital nerve

w. Sciatic nerve (L4–S3)

y. 1st to 10th proper plantar digital nerve

z. Medial plantar nerve

aa. Infracalcaneal nerve (nerve to the abductor digiti minimi), aka Baxter nerve

bb. Lateral plantar nerve

cc. Superficial branch of lateral plantar nerve

dd. Deep branch of lateral plantar nerve

ee. Communicating branch

gg. 1st to 4th common plantar digital nerve

Nerves of the foot

Medial Plantar n. (L4, L5)

Deep Peroneal n. (L4, L5)

Lateral Plantar n. (L4, L5)

Sural n. (L3, L4)

Saphenous n. (L3, L4)

Superficial Peroneal n. (L4, L5, L6)

Medial Calcaneal branch of Tibial n. (S1, S2)

BLOOD SUPPLY TO THE LOWER EXTREMITY

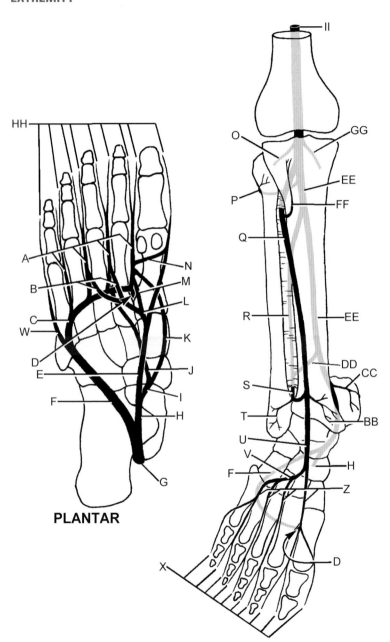

PLANTAR

Arteries of the Lower Extremity

A. 1st to 4th plantar metatarsal arteries

B. 2nd and 3rd common superficial plantar digital arteries

C. Medial or deep branch of the lateral plantar artery (deep plantar arch)

D. Deep plantar artery

E. Superficial branch of medial plantar artery

F. Lateral plantar artery

G. Posterior tibial artery

H. Medial plantar artery

I. Deep branch of the medial plantar artery

J. Lateral branch of the deep branch of the medial plantar artery

K. Medial branch of the deep branch of the medial plantar artery

L. Lateral branch of the superficial branch of the medial plantar artery

M. 1st common superficial plantar digital artery

N. Digital branch of the 1st plantar metatarsal artery

O. Lateral sural artery (an end artery)

P. Circumflex fibular artery

Q. Anterior tibial artery

R. Peroneal artery

S. Perforating branch of peroneal artery

T. Anterior lateral malleolar artery

U. Dorsalis pedis artery

V. Arcuate artery

W. Superficial branch of the lateral plantar artery

X. 1st to 10th dorsal digital proper arteries

Z. 1st to 4th dorsal metatarsal arteries

BB. Anterior medial malleolar artery

CC. Medial calcaneal artery

DD. Communicating branch of the peroneal artery

EE. Posterior tibial artery

FF. Anterior tibial recurrent artery

GG. Medial sural artery (an end artery)

HH. 1st to 4th plantar digital proper artery

II. Femoral artery

FOOT LIGAMENTS

Long Plantar Ligament (Long Calcaneocuboid Ligament)

This is not the same as the plantar fascia. The long plantar ligament originates on the plantar surface of the calcaneus just anterior to the tuberosity. It covers most of the plantar surface of the calcaneus and then divides into deep fibers, which insert into the peroneal ridge of the cuboid while longer superficial fibers continue over the peroneus longus tendon and insert into the base of the 2nd, 3rd, 4th, and 5th metatarsal bases. The superficial fibers complete the plantar portion of the osseofibrous canal called the peroneal canal through which the peroneus longus tendon is housed.

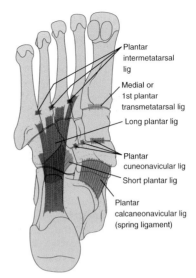

Plantar ligaments of the foot

Short Plantar Ligament (Short Calcaneocuboid Ligament)

Short plantar ligament lies deep to the long plantar ligament. It originates on the anterior tubercle of the calcaneus and inserts just proximal to the deep fibers of the long plantar ligament. The insertion of the short plantar ligament is wider than the long plantar ligament and extends onto the beak of the cuboid.

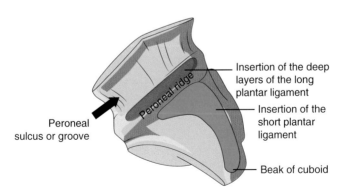

Plantar view of cuboid

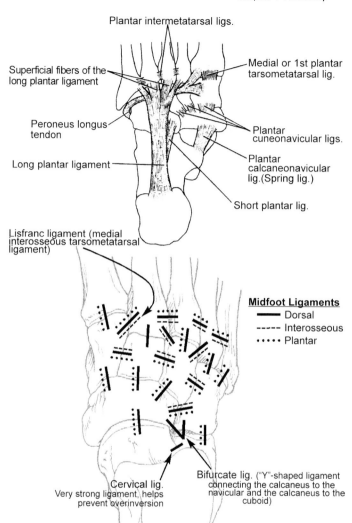

Plantar intermetatarsal ligs.

Superficial fibers of the long plantar ligament

Medial or 1st plantar tarsometatarsal lig.

Peroneus longus tendon

Plantar cuneonavicular ligs.

Long plantar ligament

Plantar calcaneonavicular lig.(Spring lig.)

Short plantar lig.

Lisfranc ligament (medial interosseous tarsometatarsal ligament)

Midfoot Ligaments
— Dorsal
----- Interosseous
····· Plantar

Cervical lig.
Very strong ligament, helps prevent overinversion

Bifurcate lig. ("Y"-shaped ligament connecting the calcaneus to the navicular and the calcaneus to the cuboid)

MIDFOOT LIGAMENTS

Retinacula and Tendon Orientation

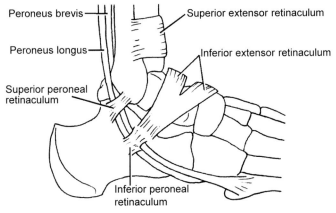

LATERAL ANKLE

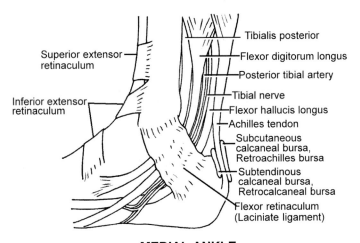

MEDIAL ANKLE

Mnemonic structures from anterior to posterior *T*om, *D*ick, *an*d *H*arry (alternative mnemonic: *T*imothy *D*oth *V*ex [Vein] *A* *N*ervous *H*orse)

*T*ibialis posterior, flexor *D*igitorum longus, (*V*ein) *A*rtery, *N*erve, flexor *H*allucis longus

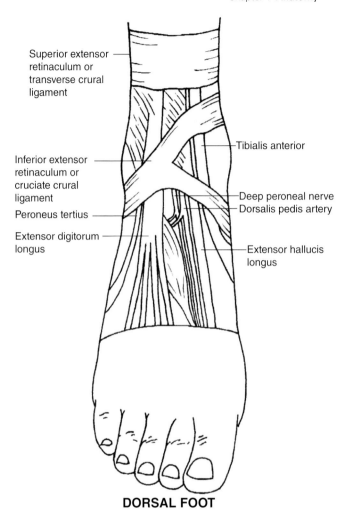

Superior extensor retinaculum or transverse crural ligament

Inferior extensor retinaculum or cruciate crural ligament

Peroneus tertius

Extensor digitorum longus

Tibialis anterior

Deep peroneal nerve
Dorsalis pedis artery

Extensor hallucis longus

DORSAL FOOT

| Mnemonic structures from medial to lateral *A HAND P* | *A*nt tib., ext. *H*allucis longus, *A*rtery, *N*erve, extensor *D*ig. longus, *P*eroneus tertius |

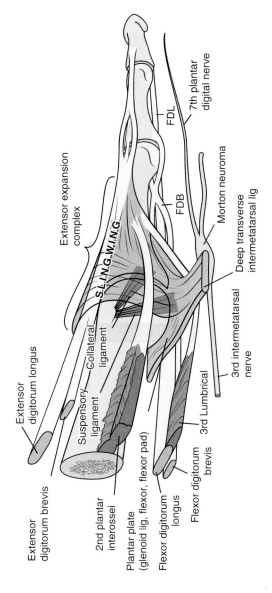

Extensor digitorum brevis

Extensor digitorum longus

2nd plantar interossei

Plantar plate (glenoid lig, flexor, flexor pad)

Suspensory ligament — Collateral ligament

Flexor digitorum longus

Flexor digitorum brevis

3rd Lumbrical

3rd intermetatarsal nerve

Extensor expansion complex

S.L.I.N.G-W.I.N.G

FDB

FDL

Morton neuroma

Deep transverse intermetatarsal lig

7th plantar digital nerve

Medial view of the 4th ray

SESAMOIDAL ATTACHMENTS

SESAMOIDAL ATTACHMENTS
(Plantar)

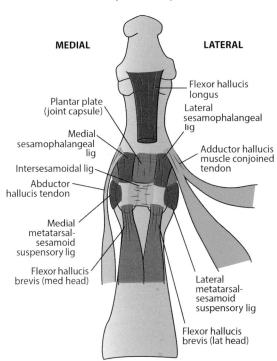

MEDIAL

LATERAL

Flexor hallucis longus

Plantar plate (joint capsule)

Lateral sesamophalangeal lig

Medial sesamophalangeal lig

Adductor hallucis muscle conjoined tendon

Intersesamoidal lig

Abductor hallucis tendon

Medial metatarsal-sesamoid suspensory lig

Flexor hallucis brevis (med head)

Lateral metatarsal-sesamoid suspensory lig

Flexor hallucis brevis (lat head)

SESAMOIDAL ATTACHMENTS
(Medial)

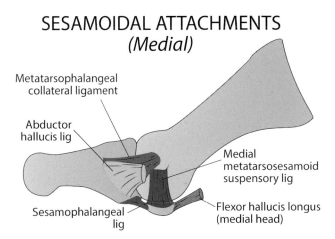

Metatarsophalangeal collateral ligament

Abductor hallucis lig

Medial metatarsosesamoid suspensory lig

Sesamophalangeal lig

Flexor hallucis longus (medial head)

Ligamentous Attachments

Intersesamoid ligament (tibial and fibular)

Medial metatarsosesamoid suspensory ligament (tibial)

Lateral metatarsosesamoid suspensory ligament (fibular)

Medial sagittal hood ligament (tibial)

Lateral sagittal hood ligament (fibular)

Medial sesamophalangeal ligament (tibial)

Lateral sesamophalangeal ligament (fibular)

Tendon Attachments

Adductor hallucis conjoined tendon (fibular)

Abductor hallucis tendon (tibial)

Flexor hallucis brevis tendon (medial head) (tibial)

Flexor hallucis brevis tendon (lateral head) (fibular)

Other Attachments

Plantar fascia (tibial and fibular)

Plantar intermetatarsal ligament (fibular)

Plantar plate (tibial and fibular)

TOENAILS

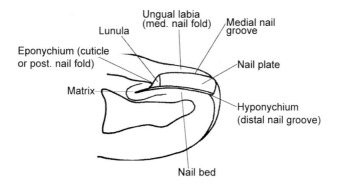

CALCANEUS

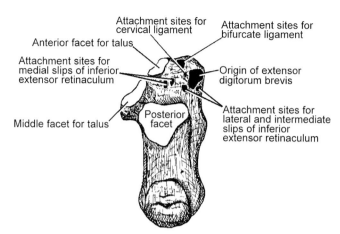

DORSAL VIEW OF CALCANEUS

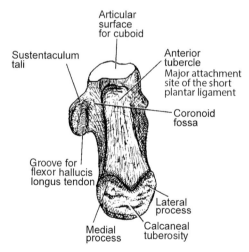

PLANTAR VIEW OF CALCANEUS

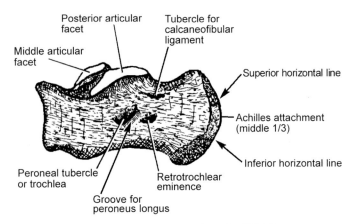

Posterior articular facet
Tubercle for calcaneofibular ligament
Middle articular facet
Superior horizontal line
Achilles attachment (middle 1/3)
Inferior horizontal line
Peroneal tubercle or trochlea
Retrotrochlear eminence
Groove for peroneus longus

LATERAL VIEW OF CALCANEUS

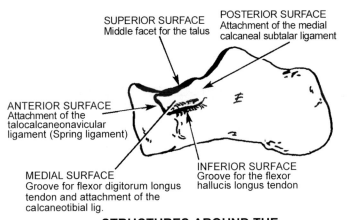

SUPERIOR SURFACE
Middle facet for the talus
POSTERIOR SURFACE
Attachment of the medial calcaneal subtalar ligament
ANTERIOR SURFACE
Attachment of the talocalcaneonavicular ligament (Spring ligament)
INFERIOR SURFACE
Groove for the flexor hallucis longus tendon
MEDIAL SURFACE
Groove for flexor digitorum longus tendon and attachment of the calcaneotibial lig.

STRUCTURES AROUND THE SUSTENTACULUM TALI

TALUS

3/5 of talus is covered by cartilage.

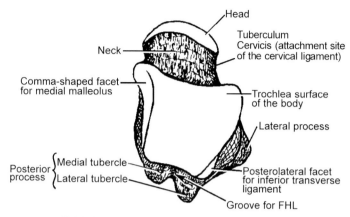

DORSAL VIEW OF THE RIGHT TALUS

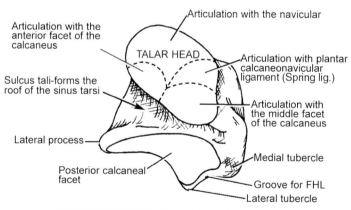

ANTERIOR VIEW OF THE RIGHT TALUS

Bone Anatomy

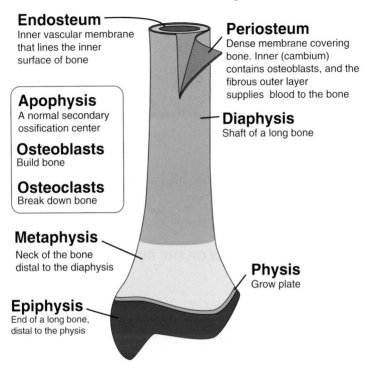

Endosteum
Inner vascular membrane
that lines the inner
surface of bone

Periosteum
Dense membrane covering
bone. Inner (cambium)
contains osteoblasts, and the
fibrous outer layer
supplies blood to the bone

Apophysis
A normal secondary
ossification center

Osteoblasts
Build bone

Osteoclasts
Break down bone

Diaphysis
Shaft of a long bone

Metaphysis
Neck of the bone
distal to the diaphysis

Physis
Grow plate

Epiphysis
End of a long bone,
distal to the physis

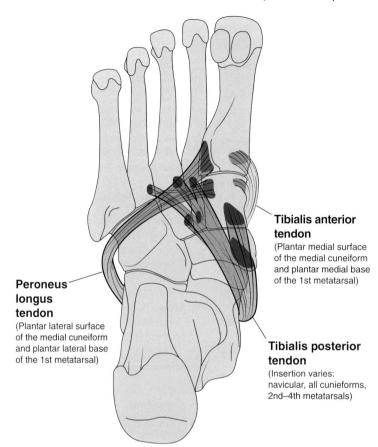

Tibialis anterior tendon
(Plantar medial surface of the medial cuneiform and plantar medial base of the 1st metatarsal)

Peroneus longus tendon
(Plantar lateral surface of the medial cuneiform and plantar lateral base of the 1st metatarsal)

Tibialis posterior tendon
(Insertion varies: navicular, all cunieforms, 2nd–4th metatarsals)

Muscle insertion sites

LEG MUSCLES

Tibialis Anterior Muscle

Origin: Lateral condyle of the tibia, the proximal lateral 1/2 of the tibial shaft, the interosseous membrane, and the deep surface of the fascia cruris

Insertion: Medial and plantar surface of the medial cuneiform and base of the 1st metatarsal

Action: Dorsiflexes ankle; adducts and inverts foot

Innervation: Deep peroneal nerve (L4, L5, S1)

Arterial supply: Anterior tibial artery

Extensor Hallucis Longus Muscle

Origin: Anterior surface of the interosseous membrane and from the middle two-fourths of the medial surface of the fibula

Insertion: Dorsal base of the distal phalanx

Action: Extension of proximal phalanx of the hallux; dorsiflexion of the ankle

Innervation: Deep peroneal artery (L4, L5, S1)

Arterial supply: Anterior tibial artery

NOTE: *Extensor hallucis capsularis* is an extra slip from the medial side of the EHL tendon. It is present in 80% to 90% of the population and inserts into the dorsomedial capsule of the 1st MPJ. Its function is believed to be to reinforce the joint and take the slack out of the joint upon dorsiflexion.

Extensor Digitorum Longus Muscle

Origin: Lateral condyle of the tibia, the upper two-thirds of the medial surface of the shaft of the fibula, the upper part of the interosseous membrane, the fascia cruris, and the intermuscular septum

Insertion: Dorsal base of the middle and distal phalanx of digits 2 to 5

Action: Extends digits 2 to 5; dorsiflexes the ankle

Innervation: Deep peroneal nerve (L4, L5, S1)

Arterial supply: Anterior tibial artery

Peroneus Tertius Muscle

Origin: Lower one-quarter of the medial surface of the fibula and the adjacent surface of the interosseous membrane

Insertion: Dorsal base and shaft of the 5th metatarsal

Action: Dorsiflexes the ankle; everts the foot

Innervation: Deep peroneal nerve (L5, S1)

Arterial supply: Anterior tibial artery

NOTE: Absent in 8% to 9% of population

Peroneus Longus Muscle

Origin: Head and upper one-half of the lateral fibula

Insertion: Plantar lateral surface of the 1st cuneiform and base of the 1st metatarsal

Action: Everts foot; plantarflexes ankle; supports the longitudinal and transverse arch of the foot

Innervation: Superficial peroneal nerve (L5, S1, S2)

Arterial supply: Anterior tibial and peroneal artery

Peroneus Brevis Muscle

Most efficient pronator of the subtalar joint

Origin: Inferior two-thirds of the lateral side of the fibula

Insertion: Styloid process of the 5th metatarsal

Action: Everts the foot; plantarflexes the ankle

Innervation: Superficial peroneal nerve (L5, S1)

Arterial supply: Peroneal artery

Gastrocnemius Muscle

Origin: Medial and lateral condyles of the femur

Insertion: Middle one-third of the posterior aspect of the calcaneus

Action: Plantarflexes ankle; flexes knee

Innervation: Tibial nerve (S1, S2)

Arterial supply: Sural artery (an end artery)

Soleus Muscle

Origin: Posterior head and upper one-third of the fibula, and soleus line of the tibia

Insertion: Middle one-third of the posterior aspect of the calcaneus

Action: Plantarflexes ankle

Innervation: Tibial nerve (S1, S2)

Arterial supply: Posterior tibial artery

Plantaris Muscle

Origin: Lateral condyles of the femur

Insertion: Medial one-third of the posterior calcaneus

Action: Plantarflexes ankle; flexes knee

Innervation: Tibial nerve (L5, S1, S2)

Arterial supply: Sural artery

NOTE: Absent in 7% of the population

Popliteus Muscle

Origin: Lateral condyle of the femur

Insertion: Superior posterior surface of the tibia

Action: Flexes the knee; medially rotates the knee

Innervation: Tibial nerve (L4, L5, S1)

Arterial supply: Medial inferior genicular artery and the posterior tibial artery

Flexor Digitorum Longus

Origin: The posteromedial aspect of the middle third of the tibial shaft

Insertion: Plantar surface of the base of phalanges 2 to 5

Action: Flexes the DIPJ, PIPJ, and MPJ of digits 2 to 5, and plantarflexes the ankle

Innervation: Tibial nerve (S2, S3)

Arterial supply: Posterior tibial artery

Tibialis Posterior Muscle

Origin: Posterior two-thirds of the interosseous membrane and the adjacent tibia and fibula

Insertion: Plantar surface of tuberosity of the navicular (major insertion site), medial, and intermediate cuneiform, and base of the 2nd, 3rd, and 4th metatarsal

Action: Inverts and adducts foot; plantarflexes ankle

Innervation: Tibial nerve (L4, L5)

Arterial supply: Sural, peroneal, and posterior tibial arteries

Flexor Hallucis Longus

Origin: Most of the inferior two-thirds of the posterior surface of the fibular and the lower part of the interosseous membrane

Insertion: Plantar surface of the base of the distal phalanx of the hallux

Action: Flexes the IPJ and 1st MPJ; plantarflexes ankle
Innervation: Tibial nerve (S2, S3)
Arterial supply: Peroneal and posterior tibial arteries

INTRINSIC MUSCLES OF THE FOOT

Extensor Digitorum Brevis

Origin: Superolateral aspect of the calcaneus, just anterior to the sinus tarsi
Insertion: Dorsal base of the 1st to 4th proximal phalanx
Action: Extension of the 1st to 4th MPJ and IPJ
Innervation: Lateral terminal branch of the deep peroneal nerve (S1, S2)
Arterial supply: Dorsalis pedis

NOTE: The most medial slip of this muscle is relatively distinct and called the *extensor hallucis brevis.*

Abductor Hallucis

Origin: Medial process of the calcaneal tuberosity
Insertion: The tendons of abductor hallucis and the medial head of the flexor hallucis brevis insert together on the medial side of the plantar aspect of the base of the proximal phalanx. Some fibers also attach to the medial sesamoid.
Action: Abducts the hallux
Innervation: Medial plantar nerve (L5, S1, S2)
Arterial supply: Medial plantar artery

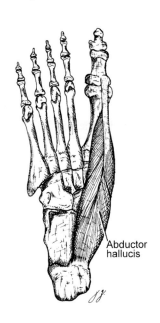

Abductor hallucis

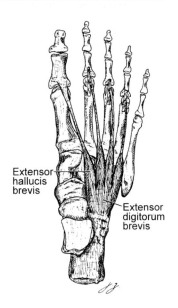

Extensor hallucis brevis

Extensor digitorum brevis

Flexor Digitorum Brevis

Origin: Plantar aponeurosis, medial intermuscular septa, lateral intermuscular septa, and the medial process of the calcaneal tuberosity

Insertion: Inserts by two tendinous slips onto each side of the shaft of the 2nd to 5th middle phalanx

Action: Flexion of the 2nd to 5th PIPJ, with continued contraction flexion of the 2nd to 5th MPJ

Innervation: Medial plantar nerve (L5, S1, S2)

Arterial supply: Medial plantar artery

Abductor Digiti Minimi Quinti

Origin: Lateral process of the calcaneal tuberosity

Insertion: Lateral side of the plantar aspect of the base of the 5th proximal phalanx

Action: Abducts the 5th toe and assists with flexion

Innervation: Lateral plantar nerve S1, S2

Arterial supply: Lateral plantar nerve

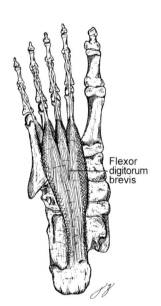

Flexor digitorum brevis

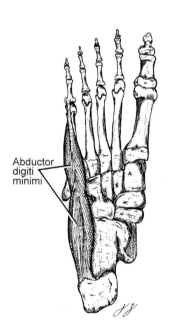

Abductor digiti minimi

Lumbricals

Origin: Tendon of the flexor digitorum longus after its separation into four slips

Insertion: Medial aspect of the extensor expansion, slightly more dorsally than plantarly

Action: Flexes the 2nd to 5th MPJ and extends the IPJs of these same toes

Innervation: The 1st (medial) lumbrical is innervated by the medial plantar nerve L5, S1. The lateral three lumbricals are innervated by the deep branch of the lateral plantar nerve S1, S2.

Arterial supply: Plantar metatarsal arteries

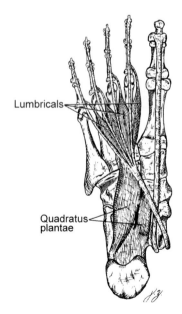

Lumbricals

Quadratus plantae

Quadratus Plantae

Origin: Arises from two heads of origin, which are separated from one another by the calcaneal attachment of the long plantar ligament. The medial head originates from the medial plantar surface of the calcaneus. The lateral head originates from the lateral plantar surface of the calcaneus.

Insertion: Tendon of the flexor digitorum longus

Action: Aids the flexor digitorum longus in the flexion of the 2nd to 5th toes by straightening the line of pull to the tendon

Innervation: Lateral plantar nerve S2, S3

Arterial supply: Lateral plantar artery

NOTE: This muscle is also called *flexor digitorum accessorius.*

Flexor Hallucis Brevis

Origin: Plantar surface of the cuboid and lateral cuneiform

Insertion: The medial (larger) head inserts on the medial side of the plantar aspect of the base of the proximal phalanx, the medial sesamoid, and the medial aspect of the plantar pad of the hallux. The lateral (smaller) head inserts on the lateral side of the plantar aspect of the base of the proximal phalanx, the lateral sesamoid, and the lateral aspect of the plantar pad of the hallux.

Action: Flexes the 1st MPJ
Innervation: Medial plantar nerve
  L5, S1
Arterial supply: The 1st plantar
  metatarsal artery

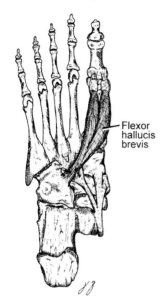

Flexor
hallucis
brevis

Adductor Hallucis

Origin: The oblique head originates
  from the bases of the plantar–
  medial aspects of the 2nd, 3rd,
  and 4th metatarsals and from
  the mid-portion of the tendinous sheath of the peroneus
  longus tendon. The transverse
  head originates from the plantar
  plates and the plantar metatarsophalangeal ligaments of the
  3rd, 4th, and 5th toes and from
  the deep transverse metatarsal
  ligament.
Insertion: The two heads come
  together and insert proximally
  along with the lateral head of
  the flexor hallucis brevis on

the lateral, plantar area of the
  proximal phalanx. The tendons
  enclose the lateral sesamoid.
Action: The oblique head functions
  to adduct and help flex the hallux. The transverse head acts to
  adduct the hallux and bring the
  metatarsals closer together and
  maintain the transverse arch of
  the foot.
Innervation: Deep branch of the lateral plantar nerve S1, S2, (S3)
Arterial supply: 1st plantar metatarsal artery

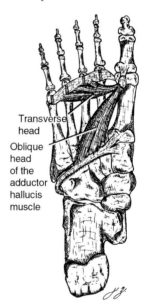

Transverse
head

Oblique
head
of the
adductor
hallucis
muscle

Flexor Digiti Minimi

Origin: Base of the 5th metatarsal
  on its medial plantar surface, the
  sheath of the tendon of the peroneus longus, and the plantar
  aponeurosis
Insertion: Lateral side of the plantar aspect of the base of the 5th
  proximal phalanx

Action: Flexes and helps abduct the 5th digit

Innervation: Superficial branch of the lateral plantar nerve S1, S2, (S3)

Arterial supply: Lateral plantar artery

superficial branch of the lateral plantar nerve.

Arterial supply: 2nd, 3rd, and 4th plantar metatarsal arteries

NOTE: Mnemonic—PAD, *P*lantar-*Ad*duction

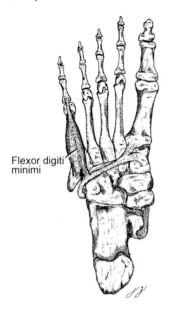

Flexor digiti minimi

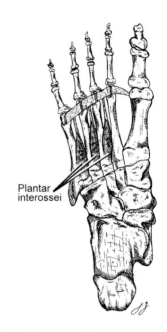

Plantar interossei

Plantar Interossei

Origin: Medial side of the bases of the 3rd, 4th, and 5th metatarsal bones

Insertion: Medial side of the bases of the proximal phalanges, the MPJ capsules, and the extensor expansion of the same digit on which they originate

Action: Adducts the 3rd, 4th, and 5th toes toward the midline of the foot

Innervation: The 1st and 2nd are innervated by the deep branch of the lateral plantar nerve. The 3rd is innervated by the

Dorsal Interossei

Origin: Originates from adjacent sides of adjacent metatarsal bones

Insertion: The base of the proximal phalanx and the extensor expansion

Action: Abducts the toes away from the midline of the foot (the 2nd toe)

Innervation: 1st deep branch of the lateral plantar nerve and an extra branch, the medial branch of the deep peroneal nerve. 2nd deep branch of the lateral plantar nerve and an extra branch, the lateral branch of the deep peroneal nerve. 3rd deep branch of the lateral plantar nerve. 4th superficial branch of the lateral plantar nerve.

Arterial supply: Dorsal metatarsal artery

NOTE: Mnemonic—DAB, *Dorsal-Ab*duction

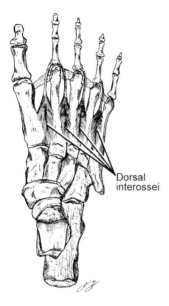

Dorsal interossei

PLANTAR LAYERS OF THE FOOT

First Layer (Superficial)

Abductor hallucis muscle
Flexor digitorum brevis muscle
Abductor digiti minimi (quinti)

Second Layer

Quadratus plantae muscle
Lumbricals
Flexor hallucis longus tendon
Flexor digitorum longus tendon

Third Layer

Adductor hallucis brevis muscle
Flexor hallucis brevis muscle
Flexor digiti minimi brevis muscle

Fourth Layer (Deep)

Plantar interossei
Dorsal interossei
Tibialis posterior tendon
Peroneus longus tendon

TYPES OF JOINTS

Spheroidal (ball and socket)— examples: Hip, shoulder
Ellipsoid (ellipsoid)—examples: Wrist, metatarsophalangeal joints
Sellar (saddle)—example: Calcaneocuboid joint
Ginglymus (hinge)—examples: Interphalangeal joints
Trochoid (ring and pivot)—examples: Atlantoaxial (C1 and C2), there are none in the low extremity
Planar (gliding or plane)—examples: Lisfranc joint, intercarpal joints

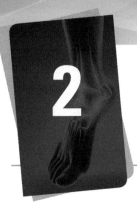

2 PHARMACOLOGY

ANTIFUNGALS (TOPICAL)

Definitions: Fungi is neither plant nor animal, although genetically it is closer to animal. It does not perform photosynthesis and must grow on organic matter to sustain itself. Yeast and mold are two different types of fungi.

Fungus		
	Mold	**Yeast**
Structure	Multicellular, filamentous (hyphae)	Unicellular, round or oval
Color	Wide variety	Monochromatic (white)
Appearance	Fuzzy	Smooth and waxy
Metabolism	Secretes hydrolytic enzymes to external food sources and absorbs nutrients	Converts carbohydrates to EtOH during fermentation
Environment	Dark, damp, moist environment	Common in the environment, rotten foot
Reproduction	Sexual or asexual: Spore formation	Asexual: Budding or binary fission
Commercial Uses	Production of cheese, ABX production	Baking, EtOH
Examples	*Mucor, Penicillium, Rhizopus* and *Aspergillus, Dermatophytes*	*Saccharomyces cerevisiae* and *Cryptococcus neoformans, Candiditis*

Antifungal Classification

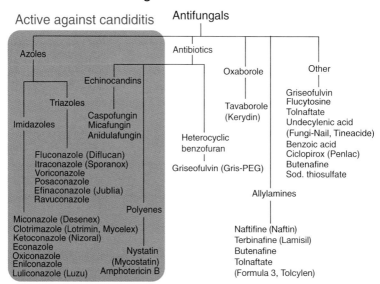

Active against candiditis

Antifungals

Azoles
Triazoles
Imidazoles

Fluconazole (Diflucan)
Itraconazole (Sporanox)
Voriconazole
Posaconazole
Efinaconazole (Jublia)
Ravuconazole

Miconazole (Desenex)
Clotrimazole (Lotrimin, Mycelex)
Ketoconazole (Nizoral)
Econazole
Oxiconazole
Enilconazole
Luliconazole (Luzu)

Antibiotics
Echinocandins
Caspofungin
Micafungin
Anidulafungin

Polyenes
Nystatin
(Mycostatin)
Amphotericin B

Oxaborole
Tavaborole
(Kerydin)

Heterocyclic benzofuran
Griseofulvin (Gris-PEG)

Allylamines
Naftifine (Naftin)
Terbinafine (Lamisil)
Butenafine
Tolnaftate
(Formula 3, Tolcylen)

Other
Griseofulvin
Flucytosine
Tolnaftate
Undecylenic acid
(Fungi-Nail, Tineacide)
Benzoic acid
Ciclopirox (Penlac)
Butenafine
Sod. thiosulfate

Efinaconazole (Jublia) 10% solution
  Apply to nails daily.
Tavaborole (Kerydin) 5% solution
  Apply to nails daily.
  Kills only *Trichophyton rubrum* and *Trichophyton mentagrophytes*
Ciclopirox (Penlac)
  Apply to nails daily.
  Penlac use develops a film over the nails that must be removed with alcohol every 7 days.
Tolnaftate (Formula 3, Formula 7, Tolcylen) 1% solution
  Apply to nails daily.
Undecylenic Acid (Tineacide, Fungi-Nail)
  Apply to nails daily.
Naftifine (Naftin)
  Topical for (tinea pedis) athlete's foot, (tinea cruris) jock itch, and (tinea corporis) ringworm
Miconazole (Desenex)
  Topical (powder) for (tinea pedis) athlete's foot, (tinea cruris) jock itch, and (tinea corporis) ringworm
Luliconazole (Luzu)
  Topical for (tinea pedis) athlete's foot, (tinea cruris) jock itch, and (tinea corporis) ringworm
Ketoconazole (Nizoral)
  Topical for (tinea pedis) athlete's foot, (tinea cruris) jock itch, and (tinea corporis) ringworm
Clotrimazole (Mycelex, Lotrimin)
  Most commonly used to treat vaginal yeast infections. Topical treatment for (tinea pedis) athlete's foot, (tinea cruris) jock itch, and (tinea corporis) ringworm. Also available as an oral lozenge for thrush.

ANTIFUNGALS (ORAL/IV)

Itraconazole (Sporanox, Onmel) 100 mg PO bid ×12 weeks for fungal toenails or ×6 weeks for fungal fingernails. "Pulse dosing" 200 mg PO bid ×1 week then 3 weeks off, 3 pulses for toenails and 2 pulses for fingernails. Onmel taken 200 mg qd ×12 weeks [100 mg, 200 mg]
  Imidazole derivative
  Active against dermatophytes and *Candida*
  Contraindicated with astemizole, terfenadine, cisapride
  Possible hepatotoxicity; monitor hepatic function before treatment and at 1 month
  Absorption increases with acids; orange juice, Coke. Decreases with antacids
Ketoconazole (Nizoral) 200 to 400 mg PO daily [200 mg]
  Imidazole derivative
  Available parenterally and topically
  Active against dermatophytes, *Candida*, and some G+, and has also shown to have some antiviral properties
  Can cause hepatotoxicity
  Contraindicated with cisapride, terfenadine
Amphotericin B (Abelcet, Amphotec, Fungizone) Test dose of 1 to 5 mg IV over 15 to 30 minutes, then wait 30 minutes. If there are no adverse reactions such as fever, chills, or muscle spasms, begin IV infusion. Dosage varies based on suspension.
  Antibiotic antifungal
  Used mostly for life-threatening fungal infections after other antifungals have failed

Active against fungus and *Candida*; does not affect bacteria or dermatophytes

Not effective orally

Can cause nephrotoxicity

Terbinafine HCL (Lamisil) 250 mg PO daily for 6 weeks for fingernails and for 12 weeks for toenails

Available orally and topically

Fluconazole (Diflucan) Oropharyngeal candidiasis (thrush): 200 mg IV/PO first day, then 100 to 200 mg daily for at least 2 weeks. Cryptococcal meningitis: 400 mg IV first day, then 200 to 800 mg daily. Vaginal candidiasis: 150 mg PO single dose [tabs 50, 100, 150, 200 mg, susp 10 and 40 mg per mL]

Imidazole derivative

Most common antifungal used to treat candidiasis

Can cause renal toxicity

Griseofulvin (Fulvicin, Grifulvin, Grisactin, Gris-PEG) For tinea corporis, tinea cruris, and tinea capitis 375 mg daily. For tinea pedis and tinea unguium 375 mg bid [tabs 125, 250, 500 mg, susp 125 mg per 5 mL]

Active against dermatophytes; does not kill *Candida*

Fungistatic, not fungicidal

Renal and hepatic function should be monitored.

Hastens warfarin metabolism

Gentian Violet

Topically bid for 3 days

Active against dermatophytes, *Candida*, and G+ (color is due to crystal violet, hence G+ activity)

Not commonly used for dermatophyte infections due to low efficacy, and has local irritant and staining properties

Solution 0.5%, 1%, 2%

Drying properties; so use on macerated infections

TOPICAL KERATOLYTICS

Keratolytics are topical agents that remove layers of skin. They are used as treatments for warts, callus, and thick skin.

Salicylic Acid (Duofilm, Duoplant)

Topically daily

Used for scaling dermatosis and localized hyperkeratosis

Also used for seborrheic dermatitis, psoriasis, and dandruff 12% to 17.6%

Urea (Ureacin, Carmol, Vanamide, Keralac)

Topically daily tid

Cream/lotion 5% to 40%

Sulfur (Sulforcin, Sulfron)

Cream/lotion/ointment 2% to 5%

CONTROLLED SUBSTANCE ACT

Schedule I (CI)

Drugs with no accepted medical use and with high abuse potential

Examples include heroin, LSD, ecstasy, methaqualone.

Schedule II (CII)

High potential for abuse

Examples include fentanyl, oxycodone (OxyContin, Percocet), hydrocodone (Vicodin, Norco), methadone, hydromorphone (Dilaudid), meperidine (Demerol), amphetamine (Dexedrine, Adderall), methylphenidate (Ritalin), codeine (>90 mg per dosage unit)

Schedule III (CIII)

Moderate abuse potential
Examples include codeine (with
    <90 mg per dosage unit), Trezix,
    anabolic steroids, testosterone.

Schedule IV (CIV)

Low abuse potential
Examples include benzodiazepines
    (Valium, Xanax), *d*-propoxyphene,
    Ambien, tramadol (Ultram), Soma.

Schedule V (CV)

Rx not required when provided in
    low doses
Examples include products with
    <200 mg of codeine per 100 mL
    (Robitussin AC, Phenergan with
    Codeine), Lyrica.

TYPES OF PAIN

Nociceptive

Results from activation of
    sensory (afferent) receptors
    (nociceptors) by mechanical,
    thermal, or chemical stimuli.
    This is "normal" pain.

Neuropathic

Results from activation of
    damaged peripheral or central
    nervous system (CNS) from
    altered processing of pain
    receptors.

PAIN RECEPTORS

Pain receptors consist of $A\delta$ and C
fibers.

Types of Nerve Fibers

	Type of Nerve Fiber	Information Carried	Myelin Sheath	Diameter (micrometers)	Conduction Speed (m/s)
	$A\alpha$ (A-alpha)	Proprioception	Yes	13–20	80–120 (fastest)
	$A\beta$ (A-beta)	Touch	Yes	6–12	35–90 (faster)
Pain Receptors	**$A\delta$** (A-delta)	**Pain** (mechanical, thermal)	Yes	1–5	5–40 (**fast**)
	C	**Pain** (mechanical, thermal, chemical)	No	0.2–1.5	0.5–2 (**slow**)

OPIOIDS

Opioid Receptors

There are three types of opioid receptors: mu (μ), kappa (κ), delta
(δ). Mu (μ) receptors are the most
clinically relevant with regard to
opioids.

Mu (μ)

Mediates analgesia, respiratory depression, euphoria, addiction
DEAR (Dependence, Euphoria, Analgesia, Respiratory depression)

Kappa (κ)

Mediates spinal analgesia, miosis, sedation
SAM (Sedation, Analgesia [spinal], Miosis)

Miosis
(pinpoint pupils)

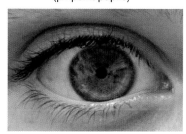

Delta (δ)

Mediates dysphoria, hallucinations, delusions

Opioid Effects

Analgesia, sedation and euphoria, cough suppression

Opioid Adverse Reactions

Respiratory depression, nausea/vomiting, constipation, miosis, urinary retention, bradycardia, syncope, xerostomia (dry mouth), histamine release—caution in asthmatics, urinary urgency but difficulty urinating. Rise in intracranial pressure—avoid in head trauma
Allergies to opioids are uncommon. Generally, allergies to one opioid do not mean the patient is allergic to all opioids. Switching to another opioid class may be effective.

Classification	Phenanthrenes	Benzomorphan	Phenylpiperidines	Diphenylheptanes	Phenylpropylamines
Cross-sensitivity	Likely	Possible	Low risk	Low risk	Low risk
Drug	Codeine Heroin Hydrocodone (Vicodin, Norco) Morphine Naloxone Oxycodone (Percocet) Hydromorphone (Dilaudid) Oxymorphone	Pentazocine	Fentanyl (Sublimaze) Sufentanil Meperidine (Demerol)	Methadone Propoxyphene	Tramadol (Ultram)

Opioid agonists—Activate some or all opioid receptors and do not block any
  Natural opium alkaloids: Morphine, Codeine
  Semisynthetic opiates: Diacetylmorphine (Heroin), Hydromorphone, Oxymorphone
  Synthetic opioids: Pethidine (Demerol), Tramadol, Methadone, Fentanyl, Alfentanil, Remifentanil

Opioid agonist–antagonists—Activate some receptor subtypes and blocks some other subtypes
  Pentazocine, Nalorphine, Butorphanol, Nalbuphine

Partial μ-receptor agonists—Activate opioid receptor, but the response is submaximal.
  Buprenorphine

μ-receptor antagonists—Block all receptor subtypes.
  Naltrexone

Naloxone

For acute morphine poisoning. 0.4 mg IV q2–3 min. No analgesic activity. Competes for μ, κ, and σ receptors. Displaces and quickly reverses all actions of opioids. It will precipitate withdrawal.

Naltrexone

Tablet 50 mg qd. Same effect as Naloxone but is used orally so it can't be used for acute toxicity. Used to decrease the sensation of craving during treatment of addition. A single dose blocks heroin effects for 24 hours so provides a negative reinforcement for taking heroin; also used to treat alcoholism.

Treating morphine dependence
Pure antagonist
Substitute an agonist. This will be less potent than the original drug and will have a longer duration. This will give similar pleasure and withdrawing effects but easier to manage. Withdrawal symptoms will be less severe. Methadone (long duration of action) or Buprenorphine (for mild withdrawal)
Side effects include hypotension, respiratory depression, nausea, urinary retention, and constipation.
Low-dose opioids suppress the cough reflex.
Contraindicated in cases of head trauma; opioids cause an increase in intracranial pressure.
All opioids cause tolerance and dependence when used for chronic pain management in all patients and addiction in some patients.

Opioid Agonists

Fentanyl (Sublimaze) CII
  IV fentanyl is often used for anesthesia due to its quick onset and short-acting properties.
  Used during anesthesia as analgesic, also for post-op pain
  Comes in a patch form for chronic pain and cancer patients
  A wide range of fentanyl preparations are available for analgesia, including buccal tablets, lollipops, nasal sprays, inhalers, and transdermal patches.

Dosage:	IV analgesia/procedural sedation:	50–100 mcg slow IV over 1–2 min, titrate to effect
	IM analgesia:	50–100 mcg IM q1–2h prn
	Transdermal patch (Duragesic):	1 patch q72h [12, 25, 50, 75, 10 mcg per hour]

Codeine CII
  Used to treat mild to moderate
    pain
  One-tenth the potency of
    morphine
  Antitussive drug for cough

Dosage:	0.5 mg per kg up to 15–60 mg PO/IM q4–6h [15, 30, 60 mg. Oral soln: 15 mg per 5 mL]
	Low dose suppresses a cough (15–20 mg q4–6h, max 120 mg per day).

Hydrocodone CII
  A semisynthetic opioid derived
    from codeine
  Used to treat moderate to severe
    pain and as an antitussive to
    treat cough
  **Hydrocodone + Acetamino-
    phen** (Norco, Vicodin, Lortab)
    Norco (5/325, 7.5/325,
      10/325)
    Vicodin (5/300)
    Vicodin ES (7.5/300)
    Vicodin HP (10/300)
    Lortab (5/325, 7.5/325,
      10/325)
    Lorcet (5/325)
    Lorcet Plus (7.5/325)
    Lorcet HD (10/325)
    Lortab Elixir (10 to 300 mg
      per 15 mL oral solution)
Oxycodone CII
  Oxycodone + Acetaminophen
    (Percocet)
    Percocet (2.5/325, 5/325,
      7.5/325, 10/325)
    1 tab PO q4–6h prn
    Xartemis XR (7.5/325)

    Controlled release: 2 tabs PO
      bid prn
  Oxycodone + Aspirin
    (Percodan)
    Percodan (4.84/325)
    1 tab PO q4–6h prn
Hydromorphone (Dilaudid)
  CII—Agonist
A derivative of morphine; used for
the management of moderate to
severe pain

Dosage:	PO:	2–4 mg q4–6h prn
	IM/SC:	0.5–2 mg or slow IV q4–6h

Meperidine aka **Pethidine**
  (Demerol) CII—Agonist
  Management of severe pain
  An opioid receptor agonist
  Anticholinergic agent
    (Atropine-like)
  Unlike other opioids that cause
    pupil constriction, meper-
    idine causes pupil dilation
    (mydriasis).

Dosage:	PO/IM/SC:	1–1.8 mg per kg q3–4h up to 150 mg prn
	IV:	1–1.8 mg per kg slow infusion q3–4h up to 150 mg prn

Methadone (Dolophine)
  CII—Agonist
  Used as an oral replacement
    for heroin and morphine
    addiction. It does not "de-
    toxify" but has a slow onset
    and slow offset so helps with

sudden and intense with-
drawals and decreases abuse
potential.
Management of moderate to
severe pain

Dosage:	PO/IM/SC:	2.5–10 mg q8–12h prn pain
	PO:	20 mg daily for treatment of opioid dependence

Morphine (MS Contin, Kadian)
  CII—Agonist
  Management of moderate to
  severe pain

Dosage:	PO:	(Controlled-release tabs: MS Contin) 30 mg q8–12h
	PO:	(Controlled-release caps: Kadian) 20 mg q12–24h
	IM/SC:	0.1–0.2 mg per kg up to 15 mg q4h prn
	IV:	0.1–0.2 mg per kg infused slow up to 15 mg q4h prn

Oxymorphone (Opana)
  CII—Agonist

Dosage:	PO:	10–20 mg q4–6h
	IM/SC:	1–1.5 mg q4–6h prn
	IV:	0.5 mg q4–6h prn

Tramadol (Ultram, Ultram ER)
  Management of moderate to
    moderately severe pain
  Avoid in epileptics. It can de-
    crease seizure threshold.
  Tramadol is a weak opioid ago-
    nist with strong norepineph-
    rine and serotonin reuptake
    inhibitor properties.

Dosage:	50–100 mg PO q4–6h, max 400 mg per day [50 mg]
	100–300 mg PO daily [100, 200, 300 mg]

Opioid Agonist–Antagonists

Pentazocine (Talwin) CIV
  Used for moderate to severe
    pain
  μ antagonist, κ agonist
  Can precipitate withdrawal in
    a morphine addict due to μ
    antagonistic effect
  Short duration of action
  Contraindicated in patients
    with ischemic heart disease
    and hypertension

Dosage:	IV/IM:	30 mg q3–4h prn
	PO:	Talwin: 1 tab PO q3–4h

Acetaminophen (Tylenol)
Inhibits μ, δ, and κ receptors

NONOPIOID ANALGESICS

Acetaminophen (Tylenol)
  Acetaminophen is not a non-
    steroidal anti-inflammatory
    drug (NSAID) and has no
    anti-inflammatory action.
    Acetaminophen is an anal-
    gesic and antipyretic drug
    (lowers a fever). 325 to
    650 mg q4–6h or 1,000 mg
    tid–qid. Not to exceed 4 g
    per day. Use caution in liver
    disease.

NONSTEROIDAL ANTI-INFLAMMATORY DRUGS

NSAIDs are used to treat inflammation, fever, and pain.
  They block prostaglandin

production by inhibiting cyclo-oxygenase (COX). Prostaglandins are chemicals that cause inflammation, pain, and fever. Prostaglandins are also involved in platelet aggregation, and they protect the gastrointestinal (GI) tract. Therefore, NSAIDs have the potential side effects of GI problems and increased bleeding. Caution should be taken with patients with stomach ulcers or on blood thinners. NSAIDs may be taken with food to reduce GI irritation. NSAIDs should be discontinued at least a week before elective surgery to decrease the risk of excessive bleeding. NSAIDs, especially aspirin, can precipitate an asthmatic attack by diverting the arachidonic acid pathway to produce more leukotrienes.

Arachidonic Acid Cascade

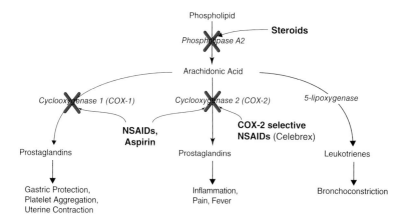

Over-the-Counter NSAIDs

Ibuprofen (Motrin, Advil)
    200 mg q4–6h prn. Maximum over-the-counter (OTC) dose 1,200 g per day
    Prescription strength (300, 400, 600 mg), maximum prescription dose 3,200 g per day. Ibuprofen is also available with a proton pump inhibitor (PPI; Duexis) to decrease GI problems.
    Ibuprofen is a more potent anti-inflammatory drug than aspirin, but it reversibly binds to COX-2 enzyme. Like aspirin, it can be used to treat a patent ductus arteriosus in premature babies.
Naproxen (Aleve)
    220 mg q8–12h prn. Maximum OTC dose 600 mg qd. Prescription strength Naproxen (Naprosyn) comes as 375, 500, and 550 mg.
Acetylsalicylic acid (ASA; Aspirin, Bayer, Ecotrin, Bufferin)
    Regular tablets 325 mg, baby aspirin 81 mg. 1 to 2 tablets PO q4–6h prn
    Aspirin differs from other NSAIDs in that it irreversibly inhibits COX.

Analgesic, antipyretic, and antiplatelet action occurs at lower doses, 81 to 1,000 mg per day (1 to 4 pills). The anti-inflammatory action of aspirin requires a higher dose, 5,000 to 8,000 mg per day (15 to 25 pills). This high dose is close to toxic levels that some patients cannot tolerate.

Contraindicated in gout because it inhibits uric acid excretion. Use caution in asthma patients, aspirin can trigger an attack.

Aspirin dosing

Respiratory/ cardiovascular failure	Lethal	150,000 mg
	Severe	
	Mild	
Tinnitus Hyperventilation		5,000 mg (~15 pills/day)
	Anti-inflammatory range	
		1,000 mg (~3–4 pills/day)
	Analgesic Antipyretic	160 mg
	Antiplatelet	81 mg
		0 mg

(TOXIC LEVELS)

Other uses of Aspirin:

Blood Thinner: Prophylactically to prevent blood clots, myocardial infarction (MI), and stroke. Usual dose 1 baby aspirin per day.

Corn Remover: Topical ASA is used as a keratolytic to remove corns.

Ductus Arteriosus: Aspirin can cause premature closure of the ductus arteriosus and should be avoided in the third trimester of pregnancy. However, it is used as a treatment for a patent ductus arteriosus in neonates.

Reye Syndrome: Occurs in infants and children when aspirin is given during viral infections. Characterized by liver damage and encephalopathy

Salicylism: Aspirin overdose more common in children. Causes the blood to become acidic. Results in nausea, vomiting, hyperventilation, headache, mental confusion, dizziness, and tinnitus. Severe salicylate intoxication results in confusion, coma, respiratory and metabolic acidosis, and death from respiratory and cardiovascular failure.

Diflunisal (Dolobid)

Salicylic acid derivative. Low GI irritation, little antipyretic activity

Prescription NSAIDs

Ketorolac (Toradol, Sprix)
30 mg IV/IM q6h. First IM dose may be 60 mg. 10 mg PO q4–6h. Sprix is an intranasal spray. Indicated for short-term (<5 days) management of moderate to severe post-op pain when opioid level analgesia is desired.

Etodolac (Lodine)
200 to 400 mg PO tid/qid
Preferential COX-2 inhibitor

Indomethacin (Indocin)
- 25 to 50 mg PO tid
- One of the most potent NSAIDs
- Commonly used to treat gout
- Increased risk of side effects; abdominal pain, diarrhea, GI bleeding

Sulindac (Clinoril)
- 100 to 200 mg bid
- Fluorinated derivative of indomethacin
- Longer duration of action than indomethacin and less GI irritation

Ketoprofen (Orudis)
- 50 to 75 mg PO tid

Diclofenac (Voltaren)
- 50 mg PO bid/tid
- More potent as an anti-inflammatory than as an analgesic or antipyretic
- Accumulates in synovial fluid
- Also available as an OTC topical gel

Piroxicam (Feldene)
- 20 mg PO qd
- Side effects include GI and CNS disturbances.
- No advantages except a longer duration of action

Celecoxib (Celebrex)
- 200 mg qd–bid
- COX-2 inhibitor, which means it selectively inhibits COX-2, making it safer on the GI.
- Contraindicated in patients with Sulfa allergy
- May have increased risk of cardiovascular side effects

Meloxicam (Mobic, Vivlodex)
- 7.5 to 15 mg PO qd
- Meloxicam is a preferential COX-2 inhibitor.
- Contraindicated in coronary artery bypass graft (CABG) patients

DISEASE-MODIFYING ANTIRHEUMATIC DRUGS

Disease-modifying antirheumatic drugs (DMARDs) are rheumatoid arthritis (RA) medications that slow the disease's progression by stopping the inflammation caused by autoimmune attacks.

Hydroxychloroquine (Plaquenil)

Dosage:	RA:	Start 400–600 mg PO daily, then taper to 200–400 mg daily
	Systemic lupus erythematosus (SLE):	400 mg PO 1–2 times per day to start, then taper to 200–400 mg daily

Used to treat malaria, severe RA, and SLE

Methotrexate (Rheumatrex, Trexall) Start with 7.5 mg PO single dose once a week or 2.5 mg PO q12h for three doses given once a week. Max dose 20 mg per week. Supplement with 1 mg per day of folic acid.
Used to treat RA, psoriasis, and several kinds of cancer

ANTICOAGULANTS

Anticoagulants, also called blood thinners, are a group of drugs that prevent blood clots. Anticoagulants DO NOT DISSOLVE BLOOD CLOTS; they prevent clots from forming. There are several different categories of anticoagulants including the following:

Anticoagulants | Antiplatelet agents

Category	VKA (Warfarin)	UFH	LMWH	Fondaparinux	Idrabiotaparinux	Rivaroxaban	Apixaban	Edoxaban	Betrixaban	Dabigatran	Bivalirudin	Desirudin	Argatroban	Lepirudin	Aspirin	Clopidogrel	Ticlopidine	Glycoprotein (IIb/IIIa) Platelet Inhibitors
Mechanism of Action (MoA)	VKA (Vitamin K Antagonist)z — Inhibits Vit K-dependent factors (II, VII, IX, and X)	Indirect Thrombin Inhibitor	Indirect Thrombin Inhibitor	Indirect Thrombin Inhibitor	Indirect Thrombin Inhibitor	Direct Factor Xa Inhibitor	Direct Factor Xa Inhibitor	Direct Factor Xa Inhibitor	Direct Factor Xa Inhibitor	Direct Thrombin Inhibitor	Direct Thrombin Inhibitor	Direct Thrombin Inhibitor	Direct Thrombin Inhibitor	Direct Thrombin Inhibitor	COX Inhibitor	ADP Inhibitor	Inhibits ADP-Mediated Aggregation	Glycoprotein (IIb/IIIa) Platelet Inhibitors
Factors Affected	II, VII, IX, X	X and II (Thrombin) XII (11)	X and II (Thrombin) X>>II	X		X		X		II			X		n/a	n/a	n/a	n/a
Drug	Warfarin	UFH (Unfractionated Heparin)	LMWH (Low molecular weight heparin)	Fondaparinux	Idrabiotaparinux	Rivaroxaban	Apixaban	Edoxaban	Betrixaban	Dabigatran	Bivalirudin	Desirudin	Argatroban	Lepirudin	Aspirin	Clopidogrel	Ticlopidine	Abciximab Eptifibatide Tirofiban
Examples	Coumadin		Enoxaparin (Lovenox) Tinzaparin (Innohep) Dalteparin (Fragmin)	Arixtra		Xarelto	Eliquis	Savaysa	Bevyxxa	Pradaxa	Angiomax	Iprivask	Acova	Refludan	Aspood	Plavix	Ticlid	Abciximab (ReoPro) Eptifibatide (Integrilin) Tirofiban (Aggrastat)
Route	Oral	SQ/IV	SQ	SC	SC	PO	PO	PO	PO	PO	IV	SC/IV	IV	IV	PO	PO	PO	IV
Monitoring	INR/PT	PTT	No	No	No	No	No	No	No	No	aPTT, ACT	aPTT, ACT			No	No	No	aPTT
Prophylaxis Dosing	Loading dose 10 mg PO daily for 2–4 days Maintenance dose 2–7.5 mg PO daily Maintain PT about 2–2.5 normal	Full dose: 5–10K U bolus then 1K U/hr IV Mini dose: 5K U SC bid	Lovenox dosing prophylaxis 40 mg SC qd or 30 mg SC bid	2.5 mg qd	3.0 mg weekly	20 mg qd	2.5 mg bid Prophylaxis	60 mg PO	Initial dose: 160 mg Maintain 80 mg PO qd	150 mg bid	0.15–2 mg/k/h IV	15 mg SC bid	2 μg/kg/min IV	Initial 0.4 mg/kg IV, 0.15 mg/kg/hr	81–160 mg qd	75 mg qd	250 mg bid	None
Antidote	KCentra (Vitamin K)	Protamine sulfate	Partial reversal with protamine sulfate	None	Avidin	Andexanet alfa (Andexxa)	Andexanet alfa (Andexxa)	Andexanet alfa (Andexxa)	Andexanet alfa (Andexxa)	Idarucizumab (Praxbind)	None	None	None	None	None	None	None	None

NOACs aka DOACs; Novel (or New) Oral Anticoagulants Direct Oral Anticoagulantss

Heparin (Unfractionated Heparin, UFH)

Heparin is a naturally occurring anticoagulant. Heparin works by binding to the naturally occurring anticoagulant in the blood called antithrombin III (AT-III) and accelerating its activity. By potentiating AT-III, heparin deactivates factor Xa and thrombin (IIa). Heparin is classified as an indirect thrombin inhibitor because antithrombin is the actual inhibitor. To a lesser extent, heparin also affects factors XIIa, XIa, IXa. Heparin is administered IV or SC. With IV administration, onset is immediate, SC administration is about 30 minutes. Monitor heparin with activated partial thromboplastin time (aPTT), 1.5 to 2 times control being the ideal range.

HIT (Heparin-Induced Thrombocytopenia)

HIT is a potentially fatal immune-mediated adverse drug reaction to heparin. Antibodies form that activate platelets in the presence of heparin. Clots form all over the body. Fingers, hands, toes, and feet can turn black and fall off. Despite "thrombocytopenia" in the name, bleeding is rare; rather, patients have an increased propensity for arterial and venous thromboembolism. HIT occurs in 2.5% to 3.5% of patients receiving heparin. It usually occurs 3 to 15 days after starting heparin. Peak incident is day 8.

Side effects: bleeding, osteoporosis, heparin-induced thrombocytopenia (HIT)

Antidote: Protamine

Full-Dose Heparin

Full-dose heparin is given IV and is used to treat a deep vein thrombosis (DVT) or pulmonary embolism (PE).

Get baseline PTT.

5,000 to 10,000 units IV bolus, then 750 to 1,500 units per hour IV (adjust to therapeutic dose)

Monitor PTT q8h (maintain PTT at 1.5 to 2 times above control).

Mini-Dose Heparin

Mini-or low-dose heparin is given subcutaneously for DVT prophylaxis.

5,000 units SC bid starting 1 hour pre-op. Continue bid dose until ambulatory.

Monitor PTT q8h (maintain PTT at 1.5 to 2 times above control).

LMWH (low-molecular-weight heparin)

LMWH is a molecule of heparin that has been fractionated or depolymerized, making it smaller, more uniform, and predictable. LMWH has the same mechanism of action as unfractionated heparin (UH) but more preferentially binds with factor Xa vs. IIa. Due to its predictability, LMWH does not require monitoring and is partially (60%) reversible by protamine sulfate.

LMWH has advantages over UH

Does not require laboratory monitoring

Higher bioavailability 90% vs. 30% with UH

Longer half-life

Less HIT

Less inhibition of platelet function

LMWHs include Ardeparin, Dalteparin (Fragmin), Enoxaparin, Nadroparin (Fraxiparine), Reviparin, Tinzaparin (Innohep), with Enoxaparin (Lovenox) being the most common.

Enoxaparin (Lovenox)

Lovenox is a LMWH used for DVT prophylaxis. Lovenox is a SC injection into belly tissue. DVT prophylaxis 40 mg SC daily. Alternate administration sites, further away from umbilicus, pinch hold, have syringe 90° angle, don't release air bubble prior to injecting. NOTE: hold the syringe so the needle is pointed down, which causes the air bubble to float away from the needle. The small air bubble is designed to be injected after the medication, to lock the medication in and prevent it from flowing out of the needle hole when the needle is removed.

Fondaparinux (Arixtra)

Fondaparinux is an even smaller synthetic molecule than LMWH. It is sometimes called "tiny heparin." It has enhanced activity on Xa and has no direct effect on thrombin (IIa). There is no reversal agent for this medication. Protamine sulfate is ineffective.

Fondaparinux has advantages over LMWH.

Does not require laboratory monitoring

Longer half-life, qd dosing

No HIT

Idraparinux and **Idrabiotaparinux**

Very similar to Fondaparinux but has a longer half-life requiring only a once-weekly SC injection

Idrabiotaparinux is Idraparinux with a biotin molecule attached. The attachment of biotin enables reversal of the drug with Avidin.

Indirect thrombin inhibitors

Drug	Heparin (UFH)	LMWH	Fondaparinux
Origin	Naturally occurring	Processed from UFH	Synthetic
Molecule size	Large	Small	Tiny
Factors affected	Xa = Thrombin (II)	Xa >> Thrombin (II)	Xa
Side effects	HIT Osteoporosis	< HIT <Osteoporosis	No risk of HIT or osteoporosis
Administration	IV/SC	SC/IV	SC
Monitoring	aPTT (1.5–2.5)	None	None
Antidote	Protamine sulfate	Protamine sulfate (partial reversal)	No reversal *(no antidote)*
Half-life	Short	Long	Longer

HEPARIN vs. COUMADIN

Anticoag	Heparin	Coumadin (Warfarin)
Antidote	Protamine Sulfate	Vit K
Onset	Rapid	Slow
Pathway	Intrinsic	Extrinsic
Administered	IV/SC	Oral
Monitor	PTT	PT
Site of action	Blood	Liver

Warfarin (*Coumadin*)

Warfarin is a vitamin K antagonist (VKA) that was originally used as a rat poison. Indications include PE and DVT prophylaxis, atrial fibrillation, and cardiac valvular dz. Warfarin interferes with the hepatic synthesis of vitamin K–dependent clotting factors II, VII, IX, and X as well as natural anticoagulants protein C and protein S. Coumadin has a slow onset and slow offset. The earliest effects are seen around 24 hours and complete effect takes 3 to 4 days. This means that for scheduled surgeries on high-risk patients, Coumadin bridging with heparin or LMWH may be necessary.

Warfarin Bridging

Coumadin takes 3 to 4 days to take effect and 3 to 4 days for its effect to wear off. With surgery, better control of anticoagulation is preferred so patients are converted to heparin, which has a fast onset and fast offset. Coumadin should be discontinued 5 days pre-op and heparin or LMWH should be started 3 days pre-op. Discontinue heparin/LMWH 24 hours pre-op. Post-op, start both Coumadin and heparin/LMWH about 24 hours after surgery. At around 3 to 4 days after restarting both the heparin/LMWH and Coumadin, discontinue heparin/LMWH. International normalized ratio (INR) should be monitored during this bridging process to maintain INR at 2 to 3.

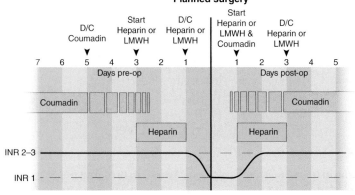

Warfarin Bridging

Warfarin interactions: Foods with high vitamin K content such as leafy greens (kale, broccoli, and spinach) lessen the effect of the Coumadin. EtOH, cranberry juice, and St. John's wort also lessen Coumadin's effects. Many herbal remedies starting with the letter "G" such as ginger, ginseng, green tea, and ginkgo biloba increase Coumadin's effect. NSAIDs, Tylenol, certain antibiotics, and vitamin E also increase Coumadin effect.

Warfarin reversal agents: Vitamin K, fresh frozen plasma (FFP), 4-factor prothrombin complex concentrate (PCC) Kcentra. Treatment is dictated by INR and bleeding.

Warfarin Reversal Protocol
INR < 10: Hold/skip Coumadin dose
INR > 10: Hold/skip Coumadin dose + oral vitamin K (2.5 mg PO)
Bleeding: Hold/skip Coumadin dose + IV vitamin K + FFP or PCC

Warfarin Dosing for DVT or PE
Loading dose 10 mg PO daily for 2 to 4 days
Maintenance dose 2 to 7.5 mg PO daily
Target INR at 2.5 times normal (range 2.0 to 3.0)
Treat 1st DVT episode for 3 months
Coumadin pills are color coded to indicate strength (mg). The color scheme is universal, although the shape may vary based on manufacturer.

Coumadin Color Scheme

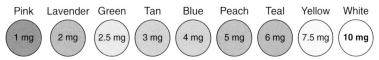

NOACs (Novel, or New, Oral AntiCoagulants), aka **DOACs** (Direct Oral AntiCoags)

This category of anticoagulants was developed as an alternative to Coumadin. NOACs work by inhibiting the conversion of only factor X to Xa. There are two classes of NOACs, direct thrombin inhibitors (Dabigatran), and direct factor Xa inhibitors (all the rest). A common suffix among this group is -xaban (i.e., Rivaro_x-aban_, Api_xaban_, Edo_xaban_, Betri_xaban_).

Antidote to direct factor X inhibitors is Andexanet alfa (Andexxa).

Antidote to direct thrombin inhibitors is Idarucizumab (Praxbind).

Advantages of NOACs over Coumadin:
  No INR monitoring
  Fewer food and drug interactions
  Effects occur faster and go away faster.

Disadvantages over Coumadin:
  Increased risk of GI bleed
  Can't be given to patients with kidney disease

Dabigatran (Pradaxa)
  Direct thrombin inhibitor
  150 mg daily bid

Rivaroxaban (Xarelto)
  Target: Factor Xa
  10 to 20 mg qd [10, 15, 20 mg]

Apixaban (Eliquis)
  Target: Factor Xa

Edoxaban (Savaysa)
  Target: Xa

Betrixaban (Bevyxxa)
  Target: Xa

Anticoagulants and the clotting factors affected

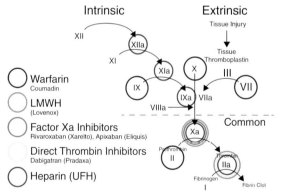

Other Hematologic Agents

Pentoxifylline (Trental) 400 mg tid with meals [400 mg]
  Decreases blood viscosity by increasing flexibility of red blood cells (RBCs)

Indicated in intermittent claudication related to chronic occlusive vascular disease

Therapeutic response may take 2 to 4 weeks.

Cilostazol (Pletal) 100 mg PO bid [100 mg]
  Indicated in intermittent claudication
  Works by causing vasodilation, increasing circulation to the legs

Platelet Aggregation Inhibitors

Aspirin
  Irreversibly binds to COX. Used to treat coronary artery disease (CAD), stroke-transient ischemic attack (TIAs)
Clopidogrel (Plavix)
  Clopidogrel is an adenosine diphosphate (ADP) receptor inhibitor. In order for platelets to aggregate, ADP must bind to receptors on each platelet. Clopidogrel blocks ADP from binding. Indications include anyone with an increased risk of blood clot such as TIAs, stroke, CAD, PVD, previous MI.
Prasugrel (Effient)
  Used to reduce the risk of heart-related events such as MI, clots in a stent, acute coronary syndrome
  Inhibits platelet aggregation
  Loading dose 60 mg PO daily
  Maintenance dose 10 mg PO daily
  Usually taken with aspirin (75 to 325 mg)

THROMBOLYTICS

Thrombolytic drugs (clot busters), unlike anticoagulants, can actually dissolve blood clots. They have a common mechanism of action by converting the proenzyme (plasminogen) to its active form plasmin. Plasmin causes lysis of fibrin clots. Thrombolytic agents are given to patients with already formed blood clots where ischemia may be fatal.

Indications

Acute MI, acute ischemic stroke, peripheral artery occlusion, PE, DVT

Timing

For arterial thrombosis (MI, stroke), the window for effective thrombolytic therapy is 3 hours.
For venous thrombosis (DVT), thrombolytic treatment can be delayed by days to weeks.

Fibrin-Specific vs. Nonfibrin-Specific Thrombolytics

Plasmin is a nonspecific protease capable of breaking down fibrin as well as other circulating proteins, including fibrinogen, factor V, and factor VIII. Thrombolytics are divided into two categories based on whether they act on plasminogen in a clot or if they act on all plasminogen in a clot and in circulating blood.

Nonfibrin-Specific Agents

Nonfibrin-specific thrombolytics bind to circulating and non-circulating plasminogen. This produces the breakdown of clots (fibrinolysis) and circulating fibrinogen (fibrinogenolysis). This causes systemic fibrinolytic state leading to bleeding.

Types of Thrombolytic Drugs

Fibrin Specific	Nonfibrin Specific
Acts on fibrin-bound plasminogen on surface of thrombus Tissue Plasminogen Activators (t-PA)	Acts on free plasminogen in the circulation
Alteplase Reteplase Tenecteplase mnemonic: ART	Urokinase Streptokinase Anistreplase mnemonic: USA

Streptokinase (SK)

A bacterial protein produced by B-hemolytic streptococci. It acts indirectly by forming plasminogen streptokinase "activator complex." It converts inactive plasminogen into active plasmin. Given IV 250,000 units, then 100,000 units per hour for 24 to 72 hours.

Anistreplase (APSAC)

Anisoylated plasminogen streptokinase activator complex (APSAC). Acylated plasminogen combined with streptokinase. It is a prodrug, deacylated in circulation into the active plasminogen streptokinase complex. IV bolus 30 units over 3 to 5 minutes. Longer duration, more thrombolytic, and greater clot selectivity than SK

Urokinase

Human enzyme synthesized by the kidney obtained from urine or cultures of human embryotic kidney cells. Acts directly to convert plasminogen to active plasmin. IV 300,000 units over 10 minutes then 300,000 units per hour for 12 hours.

Fibrin-Specific Agents

Tissue plasminogen activators (t-PAs). Clot-specific fibrin. Binds preferentially to plasminogen at the fibrin surface (noncirculating) rather than circulating plasminogen. Risk of bleeding is less than nonspecific agents. All are recombinant t-PAs, prepared by recombinant DNA technology. Directly activate fibrin-bound plasminogen rather than free plasminogen in blood. Their action is enhanced by the presence of fibrin. There is limited systemic fibrinolysis.

Alteplase

Half-life 5 minutes. 60 mg IV bolus + 40 mg infusion over 2 hours

Reteplase

Half-life 15 minutes. Given as 2 IV bolus injections of 10 units each.

Tenecteplase (TNK-tPA)

Half-life 30 minutes. Single IV bolus

Fibrinolytic Inhibitors (Antidotes)

Aminocaproic acid (Amicar),
tranexamic acid (Cyklokapron),
Aprotinin

TOPICAL ANTIMICROBIALS

Neosporin, triple antibiotic
Active ingredient: Polymyxin
B sulfate, bacitracin zinc,
neomycin
High incident of allergies to
neomycin
OTC

Polysporin
Active ingredient: Polymyxin B
sulfate, bacitracin zinc
Basically, the same as Neosporin
but the neomycin was taken
out due to high incidence of
allergic reactions.
OTC

Bactroban
Active ingredient: Mupirocin
Active against methicillin-
resistant *Staphylococcus
aureus* (MRSA)
Commonly used to treat
impetigo
This is a prescription item.

Locilex
Active ingredient: 0.8%
pexiganan
Active against G+, G−,
aerobic, anaerobic, MRSA,
vancomycin-resistant *Entero-
cocci* (VRE), and fungus

ANTIBIOTICS

All antibiotics (ABX) can decrease
efficacy of birth control pills.
Be conscious of liver and kidney
function when prescribing ABX.
Make sure the patient has no allergies to antibiotics.

MAJOR ANTIBIOTIC CLASSES

Class	Examples	Spectrum	Static/Cidal	Mode of Action
β-Lactams				
Penicillins	Penicillin, Amoxicillin/ clavulanate (Augmentin), Oxacillin, Piperacillin (Zosyn), Ticarcillin, Ticarcillin/ Clavulanate (Timentin)	G(+) G(−) synthetic forms	Bactericidal	Inhibits cell wall synthesis
Cephalosporins	Cephalexin (Keflex), Cefazolin (An-cef), Cefdinir (Omnicef)	G(+), G(−)	Bactericidal	Inhibits cell wall synthesis

Class	Examples	Spectrum	Static/Cidal	Mode of Action
Carbapenems	Imipenem/ Cilastatin (Primaxin)	G(+), G(−), *Pseudomonas*, Anaerobes	Bactericidal	Inhibits cell wall synthesis
Monobactams	Aztreonam	G(+), G(−)	Bactericidal	Inhibits cell wall synthesis
Aminoglycosides				
	Streptomycin, Amikacin, Gentamicin, Kanamycin, Tobramycin, Neomycin	G(+), G(−), *Pseudomonas*	Bactericidal	Binds to the 30S bacterial ribosome subunit and inhibits protein synthesis
Quinolones				
Fluoroquino- lones	Ciprofloxacin, Moxifloxacin, Levofloxacin (Levaquin)	G(−), *Pseudomonas*	Bactericidal	Interferes with bacterial DNA synthesis
Glycopeptides				
	Vancomycin, Teicoplanin	G(+), MRSA	Bactericidal	Interferes with cell wall synthesis
Lincosamides				
	Clindamycin (Cleocin), Lincomycin	G(+), G(−), Anaerobes	Bacteriostatic	Binds to the 50S bacterial ribosome subunit and inhibits protein synthesis
Macrolides				
	Erythromycin, Clarithro- mycin, Azithromycin	G(+), G(−)	Bacteriostatic	Binds to the 50S bacterial ribosome subunit and inhibits protein synthesis

(*continued*)

Class	Examples	Spectrum	Static/Cidal	Mode of Action
Oxazolidinones				
	Linezolid (Zyvox), Tedizolid (Sivextro)	G(+), MRSA, VRE		Binds to the 50S bacterial ribosome subunit and inhibits protein synthesis
Streptogramins				
	Quinupristin/ Dalfopristin	G(+), MRSA	Individually they are Bacteriostatic but together they are Bactericidal	Binds to the 50S bacterial ribosome subunit and inhibits protein synthesis
Sulfonamides				
	TMP/SMX, Bactrim, Sulfacetamide	G(+), G(−)	Bacteriostatic	Interferes with folate production
Tetracyclines				
	Tetracycline, Doxycycline	G(+), G(−)	Bacteriostatic	Binds to the 30S bacterial ribosome subunit and inhibits protein synthesis
Nitroimidazole				
	Metronidazole (Flagyl)	Anaerobes	Bactericidal	Disrupts bacterial DNA
Chloramphen-icol				
	Chloramphenicol	G(+), G(−)	Bacteriostatic	Binds to the 50S bacterial ribosome subunit and inhibits protein synthesis
Rifamycins				
	Rifampin	G(+), G(−) TB	Bactericidal	Inhibits DNA-dependent RNA synthesis

β-Lactam Antibiotics

β-Lactam antibiotics are antibiotics that contain a β-lactam ring in their structure. They work by inhibiting bacterial cell wall synthesis. β-Lactam antibiotics include Penicillins, Cephalosporins, Carbapenems, and Monobactams.

Many bacteria have developed enzymes called β-lactamases, also called penicillinases. These enzymes destroy the β-lactam ring, rendering the antibiotic ineffective. To combat this problem there are penicillinase-resistant antibiotics available. Additionally, there are β-lactamase inhibitors available that, when combined with certain antibiotics, protect the antibiotic from the β-lactamases.

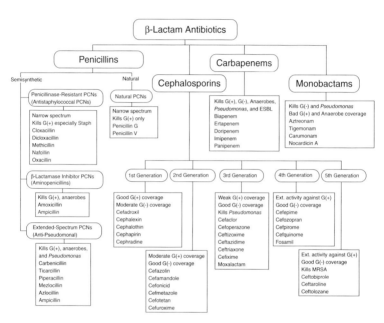

Penicillins

Natural Penicillins

Narrow spectrum
Covers G(+) only
Used mainly for strep
 Penicillin G
 Parenteral
 Penicillin V
 Oral

Penicillinase-Resistant Penicillins

Aka anti-staphylococcal Penicillins (PCNs)
Narrow spectrum, G(+) good for Staph
Not susceptible to β-lactamases (penicillinases)
 Cloxacillin
 Dicloxacillin
 Methicillin
 Nafcillin
 Oxacillin

Aminopenicillins

Aka β-lactamase inhibitor PCNs
Wider spectrum than Pen G
Active against anaerobes

Amoxicillin (Amoxil, Polymox)

Used pre-op to prophylaxis against endocarditis. Dose 2,000 mg (2 g) 30 to 60 minutes before procedure

Amoxicillin/Clavulanate (Augmentin)

Contains 125 mg of the β-lactamase inhibitor Clavulanate
Good oral ABX for dog and cat bites
Does not cover *Pseudomonas.*
Dose is 500 or 875 bid

Ampicillin (Principen, Omnipen)
Ampicillin/Sulbactam (Unasyn)

Dosing 3.0 g IV q6h
The addition of Sulbactam enhances ampicillin's resistance to β-lactamase.

Extended-Spectrum Penicillins

Aka anti-pseudomonal PCNs
Greater activity against G(−) including *Pseudomonas* and anaerobes

Carbenicillin (Geocillin)
Mezlocillin (Mezlin)
Piperacillin (Pipracil)
Piperacillin/Tazobactam (Zosyn)

Dosing 3.375 g IV q6h
Tazobactam is a β-lactamase inhibitor.
Used to treat moderate to severe diabetic foot infections

Ticarcillin (Ticar)
Ticarcillin/Clavulanate (Timentin)

3.1 g IV q4 to 6h
Clavulanic acid inactivates the β-lactamase enzyme.

Cephalosporins

5% to 10% cross-reactivity with PCN

General trends of cephalosporins

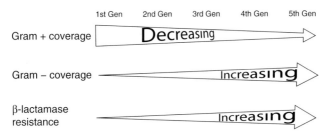

1st Generation

Good G(+) coverage
Limited G(−) coverage PECK (*Proteus mirabilis*, *E. coli*, *K*lebsiella pneumonia*)

Enterococcus and *Pseudomonas* are resistant.

Cefadroxil (Duricef, Ultracef)
Cefazolin (Ancef, Kefzol)

Most common Ceph for surgical prophylaxis

Cephalexin (Keflex, Keftab)
Cephalothin (Keflin)
Cephapirin (Cefadyl)
Cephradine (Velosef)

2nd Generation

Extended G($-$) coverage as compared to 1st Gen Cephs. HEN-PECK (*Haemophilus influenzae*, *Enterobacter*, *Neisseria*, *Proteus mirabilis*, *E. coli*, *Klebsiella pneumonia*)
  Cefaclor (Ceclor)
  Cefamandole (Mandol)
  Cefmetazole (Zefazone)
  Causes clotting impairment
  Cefonicid (Monicid)
  Ceforanide (Precef)
  Cefotetan (Cefotan)
  Cefoxitin (Mefoxin)
  Cefpodoxime (Vantin)
  Cefprozil (Cefzil)
  Cefuroxime (Zinacef, Ceftin)
  Loracarbef (Lorabid)

3rd Generation

Somewhat reduced activity against G(+), but greater G($-$) coverage including *Pseudomonas*
  Cefdinir (Omnicef)
  Cefixime (Suprax)
  Cefoperazone (Cefobid)
  Cefotaxime (Claforan)
  Ceftazidime (Fortaz, Tazidime, Ceftazidime/ avibactam-**Avycaz)**
  Best of all the Cephs against *Pseudomonas*
  Does not kill anaerobes
  Ceftizoxime (Cefizox)
  Ceftriaxone (Rocephin)
  Moxalactam (Lamoxactam, Latamoxef, Moxam)

4th Generation

Increased G(+) activity over 3rd-generation Cephs. Covers Enterobacteriaceae and *Pseudomonas*
  Cefepime (Maxipime)
  Cefpirome
  Cefquinome

5th Generation

Effective against G($-$) and G(+) including MRSA
  Ceftaroline (Teflaro)
  Novel cephalosporin covering (G$-$) and (G+) including MRSA, Vancomycin-resistant *E. faecalis* (not *faecium*)
  Ineffective against *Pseudomonas*
  Dosing: 600 mg q12h over 1 hour
Ceftobiprole (Zeftera)
  Effective against *Pseudomonas*
Ceftolozane
  Ceftolozane-tazobactam **(Zerbaxa)**

Carbapenem

Very broad-spectrum ABX, covers G(+), G($-$), *Pseudomonas*, and anaerobes. Does not cover MRSA
Cross-reactivity with PCN is similar to that of Cephs.
  Imipenem/Cilastatin (Primaxin)
  Dosing: 500 to 1,000 mg IV q6–8h
May be used as the drug of choice in severe, limb-threatening diabetes.
Biapenem
Meropenem
Ertapenem (Invanz)
  This is the only carbapenem not active against *Pseudomonas*.

Once-daily dosing
Doripenem
Panipenem

Monobactams

Spectrum differs from other
β-lactams and more closely re-
sembles that of aminoglycosides.
Resistant to β-lactamases
  Aztreonam (Azactam)
  Active against G(−) aerobes in-
    cluding *Pseudomonas*
  No activity against G(+) or
    anaerobes
  Dosing: 1 to 2 g IV q8h
  No cross-reactivity with PCN
    or Cephs (one exception is
    ceftazidime)
  Tigemonam
  Carumonam
  Nocardicin A

Aminoglycosides

Poorly absorbed orally
Good treatment for G(−) rods
Require oxygen for uptake into bac-
  teria, therefore they do not kill
  anaerobes.
Nephrotoxic and ototoxic
IV infusion over 30 to 60 minutes to
  avoid neuromuscular blockade.
  Neuromuscular blockade can
  cause paralysis and fatal respira-
  tory arrest.
Necessary to monitor serum con-
  centration (peaks and troughs)
Peaks are taken 60 minutes after
  IM injection or 30 minutes after
  IV infusion.
Troughs are taken 30 minutes be-
  fore dose infusion.
Dose is adjusted based on the
  peaks and the intervals are ad-
  justed based on the troughs.
  Gentamicin (Garamycin)
  Covers *Pseudomonas* and
    Serratia

3 to 5 mg per kg q8h (peak 6 to
  10, trough 2)
Tobramycin (Nebcin)
Covers *Pseudomonas*
3 to 5 mg per kg q8h (peak 6 to
  10, trough 2)
Netilmicin (Netromycin)
Covers *Pseudomonas*
Amikacin (Amikin)
Used for organisms resistant to
  other aminoglycosides
15 mg per kg q8h (peak 20 to 30,
  trough <10)
Streptomycin
Limited use due to resistance
Used to treat plague, tularemia,
  and TB
Kanamycin (Kantrex)
Usually limited to topical or oral
  use due to toxicity
Commonly used to irrigate
  wounds and surgical sites
Neomycin (Mycifradin)
Usually limited to topical or oral
  use due to toxicity
Spectinomycin (Trobicin)

Antiprotozoal

**Pentamidine (Nebupent, Pentam
300)**
For treating pneumonia from *Pneu-
mocystis carinii*

Quinolones (Fluoroquinolones)

Covers G(−) and *Pseudomonas*
May cause tendon ruptures
Contraindicated in children, may
  cause cartilage degeneration
  Ciprofloxacin (Cipro, Ciloxan)
  Dosing: 250 to 750 mg PO q12h.
    200 to 400 mg IV q12h
  Use caution in asthmatics, can
    increase theophylline levels.
  Often combined with Clindamy-
    cin or Metronidazole to treat
    diabetic foot infections
  Enoxacin (Penetrex)

Levofloxacin (Levaquin)
Dosing: 250 to 500 mg PO/IV q24h
Better G(+) coverage than Cipro
Moxifloxacin (Avelox)
Dosing: 400 mg PO/IV q24h
Lomefloxacin (Maxaquin)
Norfloxacin (Noroxin)
Ofloxacin (Floxin)

Sulfonamides

Broad-spectrum G(+) and many G(−)

Approximately 3% of the population is allergic to sulfonamides.

Sulfonamides can achieve high concentrations in the kidneys and are commonly used for urinary tract infections (UTIs).

> **Other Non-ABX Sulfa Drugs**
> Celecoxib (Celebrex)
> Furosemide (Lasix)
> Glyburide (Diabetic medication)
> Probenecid (Gout medication)

Sulfonamides are bacteriostatic.

Commonly used for UTIs and nocardiosis

Sulfonamides act as a competitive inhibitor of *p*-aminobenzoic acid in the folic acid metabolic cycle. Bacteria use folic acid to synthesize their DNA.

> **Trimethoprim–Sulfamethoxazole (TMP-SMX, Co-trimoxazole, Bactrim, Septra)**
> Bactrim: TMP 80 mg–SMX 400 mg
> Bactrim DS: TMP 160 mg–SMX 800 mg
> Dosing: one tablet PO bid

Trimethoprim inhibits dihydrofolate reductase and when used with sulfonamides there is a sequential blockage of the folic acid metabolic cycle giving it a one-two-punch and making the drug bactericidal.

Active against MRSA

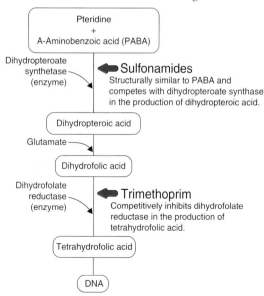

Sulfamethoxazole-Trimethoprim's synergistic inhibition of folic acid synthesis in bacteria

Sulfacetamide (Ak-sulf, Bleph-10, Cetamide, Ocu-Sul)
Used to treat ocular infections
Sulfadiazine
Silver sulfadiazine (Silvadene, SSD) topical antimicrobial used for burns
Sulfamethizole
Sulfamethoxazole
Sulfasalazine
Sulfisoxazole

Tetracyclines

Due to resistance and toxicity, Tetracyclines are rarely a first-choice drug.
Remain a good coverage for *Rickettsia*, *Mycoplasma*, *pneumoniae*, *Chlamydia*
Take on empty stomach, some foods, specifically dairy products and antacids, impair absorption.
Contraindicated during pregnancy, or children <8 years due to permanent gray or yellow staining of the teeth.

Omadacycline (Nuzyra)
Indicated for community-acquired bacterial pneumonia (CABP) and complicated skin and skin structure infection (CSSSI)
Demeclocycline (Declomycin)
Doxycycline (Vibramycin, Monodox)
Methacycline (Rondomycin)
Minocycline (Minocin)
Oxytetracycline (Terramycin)
Tetracycline (Achromycin, Tetracyn)
Used for Lyme Dz, Rocky Mountain spotted fever, and *Helicobacter pylori*.

Tigecycline (Tygacil)
A broad-spectrum Glycylcycline (minocycline derivative) antibiotic
Active against most bacteria that are resistant to traditional tetracyclines.
Covers: Strep, Staph, MRSA, VRSA, VISA, VRE, extended spectrum beta-lactamase (ESBL), and anaerobes.
Does not cover "P P P"— *Pseudomonas*, *Proteus*, or *Providencia*.
Dosing: 100 mg IV initial dose, then 50 mg IV bid

Oxazolidinones

Linezolid (Zyvox)
Dosing: 400 to 600 mg PO/IV q12h ×10 days
Indicated for MRSA and VRE
Poor G($-$) and anaerobic coverage
Tedizolid (Sivextro)
Dosing: 200 mg PO/IV qd ×6 days
Indicated for MRSA and VRE

Lipoglycopeptides

G(+) including MRSA
Vancomycin (Vancocin, Vancoled)
Dosing: 1 g IV q12h with slow infusion to prevent Red Man Syndrome, now more politically correct term is Vancomycin Flushing Syndrome.
Monitor peaks and troughs: Peaks are taken 30 minutes after 3rd dose (ideal 15 to 30 mg per mL), troughs

are taken 30 minutes before 4th dose (ideal <10 mg per mL).

Dose is adjusted based on the peaks and the intervals are adjusted based on the troughs.

Good G(+) and MRSA and methicillin-resistant *Staphylococcus epidermidis* (MRSE) coverage

Used in PCN allergic

Only use orally to treat pseudomembranous colitis, 125 mg PO q6h.

Telavancin (Vibativ)
  Dosing:
  Active against G(+) including MRSA, VISA, but not VRSA or VRE

Teicoplanin

Dalbavancin (Dalvance)
  Dosing: 1,500 mg IV, single dose for skin infections, two doses 8 days apart for osteomyelitis
  G(+) including MRSA and VRE (VanB only)
  Extended half-life

Oritavancin (Orbactiv)
  G(+) including MRSA, VRSA, and VRE

Vancomycin has become a gold standard for many infectious organisms. As a result, nomenclature of resistant bugs has evolved around its name.

VRE	Vancomycin-resistant *Enterococci*
	Can include *E. faecalis* or *E. faecium*
VREF	Vancomycin-resistant *Enterococcus faecium*
VISA	Vancomycin-intermediate-resistant *Staphylococcus aureus*
VRSA	Vancomycin-resistant *Staphylococcus aureus*
VSEF	Vancomycin-sensitive *E. faecalis*

Macrolides

Covers G(+)

Used in PCN allergic

Inhibits protein synthesis by attaching to the 50S ribosome of bacteria.

Azithromycin (Z-pak, Zithromax)

Clarithromycin (Biaxin)

Erythromycin
  Good G(+) coverage
  Used in PCN allergic patients
  Better absorbed on an empty stomach (inactivated by stomach acid)

Streptogramins

Quinupristin and **Dalfopristin (Synercid)**

Administered together, Quinupristin (70%) + Dalfopristin (30%) under the brand name **Synercid**

Quinupristin inhibits bacterial polypeptide elongation and Dalfopristin enhances Quinupristin binding.

Indicated for MRSA and VRE

Nitroimidazole

Metronidazole (Flagyl)

500 mg PO tid

Good anaerobic coverage

Contraindicated during pregnancy due to teratogenic effects

Cyclic Lipopeptide

Daptomycin (Cubicin)

Indicated for G(+) infections including staph, strep, MRSA, and VSEF

Ineffective against G(−) bugs

Dosing: 4 to 6 mg per kg q24–48h

Can cause muscle damage, monitor creatine phosphokinase at baseline and weekly

Ineffective for pneumonia

Lincosamides

Clindamycin (Cleocin, Dalacin C)

G(+) and anaerobic coverage

Used in PCN allergic patients

Metabolized in the liver

300 mg qid PO

600 to 900 mg IV q8h

Side effects: Pseudomembranous colitis

Rifamycins

Rifampin (Rimactane)

Good G(+), *Legionella*, and tuberculosis (TB) coverage

An anti-TB agent

Often administered along with other antibiotics (TMP/SMX, doxycycline, minocycline, clindamycin, or fluoroquinolone) as part of a rifampin-based combination therapy for MRSA

Stains body fluids (tears, sputum, sweat, urine) red-orange

Rarely used alone because of rapid resistance development

Penetrates bone

Miscellaneous

Chloramphenicol (Chloromycetin)

Good G(−) coverage including anaerobes

Not a first line ABX due to side effects

Rarely used due to serious side effects including aplastic anemia (bone marrow suppression) and liver damage

Can cause Grey Baby Syndrome

Dapsone

Drug of choice for leprosy

Nitrofurantoin (Macrobid)

Commonly used for UTIs

Bacteriostatic

Pleuromutilin

Lefamulin (Xenleta)

Indicated for CABP

150 mg bid ×5–7 days

600 mg PO bid ×5 days

Hypersensitivity Reactions

Types of allergic reactions

Type	Reaction	Mediator	Example	Action
I	Anaphylactic (Immediate)	IgE	Anaphylaxis, urticaria, food/drug allergies, hay fever, asthma	Mast cell degranulation releasing histamine
II	Cytotoxic	IgG or IgM	Hemolytic anemia, thrombocytopenia, interstitial nephritis, blood transfusion mismatch	Formation of antigen–antibodies resulting in lysis of cells harboring the antigen
III	Immune Complex	Ag–Ab	Serum sickness, drug fever, rashes, vasculitis, RA, SLE	Due to elevated level of antigen–antibody complexes resulting in an inflammatory response
IV	Cell mediated (Delayed)	T cells*	Contact dermatitis, Tb skin test	T cells activate macrophages and neutrophils causing copious amount of enzymes that contribute to tissue damage.

Type IV is cell mediated, all other types are antibody mediated.

TOPICAL CORTICOSTEROIDS

Side effects: striae, atrophy, acne, rosacea, periorbital dermatitis, pigmentation abnormalities, glaucoma, systemic absorption

GLUCOCORTICOSTEROIDS

Steroids exert a negative feedback control over their own secretion. Therefore, when administering steroids, the body stops producing its own steroids. Patients must be weaned off steroids to prevent complications such as Addison-like symptoms.

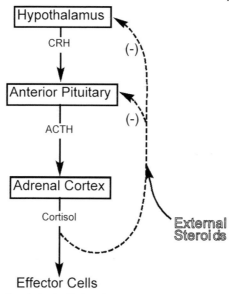

Hypothalamic–Pituitary Negative Feedback

TOPICAL CORTICOSTEROIDS

Class	Product	Generic	Formulation	Sizes
Superpotent				
I	Diprolene	Betamethasone dipropionate	Cream, 0.05%	15, 50 g
			Ointment, 0.05%	15, 50 g
			Gel, 0.05%	15, 50 g
			Lotion, 0.05%	30, 60 mL
	Psorcon	Diflorasone diacetate	Ointment, 0.05%	15, 30, 60 g
	Temovate	Clobetasol propionate	Cream, 0.05%	15, 30, 45, 60 g
			Ointment, 0.05%	15, 30, 45, 60 g
			Scalp application, 0.05%	25, 50 mL
	Ultravate	Halobetasol propionate	Cream, 0.05%	15, 50 g
			Ointment, 0.05%	15, 50 g

(*continued*)

Class	Product	Generic	Formulation	Sizes
Potent				
II	Cyclocort	Amcinonide	Ointment, 0.1%	15, 30, 60 g
	Diprolene AF	Betamethasone dipropionate	Cream, 0.05%	15, 50 g
	Elocon	Mometasone furoate	Ointment, 0.1%	15, 45 g
	Florone	Diflorasone diacetate	Ointment, 0.05%	15, 30, 60 g
	Halog	Halcinonide	Cream, 0.1%	15, 30, 60, 240 g
	Lidex	Fluocinonide	Cream, 0.05%	15, 30, 60, 120 g
			Gel, 0.05%	15, 30, 60, 120 g
			Ointment, 0.05%	15, 30, 60, 120 g
	Maxiflor	Diflorasone diacetate	Ointment, 0.05%	30, 60 g
	Topicort	Desoximetasone	Cream, 0.25%	15, 60, 120 g
			Gel, 0.05%	15, 60 g
			Ointment, 0.25%	15, 60 g
III	Aristocort A	Triamcinolone acetonide	Ointment, 0.1%	15, 60 g
	Cutivate	Fluticasone propionate	Ointment, 0.005%	15, 30, 60 g
	Cyclocort	Amcinonide	Cream, 0.1%	15, 30, 60 g
			Lotion, 0.1%	20, 60 mL
	Halog	Halcinonide	Ointment, 0.1%	15, 30, 60, 240 g
			Solution, 0.1%	20, 60 mL
	Lidex-E	Fluocinonide	Cream, 0.05%	15, 30, 60, 120 g
	Maxiflor	Diflorasone diacetate	Cream, 0.05%	15, 30, 60 g
	Topicort LP	Desoximetasone	Cream, 0.05%	15, 60 g
Midstrength				
IV	Aristocort	Triamcinolone acetonide	Ointment, 0.1%	15, 60, 240, 2,400 g
	Elocon	Mometasone furoate	Cream, 0.1%	15, 45 g
			Lotion, 0.1%	30, 60 mL
	Kenalog	Triamcinolone acetonide	Cream, 0.1%	15, 60, 80, 240 g
			Ointment, 0.1%	15, 60, 80, 240 g
	Synalar	Fluocinolone acetonide	Ointment, 0.1%	15, 30, 60, 120, 425 g
	Westcort	Hydrocortisone valerate	Ointment, 0.2%	15, 45, 60 g
	Cloderm	Clocortolone pivalate	Cream, 0.1%	15, 45 g
V	Cordran	Flurandrenolide	Cream, 0.05%	15, 30, 60, 225 g
	Cutivate	Fluticasone propionate	Cream, 0.05%	15, 30, 60 g
	Kenalog	Triamcinolone acetonide	Ointment, 0.025%	15, 60, 80, 240 g
			Lotion, 0.1%	15, 60 mL
	Locoid	Hydrocortisone butyrate	Cream, 0.1%	15, 45 g
			Ointment, 0.1%	15, 45 g

Class	Product	Generic	Formulation	Sizes
			Solution, 0.1%	20, 60 mL
	Synalar	Fluocinolone acetonide	Cream, 0.025%	15, 30, 60, 425 g
	Desowen	Desonide	Ointment, 0.05%	15, 60 g
	Westcort	Hydrocortisone valerate	Cream, 0.2%	15, 45, 60, 120 g
			Ointment, 0.2%	15, 45, 60 g
Mild				
VI	Aclovate	Alclometasone dipropionate	Cream, 0.05%	15, 45 g
			Ointment, 0.05%	15, 45 g
	Aristocort	Triamcinolone acetonide	Cream, 0.1%	15, 60, 240, 2,520 g
	Synalar	Fluocinolone acetonide	Cream, 0.01%	15, 45, 60, 425 g
			Solution, 0.01%	20, 60 mL
	Tridesilon	Desonide	Cream, 0.05%	15, 60 g
VII	Hytone	Hydrocortisone	Cream, 2.5%	30, 60 g
			Lotion, 2.5%	60 g
			Ointment, 2.5%	30 g
	Pramosone	Hydrocortisone acetate and Pramoxine HCL 1%	Cream, 1.0%	30, 60 g
			Cream, 2.5%	30, 60 g
			Lotion, 1.0%	2, 4, 8 oz
			Lotion, 2.5%	2, 4 oz
			Ointment, 1.0%	30 g
			Ointment, 2.5%	30 g

Addison Disease

Due to decreased adrenocortical function. Signs/symptoms include hyperpigmentation, hypoglycemia, anemia, decreased Na^+ and blood pressure (BP), and increased K^+.

Cushing Disease

A condition that develops by excessive exposure to corticosteroids either by exaggerated adrenal cortisol production or by chronic glucocorticoid therapy. Signs/symptoms include hyperglycemia, polycythemia, protein wasting, decreased cellular immunity, rounded face (moon faces), buffalo hump (a lump of fat that develops at the top of the back between the shoulders), hirsutism, increased Na^+ and BP, and decreased K^+.

INJECTABLE STEROIDS

Side effects are infrequent but may include hypopigmentation of the skin over the injection site, soft tissue atrophy, and steroid flares. A steroid flare is a transient increase in pain, usually beginning several hours after the injection and subsiding in about 24 hours.

Intra-articular Injections

Amount injected is arbitrary, but as a general guideline:

Knee, ankle, and shoulder	20–40 mg
Wrist, elbow	10–20 mg
Small joints of the foot	5–15 mg

Injectable glucocorticosteroids come in two forms:

Phosphates	Acetates
Short acting	Long acting
H$_2$0 soluble	H$_2$0 insoluble (shake vial prior to use)
Injectable anywhere	Should not be injected in a jt, superficially, or in an infection
Clear	Cloudy; forms a precipitate

Use caution with acetates; they leave a precipitate that can damage the joint. Intra-articular acetate injections should be reserved for damaged joints (moderate to severe degenerative joint disease [DJD]).

A local anesthetic can be mixed in a single syringe with the glucocorticosteroids to promote immediate relief.

Triamcinolone (Kenalog)
An acetate
Long acting
Kenalog-10 (10 mg per mL);
Kenalog-40 (40 mg per mL)

Betamethasone (Celestone)
Celestone Phosphate
A phosphate (3 mg per mL)
Can be used anywhere

Celestone Soluspan
An acetate and a phosphate
3 mg per mL betamethasone sodium phosphate and 3 mg per mL betamethasone acetate

Dexamethasone (Decadron, Dexon)
Short acting
Prepared in both acetate and phosphate forms
4 to 8 mg per mL

INJECTABLE LOCAL ANESTHETICS

Injectable local anesthetics come in amines and esters (see Chart)

Lidocaine may be mixed with sterile bicarbonate in a 1:10 dilution to decrease the pain during injection by balancing the pH. Lidocaine/bicarbonate mixtures are only good for 1 to 2 weeks with refrigeration.

Local anesthetics are less effective when injected into an infected site. Infections cause a drop in local tissue pH. Local anesthetics are less effective in an acidic environment.

Systemic effects from local anesthetics may include anxiety, anaphylaxis, overdose toxicity, or allergic reaction.

Epinephrine mixed with local anesthetics (in a concentration of 1:200,000 to 1:400,000) results in vasoconstriction, resulting in:

1. decreased bleeding;
2. increased duration of block by reducing absorption of anesthetic.

The use of Marcaine in children under 12 years of age is contraindicated due to its effect on growth plates.

Diphenhydramine (Benadryl) may be used as a local anesthetic when patients are allergic to both amines and esters. It is not used much anymore because it occasionally causes skin necrosis.

INJECTABLE LOCAL ANESTHETICS

	Generic	Brand Name	Concentration (%)	Potency	Maximum Dose W/O EPI	Maximum Dose W/EPI
AMINES hydrolyzed in the liver	Lidocaine	Xylocaine	0.5, 1.0, 2.0	Intermediate	300 mg	500 mg
	Mepivacaine	Carbocaine	0.5, 1.0, 1.5, 2.0, 3.0	Intermediate	300 mg	Not available
		Polocaine	0.5, 1.0, 1.5, 2.0, 3.0	Intermediate	300 mg	Not available
	Bupivacaine	Marcaine	0.25, 0.50, 0.75	High	175 mg	225 mg
		Sensorcaine	0.25, 0.50, 0.75	High	175 mg	225 mg
		Exparel[a]	1.3	High	20 mg	Not available
	Etidocaine	Duranest	1.0, 1.5	High	300 mg	400 mg
ESTER hydrolyzed in the blood (pseudocholinesterase)	Benzocaine		Topical only			
	Cocaine	Tetracaine, adrenaline, cocaine	Topical only			
	Procaine	Novocaine	0.5, 1.0, 2.0	Low	750 mg	1,000 mg
	Chloroprocaine	Nesacaine	1.0, 2.0, 3.0	Low	800 mg	1,000 mg
	Tetracaine	Pontocaine	0.1, 0.25	High	75 mg	100 mg

[a]Encapsulated in a liposome, which breaks down over time.

To prevent complications/side effects from local anesthetics, it is important not to exceed the maximum dosage. Milligrams of local anesthetics injected can be determined by the following conversion.

Conversion of % Solution to mg

Step 1: Multiply the concentration (%) by 10

Step 2: Change % to mg/cc

Step 3: Multiply by the # of cc's injected

Example: 10 cc's of 0.25% Marcaine is how many mg?

$0.25\% \times 10 = 2.5$ mg/cc $\times 10$ cc $= 25$ mg

ANESTHESIA MEDICATIONS

Fentanyl (Sublimaze)
  Opioid
  Used for induction of anesthesia
  Has the advantage of no cardiac effects

Ketamine (Ketalar)
  Used to start and maintain anesthesia
  Produces "dissociative anesthesia"; patient cooperates but with analgesia and amnesia
  Often used with benzodiazepines (BDZ) due to "emergence reaction," adverse hallucinations
  Used topically in compounded medications for pain

Midazolam (Versed)
  Shortest-acting IV BDZ
  Primarily used IV for preoperative anxiety, not typically used to maintain anesthesia

Propofol (Diprivan)
  Hypnotic/amnestic; used for the indication and maintenance of anesthesia
  White IV liquid

Sevoflurane
  An inhalational anesthetic
  Only agent approved for anesthesia induction
  Joins isoflurane, desflurane, and succinylcholine as the only group of drugs that can cause malignant hyperthermia

Isoflurane
  An inhalational anesthetic
  Decreases BP by vasodilation only, no cardiodepressant activity
  Joins sevoflurane, desflurane, and succinylcholine as the only group of drugs that can cause malignant hyperthermia

Desflurane
  An inhalational anesthetic
  Low solubility in blood/tissue allows very rapid wake-up.
  Joins isoflurane, sevoflurane, and succinylcholine as the only group of drugs that can cause malignant hyperthermia

Nitrous oxide
  MAC is >100%, not very potent
  Least effects on cardiovascular system
  Chronic exposure (dental office staff) may lead to pernicious anemia

Succinylcholine
  Blocks nicotinic acetylcholine receptors
  Used to cause paralysis during anesthesia
  Irreversible by drug
  Short duration
  May cause fasciculations
  Joins desflurane, isoflurane, and sevoflurane as the only group of drugs that can cause malignant hyperthermia

Rocuronium

Blocks nicotinic receptors

Muscle relaxant used in anesthesia

Effects are reversible by neostigmine or physostigmine.

Longer duration than succinylcholine

Does not cause fasciculations

Atropine

Anticholinergic, muscarinic receptor antagonist

Used more in emergency medicine than routine anesthesia

Increases heart rate and decreases secretions: tears, saliva, sweat

Causes pupil dilation

Crosses the blood–brain barrier. May cause delirium, especially in the elderly

Glycopyrrolate (Robinul)

Anticholinergic, muscarinic receptor antagonist

Used in surgery to decrease secretions (tears, saliva, sweat). Keeps patients from choking on saliva while unconscious.

Does not cross blood–brain barrier

PERIPHERAL NEUROPATHY MEDICATIONS

Antiseizure Medication

Gabapentin (Neurontin, Gralise, Horizant)

Neurontin: 100 to 600 mg PO tid

Gralise: 300 mg PO once daily with evening meal. Increase to 600 mg on day 2; 900 mg on days 3 to 6; 1,200 mg on days 7 to 10; 1,500 mg on days 11 to 14; and 1,800 mg on day 15. Max 1,800 mg per day

Horizant: 600 mg qd ×3 days, then 600 mg bid

Pregabalin (Lyrica)

Lyrica: Start 50 mg PO tid; may increase within 1 week to max 100 mg PO tid

Antidepressants

Amitriptyline (Elavil) 10 to 100 mg per PO daily

Not used much anymore due to side effects and newer better drugs

Elavil brand name no longer available

Duloxetine (Cymbalta) 60 mg PO daily

ANTIGOUT MEDICATIONS

Indomethacin (Indocin) 25 to 50 mg tid [25, 50 mg, supp 50, susp 25 mg per 5 mL] (Indocin SR) 75 mg PO daily/bid

Strong NSAID

Allopurinol (Zyloprim, Purinol) 200 to 300 mg PO daily/bid [100, 300 mg]

Inhibits xanthine oxidase, which is a major enzyme in uric acid synthesis

Colchicine (Colcrys) PO 1 mg initially, 0.5 mg q1–2h until nausea/vomiting or diarrhea occurs to a maximum dose of 7 to 8 mg [0.5, 0.6 mg], IV 2 mg initially, then 0.5 mg q6h to a maximum dose of 4 mg.

Acts by interfering with white blood cell (WBC) ability to phagocytize urate crystals, thus reducing inflammation

Very effective for acute attacks, but side effects often outweigh the advantages.

Can be used as a diagnostic tool
for acute gout; if symptoms
are relieved, it confirms gout.
Febuxostat (Uloric) 40 to 80 mg
PO daily
Works by stopping the body
from turning purines into
uric acid
Probenecid (Benemid) 250 mg
PO bid for 7 days, then 500 bid
[500 mg]
Inhibits the reabsorption of uric
acid in the proximal tubules
Increases the plasma concentration of penicillins and is
sometimes given in conjunction with penicillins to make
them more effective.
Sulfinpyrazone (Anturane) 100 to
200 mg PO bid [100, 200 mg]
Competitively inhibits uric acid
reabsorption in the kidneys
Pegloticase (Krystexxa) 8 mg IV
q2 weeks
Indicated for chronic gout in
adults
Contraindicated in patients
with glucose-6-phosphate
dehydrogenase (G6PD)
deficiency

ANTIEMETICS

Dimenhydrinate (Dramamine)
50 mg PO/IM/IV q4h [50 mg]
Indicated for N/V associated
with motion sickness
Ondansetron (Zofran)

Post-op nausea and vomiting:	IV/IM:	4 mg before induction of anesthesia or post-op
	PO:	16 mg PO 1 h before anesthesia

Promethazine (Phenergan) 12.5
to 25 mg PO/Rect/IM/IV, q4–6h.
Peds 0.25 to 1 mg per kg PO/
Rect/IM/PR (not to exceed
25 mg) q4–6h [12.5, 25, 50 mg,
syrup 6.25, 25 mg per 5 mL, supp
12.5, 25, 50 mg].
Indicated for post-op N/V associated with anesthesia, motion sickness, as an adjunct
to analgesics for control of
post-op pain. Promethazine
potentiates Demerol.
Scopolamine (Transderm-Scop,
Scopace) Apply one circular disk
(1.5 mg) behind ear 4 hours prior
to event, replace q3 days
Indicated for N/V associated
with motion sickness
Wash hands after handling;
causes dilation of pupils and
blurred vision if chemicals
come in contact with the
eyes.

ANTIDOTES

Poison	Antidote
Acetaminophen	N-Acetylcysteine
Anticholinesterase inhibitors	Atropine or pralidoxime
Benzodiazepine	Flumazenil (Romazicon)
Digoxin, digitoxin	Digoxin immune Fab
Epinephrine	Phentolamine (Regitine)
Heparin	Protamine sulfate
Iron	Deferoxamine
Lead	Succimer
Methanol	Ethanol
Methotrexate	Leucovorin calcium

Poison	Antidote
Opioids, Heroin	Naloxone
Dabigatran (Pradaxa)	Idarucizumab (Praxbind)
Tricyclic Antidepressants	Physostigmine
Warfarin	Phytonadione (vitamin K)
Rivaroxaban (Xarelto)	Andexanet alfa (Andexxa)
Apixaban (Eliquis)	Andexanet alfa (Andexxa)
Idrabiotaparinux	Avidin

TETANUS/TETANUS PROPHYLAXIS

General

The causative organism is *Clostridium tetani* (anaerobic, G+, slender, motile rods), which is ubiquitous in soil and stool. The sporulated form has a characteristic drumstick or tennis racket shape. This bacterium produces an exotoxin called tetanospasmin. Any injury that violates the integrity of the skin, including burns, is at risk for developing tetanus. Incubation period is 2 to 54 days (average 12 to 14 days), and mortality rate is around 50%. Natural infection does not result in immunity against future infections.

Symptoms

- Trismus (lock jaw)
- Muscle spasm
- Irritability
- Dysphagia
- Neck stiffness

NOTE: Strychnine poisoning and the use of phenothiazines may produce similar symptoms.

Immunization

DTaP (diphtheria, tetanus, pertussis)
Part of the standard primary immunization given to children under 7 years of age. Immunization consists of five doses given at 2, 4, 6, and 15 to 18 months, and between 4 and 6 years. DT can be given instead of DTaP in children who cannot tolerate the pertussis vaccine. Thereafter, a booster of Td or Tdap is necessary every 10 years.
DTaP is used in patients <7 years of age unless history of hypersensitivity to pertussis, then use DT. The DTaP vaccine has replaced DTP. The "a" stands for acellular and pertains to a modification in the pertussis vaccine that has fewer side effects.

Tdap Same ingredients as DTaP but lower concentration. Used for the booster shot given at age 11 and then throughout life after roughly every 10 years to ensure continued immunity.
TT (tetanus toxoid)
TT is given instead of DT or Td in patients who cannot tolerate the diphtheria vaccine.
0.4 mL dose given IM
DT (diphtheria, tetanus)
Same dosage as Td (0.5 mL)
Used in patients <7 years old
Td (diphtheria-*adult dose*, tetanus)
Contains 25% less diphtheria toxoid than DTaP and DT to reduce side effects
Used in adults and children >7 years of age

Used in place of Tdap for patients who cannot tolerate the pertussis vaccine

Dosage for boosters and for immunization series is the same 0.5 mL IM

NOTE: Uppercase letters in these abbreviations denote full strength doses of diphtheria (D) and tetanus (T) toxoid and pertussis (P) vaccine. Lowercase "d" and "p" denote reduced doses of diphtheria and pertussis used in the adolescent/adult formulations.

Tetanus immunoglobulin (given postexposure to neutralize the toxin)

TIG (tetanus, immune globin)

Given postexposure

Dose 250 units IM

If tetanus toxoid and tetanus immunoglobulin are both administered, they should be given in separate arms in case of allergic reaction.

Tetanus Vaccines and TIG for Wound Management

Age	Vaccination History	Clean, Minor Wounds	All Other Wounds
0–6 y	Unknown or less than full series	DTaP	DTaP TIG
	Up to date based on age	No indication	No indication
7–10 y	Unknown or less than full series	Tdap and catch-up vaccination	Tdap and catch-up vaccination TIG
	Up to date and <5 y since last dose	No indication	No indication
	Up to date and at least 5 y old	No indication	Td, but Tdap preferred if child is 10 y
11 y and older	Unknown or less than full series	Tdap and catch-up vaccination	Tdap and catch-up vaccination TIG
	3 or more doses and <5 y since last dose	No indication	No indication
	3 or more doses and 5–10 y since last dose	No indication	Tdap or Td
	3 or more doses and >10 y since last dose	Tdap or Td	Tdap or Td

WART TREATMENT

Regardless of treatment, when using topical modalities, everything works better if you first pare the wart down to the bleeding point.

I. **Salicylic acid** (Duofilm, Duoplant, Occlusal-HP, Viranol, Compound-W)

- Concentrations >6% are destructive to tissue.

- Some formulations contain lactic acid for additional keratolytic effects.

II. Mono-, di-, trichloroacetic acids

- 80% monochloroacetic acid penetrates the skin, causing blister formation.
- 50% to 80% dichloroacetic acid or trichloroacetic acid are less powerful but still effective therapies.

III. Cantharidin

- Due to a lack of controlled studies, this product is no longer commercially available in the United States. However, some pharmacies still make it available by compounding it from its ingredients.
- Cantharidin requires occlusion for anywhere from 1 to 24 hours depending on thickness of skin.

IV. Cryotherapy

- Mainstay in most dermatologist offices
- Freezing destroys the cells that harbor the virus.
- Retreatment is usually at 2- to 4-week intervals.

V. Electrodesiccation and curettage

- Creates plume and can leave a scar
- Requires local anesthesia

VI. Laser (CO_2)

- Creates plume and can be technically difficult

VII. Excision with suturing

- Leaves a scar
- Requires local anesthesia

VIII. Podophyllum

- An antimitotic agent by preventing the formation of mitotic spindles
- Podofilox 0.5% solution is a pure form of podophyllin applied to the warts bid for 3 days, followed by a rest for 4 days, and the cycle repeated until resolution
- Problem is the shelf life is only 6 months.

IX. Imiquimod

- An immune-response modifier applied topically bid, causing the patient's cells to produce interferon

X. Bleomycin

- Injected into wart, usually takes several injections
- Extremely painful and causes local tissue necrosis

XI. Cimetidine

- Generally accepted to be of placebo value only
- The bulk of evidence shows that it does not work effectively for treating wart

XII. Benzalkonium

- Antiseptic agent is also used as a 25% solution to treat warts

XIII. 5-Fluorouracil

- A pyrimidine analog that inhibits thymidylate synthase, thereby preventing the conversion of deoxyuridylic acid to thymidylic acid and inhibiting DNA synthesis.

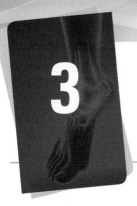

3 MICROBIOLOGY

BACTERIA FLOW SHEET

*GAS PRODUCING ORGANISMS

BACTERIA

RODS

GRAM +

NONSPORFORMING

CATALASE –
Lactobacillus

CATALASE +

NONMOTILE

Corynebacterium diphtheriae
- "diphtheroids"
- lipophilic
- nonlipophilic
- fluorescent

minutissimum
Erythrasma
coral-red flores-
cence under
Wood's lamp

(Acid Fast)
Mycobacterium tuberculosis
bovis
leprae Hansen's dz
ulcerans

MOTILE

Listeria monocytogenes
-tumbling

SPORFORMING

AEROBIC
MOTILE
Bacillus anthracis Woolsorter's dz
-pulmonary
cereus -fried rice

ANAEROBIC
Clostridium*
botulinum
tetani
perfringens Gas gangrene
difficile Pseudomembranous
colitis

GRAM –

ENTERIC

OBLIGATE AEROBES
Pseudomonas aeruginosa
-Postburn infection
-blue green color

FACULTATIVE

Enterobacteriaceae

LACTOSE +
Escherichia coli
UTI
-Traveler's diarrhea
aerogens
Klebsiella pneumonia
-viscous sputum
Serratia marcescens

LACTOSE –

UREASE +
Proteus -swarms

UREASE –
Salmonella Shigella

	motile	gas	H₂S
+	+	+
–	–	–

Vibrio cholerae
-rice water stool
-found in shellfish
-curved rod with
flagella
vulnificus
-found in raw
oysters

ANAEROBES
Bacteroides*
B. fragilis
-below the belt
B. melaninogenicus Fusobacterium*
-above the belt

ZOONOTIC
Brucella -undulating fever
Yersinia pestis plague
Francisella Tularemia
-from jack rabbits
Pasteurella -from cat bites

MISC.

Legionella pneumophilia
Pontiac dz
Legionnaires dz

Vibrionaceae
Campylobacter jejuni -special 42°C medium
Aeromonas hydrophilia

Neisseriaceae
Acinetobacter calcoaceticus
Moraxella lacunata

UPPER RESP. TRACT

Bordetella pertussis
-whooping cough

Haemophilus influenzae
Childhood meningitis
ducreyi Chancroid

COCCI

GRAM –
Neisseriaceae

OXIDATIVE +
Neisseria gonorrhoeae Gonarrhea
Neisseria meningitidis

OXIDATIVE –
Moraxella catarrhalis

GRAM +

CATALASE +
Micrococcaceae

AEROBES
Micrococcus
"nonpathogens"

FACULTATIVE

CATALASE –
Streptococcus

Staphylococcus

S. epidermis   S. aureus

	coag.	hem.	mannit fer.	color
–	+	
+	+	b
white		yellow

ANAEROBES
peptococcus

S. pyogenes(A)
Rheumatic fever
Scarlet fever
S. agalactiae(B)

(hemolysis)
S. faecalis(D)
(Enterococcus)

ANAEROBES
**pepto-
streptococcus**

∨ hemolysis

S. pneumoniae Viridans
-optichine +
-encapsulated
diplococci
-optichine –
-dental exams

VIROLOGY
DNA Viruses

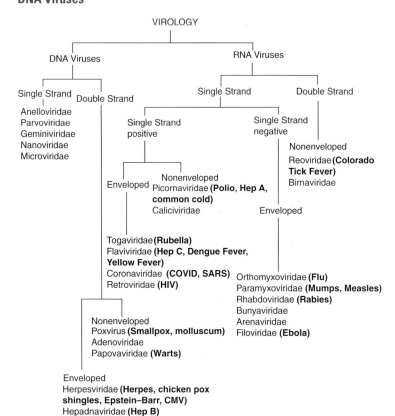

VIROLOGY

DNA Viruses | RNA Viruses

DNA Viruses:
Single Strand
- Anelloviridae
- Parvoviridae
- Geminiviridae
- Nanoviridae
- Microviridae

Double Strand

RNA Viruses:
Single Strand | Double Strand

Single Strand positive | Single Strand negative

Double Strand:
Nonenveloped
- Reoviridae **(Colorado Tick Fever)**
- Birnaviridae

Single Strand positive:
Enveloped

Nonenveloped
- Picornaviridae **(Polio, Hep A, common cold)**
- Caliciviridae

Single Strand negative:
Enveloped

Enveloped (positive):
- Togaviridae **(Rubella)**
- Flaviviridae **(Hep C, Dengue Fever, Yellow Fever)**
- Coronaviridae **(COVID, SARS)**
- Retroviridae **(HIV)**

Enveloped (negative):
- Orthomyxoviridae **(Flu)**
- Paramyxoviridae **(Mumps, Measles)**
- Rhabdoviridae **(Rabies)**
- Bunyaviridae
- Arenaviridae
- Filoviridae **(Ebola)**

Nonenveloped (DS DNA):
- Poxvirus **(Smallpox, molluscum)**
- Adenoviridae
- Papovaviridae **(Warts)**

Enveloped (DS DNA):
- Herpesviridae **(Herpes, chicken pox shingles, Epstein–Barr, CMV)**
- Hepadnaviridae **(Hep B)**

Adenoviridae (double stranded [ds], icosahedral, nonenveloped)
  Human adenoviruses
  - Found in 50% to 80% of normal human adenoid tissue (tonsils)
  - Respiratory and conjunctival infections
  - Vaccine, live attenuated
  - High incident in military
Hepadnaviridae (ds, icosahedral, nonenveloped)
  Hepatitis B
  - Parenteral route, STD

- Acute and chronic states
- Vaccine, purified HBsAg
- Incubation 4 to 12 weeks
- HBsAg is found on the surface of the viral particles, and its presence indicates that the patient has been infected with the hepatitis B virus.
- HBsAb is the hepatitis B antibody, and its presence indicates that the patient is now immune from the disease and noninfectious.

Herpetoviridae (ds, icosahedral, enveloped)
  Type I, herpes simplex 1
  - Oral herpes (cold sores, fever blisters)
  - Trigeminal ganglion cells (latency)
  Type II, herpes simplex 2
  - STD
  - Genital herpes
  - Lumbar/sacral ganglion cells (latency)
  - Intranuclear inclusion bodies
  Type III, varicella-zoster
  - Varicella (chicken pox)/skin
  - Zoster (shingles)/dorsal root ganglion
  - Multinucleated giant cells
  Type IV, Epstein–Barr
  - African Burkitt lymphoma/B-lymphoid cells
  - Nasopharyngeal carcinoma
  - Infectious mononucleosis
  Type V, cytomegalovirus (CMV)
  - Birth defects
  - Serious infection in immunocompromised
Papovaviridae (ds, icosahedral, nonenveloped)
  Papilloma
  - Common warts (verrucae)
  - Genital warts (condyloma acuminatum)
  - Associated with benign and malignant tumors
  Polyoma
  - Found in 70% of normal adults
  - Less significant in humans/ initiates tumors in mice
  Simian vacuolating (SV40)
  - Monkey virus that can initiate tumors in mice

Parvoviridae (single stranded [ss], icosahedral, nonenveloped)
  Parvoviruses
  - Transient aplastic crisis (TAC) in people with hemolytic (smallest virus) anemia (i.e., sickle cell anemia)
  - Canine parvo
  Dependoviruses
  - Adeno-associated viruses
  - Need helper virus to replicate
Poxviridae (ds, complex, enveloped)—largest virus
  Variola
  - Smallpox/skin
  - Respiratory route
  - Eliminated in 1977
  - Guarnieri inclusion bodies in cytoplasm
  - Vaccine, live attenuated
  Molluscum contagiosum
  - Benign, wart-like epidermal tumor
  - Spread by direct (STD) or indirect (towels, Jacuzzi) contact

RNA Viruses

Filoviridae (ss, helical, enveloped)
  Filovirus
  - Ebola virus
  - Acute hemorrhagic fever
Orthomyxoviridae (ss, helical, enveloped)
  Influenza A
  - Humans, animals, birds
  - Epidemic every 2 to 3 years; pandemic every 10 to 11 years
  - Vaccine, killed virus (short-term immunity)
  Influenza B
  - Humans only

- Epidemic 4 to 6 years
- Vaccine, killed virus (short-term immunity)
- Less severe than influenza A

Influenza C
- Humans only
- No epidemics
- Less severe than influenza B

Paramyxoviridae (ss, icosahedral, enveloped)

Parainfluenza
- Common respiratory infections

Mumps
- Respiratory route
- Infected parotid glands
- Complications, orchitis, encephalomyelitis
- Vaccine, live attenuated virus (part of the MMR vaccine)

Measles (Rubeola)
- Respiratory secretions/very contagious
- Complications include encephalitis.
- Vaccine, attenuated virus (part of the MMR vaccine)

Respiratory syncytial virus (RSV)
- Most important cause on lower respiratory infection in infants under 1 year

Picornaviridae (ss, icosahedral, nonenveloped)

Enteroviruses (fecal–oral route)
- *Polio*
  - Target cells CNS/flaccid paralysis—man is the only known host, and it is highly contagious
  - Tends to attack the anterior horn of the spinal cord

- Vaccine, Salk-inactivated virus particles and Sabin live attenuated
- Coxsackie
  - Mild/asymptomatic dz
  - Some diseases associated with this virus are hand/foot/mouth dz, paralysis, neonatal dz, colds, myocardiopathy, conjunctivitis, and diabetes.
- *ECHO* (enteric cytopathogenic human orphans)
  - No diseases associated with this
- *Hepatitis A*
  - Incubation period 2 to 4 weeks
  - Low fatality
  - No chronic (carrier) state

Rhinovirus
- Common cold
  - Air droplets
  - Upper respiratory infection

Reoviridae (ds, icosahedral, nonenveloped)

Arboviruses
- Orbivirus
- *Colorado tick fever*
  - Rocky Mountains
  - Vector, wood tick
  - More common in April to July

Retroviridae (ss, icosahedral, enveloped)

Oncovirinae
- Tumor viruses (leukemias, sarcomas, lymphomas)

Lentivirinae
- *HIV*
  - AIDS

- *Simian and feline immuno-deficiency viruses* (SIV, FIV)
  - AIDS-like diseases in monkeys and cats
  - *Spumavirinae*
    - Cause "foamy" degeneration of inoculated cell

Rhabdoviridae (ss, icosahedral, enveloped)

Rabies

- Bite of rabid animal
- CNS/encephalitis
- Negri bodies (inclusion bodies) in cytoplasm
- Vaccine, inactivated virus
- Incubation 10 days to 1 year

Togaviridae (ss, icosahedral, enveloped)

Arboviruses (arthropod borne)

- *Alphavirus*
  - Vector, mosquito
  - Encephalitis, febrile illnesses
- *Flavivirus*
  - Vector, mosquito
  - Dengue fever
  - Yellow fever (hemorrhagic fever)
  - Vaccine, live attenuated virus

Pestivirus

Rubivirus

- Rubella (German measles)
- Exception, not arthropod borne
- Vaccine, live attenuated virus (part of the MMR vaccine)

Flaviviridae (ss, icosahedral, enveloped)

Hepatitis C

- Non-A, non-B
- Parenteral route, also labeled as togavirus group
- Acute and chronic state
- Most common cause of posttransfusional hepatitis
- Incubation 8 weeks

Hepadnaviridae (ds, icosahedral, nonenveloped)

Hepatitis D

- Requires obligatory helper function of hepatitis B virus because there is no outer protein coat
- Transmitted same as hepatitis B
- Incubation 2 to 12 weeks

Caliciviridae (ss, icosahedral, nonenveloped)

Hepatitis E

- Fecal–oral route/waterborne

Norwalk

- Winter vomiting disease

MYCOLOGY

Cutaneous Mycosis (Dermatophytes)

- See Chapter 14

Superficial Mycosis

Superficial mycoses are found on the outer layers of the stratum corneum or on the hair.

These fungi do not elicit an immune response and do not become systemic.

Superficial mycoses cannot live in living cells.

Tissue	Disease	Etiology	Description
Skin	Tinea versicolor	*Malassezia furfur*	Superficial brownish red scaling areas Usually on the trunk Fluoresce under UV light
Skin	Tinea nigra	*Exophiala werneckii*	Light brown to black macules on the palms and soles, no scaling Tx: Keratolytics
Hair	Piedra	*Piedraia hortaes* (primarily found in the tropics)	Hard black nodules form on the hairs of the scalp & beard
		Trichosporon beigelii	Soft white/light brown nodules form on axilla, pubic, beard, and scalp hair Tx: Cut hair

Subcutaneous Mycosis

Saprophytic fungi can affect the skin, fascia, subcutaneous tissue, and, sometimes, bone and muscle. Infection is usually by way of a thorn, producing a localized abscesses and granulomata. Usually, the infection is chronic and self-limiting, but it can become systemic.

Disease	Etiology	Description
Sporotrichosis	*Sporothrix schenckii*	Lesions develop along lymphatics
Chromomycosis	*Phialophora* sp. *Fonsecaea* sp. *Cladosporium* sp.	Mostly in the tropics and form warty, tumor-like lesions
Eumycotic mycetoma (Madura foot)	*Petriellidium boydii*	Triad: 1. Swollen lesions 2. Draining sinuses 3. "Grains" of colonies draining from sinuses

Systemic Mycosis

Most infections begin in the lungs by inhalation of spores. Symptoms usually include cough, fever, and malaise.

Disease	Etiology	Description
Coccidioidomycosis (San Joaquin Valley fever)	*Coccidioides immitis*	Saprophyte More common in dark-skinned people
Histoplasmosis (Cave disease)	*Histoplasma capsulatum*	Saprophyte Found in bird and bat manure (esp. chicken and turkey) More common east of the Mississippi
Blastomycosis	*Blastomyces dermatitidis*	Saprophyte Single bud off mother cell attached by a broad base
Paracoccidioidomycosis	*Paracoccidioides brasiliensis*	Saprophyte Common in Brazil Steering-wheel appearance
Cryptococcosis	*Cryptococcus neoformans*	Predilection for brain and meninges Found in soil and bird manure (esp. pigeon)

Opportunistic Fungi

These are not pathogenic in healthy humans.

Disease	Etiology	Description
Candidiasis (Thrush)	*Candida albicans*	Oral candidiasis Vulvovaginal candidiasis
Aspergillosis	*Aspergillus fumigatus*	Caused by inhalation of spores
Zygomycosis	*Rhizopus* sp. *Mucor* sp.	Caused by inhalation of spores
Pneumocystis carinii pneumonia	*Pneumocystis carinii*	Caused by inhalation of spores Most common opportunistic infection found in AIDS patients

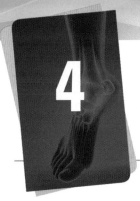

4 PERIPHERAL VASCULAR DISEASE

VIRCHOW TRIAD

Virchow triad describes the three main factors that account for the formation of blood clots (thrombosis): hypercoagulability, stasis, and endothelial injury. Virchow triad is useful when evaluating a patient for anticoagulation therapy.

Virchow Triad

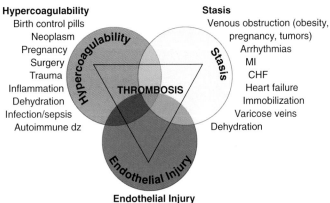

Hypercoagulability
Birth control pills
Neoplasm
Pregnancy
Surgery
Trauma
Inflammation
Dehydration
Infection/sepsis
Autoimmune dz

Stasis
Venous obstruction (obesity, pregnancy, tumors)
Arrhythmias
MI
CHF
Heart failure
Immobilization
Varicose veins
Dehydration

THROMBOSIS

Endothelial Injury
Trauma, Fractures, IV, Thrombophlebitis
Cellulitis, Atherosclerosis

STAGES OF ARTERIAL OCCLUSION

Intermittent Claudication

Bilateral pain, usually in the calf, occurs after the patient walks a distance. It can be relieved by rest and reoccurs if the patient resumes activity. The pain is due to the arteries' inability to meet the metabolic demands of the exercising muscle.

Rest Pain

As occlusion worsens, the blood supply is not sufficient to supply the demands of even the resting muscle and pain develops even when not active. Pain is constant but usually worsens at night when other distracting stimuli are at a minimum. Night pain may lessen if the legs are allowed to dangle off the bed, which allows more blood to enter the extremity. Night pain relieved by walking indicates a venous problem.

Gangrene

Gangrene is the death of tissue associated with loss of vascular supply. Dry gangrene occurs gradually as a result of occlusion of blood supply and is not usually associated with bacterial infection. Wet gangrene is the result of sudden stoppage of blood (burns, freezing, embolism) with subsequent bacterial infection.

Artery Anatomy

Tunica intima: the innermost layer of the artery consisting of endothelial cells and a basement membrane. The internal elastic lamina is also usually considered part of the intima. The intima receives oxygen from direct diffusion of blood in the lumen.

Tunica media: the middle and thickest layer of the artery. It is made up of smooth muscle cells. The media is responsible for maintaining the integrity of the artery and helps control the diameter of the artery. The very outer portion of the tunica media consists of the external elastic lamina.

Tunica externa (adventitia): the outermost layer of the artery. It is made up of elastic fibers and collagen. This layer predominately provides structure and support. Vasa vasorum are special blood vessels found in the tunica externa that supply blood to the tunica externa and tunica media of larger vessels.

Arterial wall

Vasa vasorum
a network of small blood vessels that supply the walls of large blood vessels

Tunica externa or Tunica adventitia

External elastic lamina

Smooth muscle layer

Tunica media

Internal elastic lamina
Basement membrane
Endothelial cells

Tunica intima or Tunica interna

LUMEN

NONINVASIVE VASCULAR STUDIES

Toe Pressure

Toe pressure measurements are valuable in vascular studies because they can pick up on microvascular disease not apparent on an ABI. Toe pressure also tends to be unaffected by calcified arteries (Mönckeberg dz). A toe pressure of >30 mm Hg is indicative of good healing potential.

Ankle/Brachial Index (ABI)

ABI is used to predict the severity of peripheral arterial disease by taking the ratio of the lower leg blood pressure over the arm blood pressure. The blood pressure at the ankle should be the same as the blood pressure in the arm; therefore, the ankle brachial ratio should be 1. Values ≤0.90 mm Hg are indicative of PAD. Values >1 indicate calcified vessels.

Technique

First, the brachial systolic pressure and then the ankle systolic pressure should be determined.

The BP cuff should be placed just above the ankle and elevated until no arterial pulsation can be heard through Doppler over the posterior tibial artery. The point at which arterial sound returns is the systolic pressure of the artery. This procedure should be repeated on the dorsalis pedis and peroneal artery. The highest of the three values is used as the ankle systolic pressure.

The ankle systolic should then be divided by the arm systolic.

$$\frac{\text{Ankle pressure}}{\text{Brachial pressure}} = \text{ABI}$$

Toe Brachial Index (TBI)

TBI is a beneficial index if there is arterial disease further distal than the ankle. Also, digital arteries tend to not become calcified, which affects the results of an ABI. Unlike an ABI, the pressure in the toes does not equal brachial pressures. A TBI of <0.70 mm Hg generally indicates arterial insufficiency.

$$\frac{\text{Toe pressure}}{\text{Brachial pressure}} = \text{TBI}$$

Photoplethysmography (PPG)

Photoplethysmography is an optical technique for detecting blood in the microvascular tissue bed. It works by emitting nonvisible infrared light into the skin, which is reflected by cutaneous circulation into a photodetector. This is the same technology used for pulse oximetry.

Doppler

The Doppler method uses ultrasound with an audible output, which the physician uses for interpreting the velocity and flow pattern.

Normal arteries: sharp, high-pitched sound, bi- or triphasic. The second sound represents backward flow. Small digital arteries may be monophasic because they are too small and blood flow at this level is too smooth for backward flow.

Abnormal arteries: monophasic, lower pitched, longer "swishing" sound. This indicates an occluded vessel or collateral flow.

For a more comprehensive discussion on the Doppler method, see Chapter 11.

Elevation-Dependency Test

In ischemic foot, elevation of the foot produces pallor, whereas having it in the dependent position produces erythema. Care should be taken to not note color change due to venous blood, which will produce a false positive. Patients with severe ischemia may not have erythema on dependency due to occlusion.

Exercise Test

The pedal blood pressure should be recorded with foot at heart level, and then the leg should be elevated to 30°. Against slight resistance, the foot should be dorsiflexed and plantarflexed for 1 minute (at a rate of around 1 cycle per second). Then, the leg should be returned to heart level and pedal BPs recorded again every 30 seconds for 2 minutes.

Results

A drop in ankle pressure of $>20\%$ and failure to return to normal within 2 minutes indicate arterial occlusion.

Explanation

The reason for the drop in pressure is that the blood going into the foot is diverted to the exercising calf muscles where there is less resistance to flow.

5-Minute Reactive Hyperemic Test

In this test, the patient lies supine with legs raised 30°, and the foot is dorsiflexed and plantarflexed several times to empty venous blood. Ankle cuff should be applied and inflated to 100 mm Hg above ankle systolic pressure. The foot should be placed at heart level. After 5 minutes, the cuff should be quickly deflated. The interval between cuff let-down and color return to foot should be recorded.

Results

Normal: Color returns almost instantaneously, with maximum erythema occurring at ~1 minute. The foot should be uniformly erythematous.

Vasospastic disease: Return of color is uniform, but slightly delayed especially in toes (5 to 8 seconds). Maximum erythema takes ~2 minutes and may be markedly erythematous.

Organic occlusive disease: Return of color is not uniform and requires at least 15 seconds to reach toes. Maximum erythema exceeds 2 minutes, and the amount of erythema is less than normal.

Perthes Test

The Perthes test is used to detect deep vein valvular incompetence.

A tourniquet is placed around the elevated leg and inflated to 30 to 60 mm Hg to occlude superficial venous flow. The tourniquet is placed at midthigh or proximal calf level to obstruct superficial veins.

The patient is asked to walk in order to assess muscle pumping function on the deep veins, which may help to evacuate blood or, with incompetent valves, may accentuate the abnormal flow through perforators into the varicosities.

Results

With competent valves, the blood flows through the deep veins back to the heart. With valvular incompetence, blood will reflux from deep veins through incompetent communicators to the superficial venous system and superficial veins will enlarge below the tourniquet.

If the patient feels pain on walking, this could imply deep venous claudication, meaning that the secondary varicose veins are critical collateral channels and should not be interrupted or removed.

Trendelenburg Maneuver

This test is used to differentiate between deep and superficial venous incompetence.

Technique

In this test, first, the leg should be elevated to empty venous blood. The tourniquet should be placed around the upper thigh at a pressure of 30 to 60 mm Hg to occlude superficial venous flow. Then, the patient should be made to stand.

Results

If the varicosities fill within 20 to 30 seconds, deep and perforation disease is present.

If the varicosities do not fill after about 30 seconds, the tourniquet should be released.

If the varicosities promptly return, the source of reflux is the superficial system.

INVASIVE VASCULAR STUDIES

Arteriography

Radiopaque dye is injected into an artery to better visualize blood flow within a vessel.

RAYNAUD DISEASE/ PHENOMENON

Raynaud disease is the paroxysmal vasospasm of the digits in response to cold or emotional stress, resulting in digital ischemia. Raynaud phenomenon is a condition that develops secondary to another disease such as occlusive arterial disease, connective tissue disorders especially scleroderma, neurogenic disorders, drugs, or exposure to chemicals. Raynaud disease is a primary disorder of unknown origin; it is more common in females. Raynaud disease is characterized by more gradual onset and tends to be more bilateral and symmetrical than Raynaud phenomenon.

ARTERIAL INSUFFICIENCY

Arteriosclerosis (Arteriosclerosis Obliterans, ASO)

Arteriosclerosis is a generic term meaning hardening of the arteries. There are three types of arteriosclerosis: Monckeberg dz, atherosclerosis, and arteriolosclerosis.

Arterioscleosis
hardening of the arteries

(3 types)

	Mönckeberg dz	Atherosclerosis	Arteriolosclerosis
Layer affected	Tunica media	Tunica intima	Tunica media
Vessel size affected	Medium	Large and medium (aorta, carotids, coronary arteries, iliac, popliteal)	Small arteries and arterioles (0.01-1 mm in diameter)
Pathophysiology	Calcium crystals stiffen artery	Plaque occludes lumen	Hypertrophy of the smooth muscles and/or hyaline deposits decrease lumen size
Morbidity	Low (incidental finding)	High (MI, stroke, aortic aneurysms)	Medium/high (accounts for eye, kidney, feet, and impotence issues)
Cause	Unknown, more common in older men	Age, gender (men are 5 times more likely than women until menopause), genetics, high cholesterol, HTN, smoking, diabetes, obesity, stress	Diabetes, HTN

Mönckeberg Medial Calcific Sclerosis (Mönckeberg Dz)

Mönckeberg dz is a benign arteriosclerosis, resulting in extensive deposits of calcium in the tunica media layer of medium-sized arteries. This is a sclerotic, but not an occlusive, disorder and is usually an incidental finding of x-ray. This condition does not obstruct the lumen and so does not decrease blood flow. It is only clinically significant because it may decrease pulses due to lack of distention of the vessels. Also, ABIs may be artificially elevated because the vessels require more pressure to compress.

Mönckeberg Dz

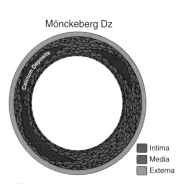

- Intima
- Media
- Externa

Mönckeberg calcifications can be seen on x-ray

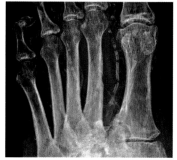

Atherosclerosis

Atherosclerosis is the worst kind of arteriosclerosis. It is responsible for heart attacks, strokes, aortic aneurysms, and occlusive disease in the legs. Atherosclerosis occurs when plaque develops in the intima (inner) layer of the arteries. Atherosclerosis affects medium-to-large arteries, specifically the aorta, carotid, iliac, popliteal, and coronary arteries. If the plaque becomes large enough, it can occlude the artery and cause infarction. As the plaque grows in size, it also begins to cause degeneration of the underlying smooth muscle. This weakens the integrity of the artery and can lead to an aneurysm.

An atherosclerosis plaque can also cause a thrombosis to form.

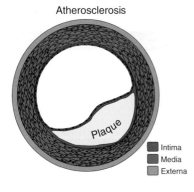

Atherosclerosis

Plaque

■ Intima
■ Media
■ Externa

Signs/Symptoms

Common symptoms include painful, cold, and numb feet. The skin presents as dry and scaly with dystrophic nails and poor hair growth. There may be atrophy of muscle and soft tissue. Edema is usually absent. Initial symptom includes intermittent claudication. Pain, usually bilateral in the calf, occurs after walking, which can be relieved by rest. Rest pain may occur as the disease advances. Severe unrelenting pain may even wake patients up at night. Elevation increases pain, and hanging the foot off the bed relieves pain. Ischemic feet may develop ulcers after minor local trauma. Ulcers are usually developed on toes or heels and occasionally on the legs. Severe ischemic feet develop gangrene.

Contributing Factors

The contributing factors include advanced age and gender, with males being five times more likely than females to develop atherosclerosis until menopause. After menopause, males and females have equal likelihood of being affected. Some other contributing factors include genetics, high cholesterol, smoking, HTN, diabetes, stress, obesity.

Treatment

Daily walking is recommended to build up collateral circulation. Patients should walk until claudication pain occurs, at which time they should rest for 3 minutes and then walk again. This should be performed at least eight times a day.

Arteriolosclerosis

Arteriolosclerosis is a type of arteriosclerosis that affects small arteries and arterioles, 0.01 to 1 mm in diameter. Arteriolosclerosis results in hardening and thickening of the tunica media. As a result of this thickening, the media layer encroaches on the lumen, making it too small for blood to pass through. HTN and diabetes are the most common causes of arteriolosclerosis. This process contributes to the reason diabetic patients are known to have small vessel disease. It contributes to diabetics-related issues with their eyes, kidneys, feet, and impotence.

Diabetes and HTN cause arteriolosclerosis in different ways. HTN increases blood pressure in the arterioles, which literally forces serum proteins out of the blood through the tunica intima and into the media. This protein forms an amorphous protein mass in the media, hyaline arteriolosclerosis.

Diabetic hyperglycemia affects the arterioles by causing the tunica intima to become leaky. This allows glucose and protein to leak into the tunica medial. This results in hyperplasia of smooth muscles.

Hyaline arteriolosclerosis: In this condition, protein in the tunica media takes on a "glassy" appearance that stains pink. Hyaline means glassy. This process of accumulating protein in the media causes sclerosing (hardening) of the arterioles and decrease in arteriole lumen size.

Hyperplastic arteriolosclerosis: Over time, protein/sugar in the media causes the smooth muscle cells to hypertrophy. This increase in smooth muscle cells thickens the media and encroaches on the lumen. Eventually, the lumen becomes too small for blood to flow. Cross-sectional microscopic evaluation of these arterioles has a classic "onion-skin" appearance. Hyperplastic arteriolosclerosis is most classically linked to malignant hypertension. The thickened tunica media is thought to be an adaptive change and frequently affects blood vessels in the kidneys.

Hyaline Arteriolosclerosis

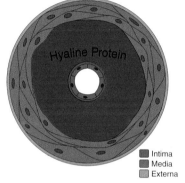

Hyperplastic Arteriolosclerosis

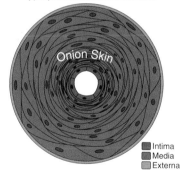

Thromboangiitis Obliterans (Buerger Disease)

Description

This disease is characterized by inflammatory changes in small- to medium-sized arteries and veins and is caused by some sort of hypersensitivity to tobacco. It occurs more in males (20:1), between 20 and 40 years of age who smoke. The disease onset begins gradually in the most distal vessels and progresses proximally, causing gangrene. It is episodic with quiescent periods of weeks, months, or years. As compared with atherosclerosis obliterans, the condition tends to be more drastic and less progressive. The disease is very similar to arteriosclerosis obliterans, and some feel that it is not a distinct clinical entity. Thrombosis of the superficial veins may also occur.

Signs/Symptoms

Some common signs and symptoms are those of arterial ischemia and superficial phlebitis.
Raynaud phenomenon is common. Intermittent claudication pain may occur, usually in the arch of the foot. Later, rest pain may occur.
Sympathetic nerve overactivity may occur. Other symptoms include coldness, hyperhidrosis, cyanosis and decreased pulses.
Inflammatory occlusions tend to be in the more distal arteries, resulting in circulatory insufficiency of the toes and fingers.
There may be a history or findings of small, red, tender cords usually in the saphenous tributaries rather than the main vessel. These findings are a migratory, superficial segmental thrombophlebitis.
Patients often have increased HLA-A9, HLA-B5.

Treatment

Treatment modality is identical to that recommended for atherosclerosis obliterans. Patients are recommended to stop smoking.

Aneurysm (Aortic, Femoral, and Popliteal)

Description

Aneurysm refers to the formation of sack by the dilatation of the wall of an artery, most of them exhibiting arteriosclerosis. Eighty percent occur in the infrarenal aorta, 20% in the iliac arteries, and 2% in the femoral and popliteal arteries.

Signs/Symptoms

Aneurysms are asymptomatic. With expansion, they may be associated with back pain or flank pain.
Abdominal aneurysms may be recognized as painless pulsatile masses during routine physical exam.

Diagnosis

Ultrasonography is the most efficacious manner to screen for these lesions.

ACUTE ARTERIAL OCCLUSION

Arterial Embolism

Description

Acute ischemia is caused by emboli thrown from somewhere else in the body. Usually, large emboli come from the heart and a history of heart disease is present (MI, rheumatic heart disease). Forty percent of embolic obstructions are in the femoral artery and 20% are in the popliteal artery. Emboli from arteries (vs. the heart) are usually small and give rise to transient symptoms in the toes and brain. Atheroembolism is an important form of embolism. Dislodged debris from aneurysms or extensive occlusive lesions become entrapped in small distal arteries. This may cause pain and focal cutaneous infarction.

Signs/Symptoms

Common symptoms include the five "p's" (pain, pallor, paresthesia, paralysis, pulseless extremity) and sudden onset of severe pain, coldness, numbness, and pallor.

Pulses are absent distal to the obstruction.

Diagnosis

Angiography (and MRI angiography) are valuable diagnostic tools. Fogarty catheter is recommended.

Treatment

Extremity is kept at or below horizontal plane.

Immediate embolectomy is the treatment of choice, best if performed within 4 to 6 hours after embolic episode.

Delayed embolectomy ($\geq$12 hours after occlusion) when there is ischemia or necrosis (mottled cyanosis, muscular rigidity, anesthesia, elevated CK) involves a high risk of acute respiratory distress syndrome or acute renal failure. Anticoagulation rather than surgery is indicated, accepting urgent or elective amputation as the necessary lifesaving procedure.

Acute Arterial Thrombosis

Description

This condition generally occurs in an arteriosclerotic artery. Blood flowing through a narrow, irregular, or ulcerative lumen may clot, leading to sudden complete occlusion. Incomplete arterial flow usually results in some collateral flow, and so when the occlusion develops, blood is shunted; however, until additional collateralization develops, the limb may be threatened.

Signs/Symptoms

Same as described in arterial embolism, differentiation is made by patient history. Thrombosis will have a history of occlusive arterial disease, absent pulses, intermittent claudication, dystrophic skin, and soft-tissue changes. With embolism, these symptoms may or may not be present, and there is more often a history of heart disease (MI, rheumatic heart disease).

Treatment

Surgery is not indicated because

1. removing embolism from an already sclerotic artery is difficult;
2. the extremity is likely to survive due to collateral circulation; and
3. the segment of occlusion may be quite long.

Treatment includes thrombolysis using streptokinase, urokinase, or tissue plasminogen activator (tPA).

VENOUS DZ

Varicose Veins

Description

This condition is characterized by dilated, tortuous superficial veins in the lower extremity, more common in women. It is caused by periods of increased venous pressure due to prolonged standing, heavy lifting, or pregnancy. The long saphenous vein and its tributaries are most commonly involved, but the short saphenous may also be affected. Thrombophlebitis may develop in the varicosities, especially in post-op patients, pregnant or postpartum women, or those taking oral contraceptives. A second type of subcutaneous varicose veins (sunburst varices) exist. These are dilations of subcutaneous venous plexuses that have a spider-like arrangement and an unsightly purple color. Although these sunburst varices are cosmetically displeasing, they are otherwise asymptomatic.

Signs/Symptoms

Itching from an associated eczematoid dermatitis may occur.

Varicose veins may be asymptomatic or associated with fatigue, aching, discomfort, fullness, or pain. In some cases, edema, pigmentation, and ulceration of the skin may develop.

Treatment

Elastic stockings and surgical excision are recommended. Cramps may occur at night that are relieved by elevation.

Thrombophlebitis of the Superficial Veins

Description

Inflammation of a superficial vein associated with thrombus formation presents as a palpable linear indurated cord possibly with variable inflammatory reaction manifested as pain, tenderness, erythema, and warmth. There may be a history of recent IV or trauma, which could be the etiology. It indicates occult, deep venous thrombosis in 20% of cases. Pulmonary embolism is rare.

Signs/Symptoms

Contributing factors include those of Virchow triad (epithelial injury, hypercoagulability, stasis).

There is no significant swelling of extremity. The long saphenous vein is most often involved.

Symptoms arise over a period of hours to 1 to 2 days. The condition is self-limiting and lasts 1 to 2 weeks. The inflammatory reaction generally subsides in 1 to 2 weeks, but a firm cord may remain for a much longer period. Edema and deep calf tenderness are absent, unless deep thrombophlebitis has developed. The linear rather than circular nature of the lesion and the course along a vein serve to differentiate it from cellulitis. Lymphangitis is also a differential diagnosis.

Treatment

Local heat, bed rest with elevation, and NSAIDs are recommended.

Venous Insufficiency

Description

This disorder usually results from deep venous thrombophlebitis, with destruction of valves in the deep venous system and reversal of normal superficial to deep flow of blood in the perforating veins. The muscular action of the calf becomes ineffective, and blood flows to the superficial veins. Valves in the superficial (saphenous) system become incompetent, resulting in retrograde venous flow. Increased pressure results in edema, fibrosis, pigmentation (hemosiderin deposits), and later dermatitis, cellulitis, and ulceration. Hemosiderin deposits are caused by venous hypertension, which distends local capillaries, allowing RBCs to leak into tissue. Hemoglobin from these cells is metabolized and results in a brawny appearance in the skin. CHF and chronic renal disease also have B/L edema of the LE, but generally there are other clinical and laboratory findings of heart and kidney dz. Dilation of superficial veins may occur, leading to varicosities. Venous insufficiency due to deep thrombophlebitis is also called postphlebitic syndrome.

Signs/Symptoms

First sign is progressive edema of the leg, followed by 2° changes in the skin and subcutaneous tissues. Usual symptoms include itching and a dull discomfort that is made worse by periods of standing. Skin is usually thin, shiny, atrophic, and cyanotic, with brownish pigmentations (hemosiderin deposits). Eczema may be present, with superficial weeping dermatitis. Other signs include dermatitis and dry, scaling skin, which may be pruritus. Subcutaneous tissue becomes thick and fibrous.

Hemosiderin deposits: Hemosiderin is a by-product of the breakdown of red blood cells forced into the interstitium by venous hypertension.

Lipodermatosclerosis: The hyperpigmentation and accompanying erythema, induration, and plaque-like structural changes that occur due to long-standing venous insufficiency.

Recurrent ulceration may occur usually just above the medial malleolus; these venous ulcers are usually not as painful as an ischemic ulcer.

Lymphedema is associated with a brawny thickening in the subcutaneous tissue as well, but lymphedema does not respond well to elevation and varicosities are absent.

Pitting edema is a sign of chronic venous obstruction or of an acute inflammatory process.

Patients may complain of fullness, aching, and tiredness in their legs when standing or walking. Symptoms are relieved by rest and elevation. Night pain is relieved by getting out of bed and walking.

Treatment

Bed rest with legs elevated and support hose are recommended.

Weeping ulcers should be treated with wet compresses containing an astringent solution such as boric acid, Burow solution, or saline.

Compresses are followed by local corticosteroids such as 0.5% hydrocortisone cream in a water-soluble base; topical antibiotics may be incorporated.

Ulcers can also be treated with wet to dry dressings. Necrotic tissue and other debris will be removed when the dry dressing is removed. This treatment is appropriate early in ulcer management when there is substantial exudate and debris to remove. Later, the dressing can be moistened before removal to avoid damage to delicate healing tissue. When an ulcer is clean or shallow, a hydrocolloid dressing or Unna boot may be appropriate.

Resolution of edema is important to ulcer management: Elevation, compression hose, and diuretics are recommended.

If an ulcer fails to heal, skin grafting may be required along with venous stripping and ligation.

Deep Venous Thrombosis (DVT)

Description

Deep venous thrombosis is the partial or complete occlusion of a vein by thrombus with secondary inflammatory reaction in the wall of the vein. It arises ~80% of the time in the deep veins of the calf. Common contributing factors include those of Virchow triad such as CHF, MI, stroke, malignancy, surgery, trauma, immobilization, previous thromboembolic disease, obesity, pregnancy, oral contraceptives, and advanced age. There is a danger of pulmonary embolism in these patients. The clot breaks free and travels to the heart, goes through the heart and becomes lodged in the pulmonary arteries. DVT often results in destruction of the venous valves, leading to veins that are incompetent, ultimately resulting in

postphlebitic syndrome (venous insufficiency).

Phlegmasia

Phlegmasia is a rare but severe form of DVT in which the clot is so big, blood is completely or almost completely unable to flow through the vein. It usually occurs at the iliofemoral junction and is considered a medical emergency. There are two types of phlegmasia: phlegmasia cerulea dolens (PCD) and phlegmasia alba dolens. Both types are a continuum of the same condition. 50% to 60% of patients with PCD are preceded by phlegmasia alba dolens. Untreated phlegmasia can lead to venous gangrene or even death.

**Phlegmasia
Cerulea Dolens**

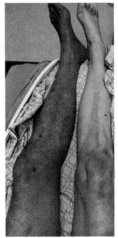

Phlegmasia cerulea dolens: It presents with a triad of significant edema, agonizing ischemic pain, and cyanotic blue extremity. Occlusion of venous drainage extends to the collateral veins, resulting in massive fluid sequestration. These patients are at high risk for a massive PE, and PCD may result in gangrene of the extremity. In addition to the usual causes of DVT, malignancy is a major contributor to the development of PCD.

Phlegmasia alba dolens: This condition is basically the same as PCD, but the superficial veins are spared, allowing some venous drainage and preventing cyanosis. There is severe pain and swelling and the leg is pale in color. The leg is pale cool with a diminished pulse due to arterial spasm. Historically, it was seen during pregnancy and postpartum and was known as "milk leg or white leg." Pregnancy causes the enlarged uterus to compress the left common iliac vein against the pelvic rim.

Signs/Symptoms

Symptoms arise over a period of hours to 1 or 2 days. The condition is self-limiting and lasts 1 to 2 weeks. Distention of superficial venous collaterals, and slight fever and tachycardia may develop. Physical exam is normal in 50% of patients.

Common symptoms include painful swollen leg with dilated superficial veins and a palpable cord.

(+)Homans sign—dorsiflexion of foot causes deep pain in calf. This test is not very sensitive or specific.

Pratt sign: squeezing of posterior calf elicits pain.

Pulses are usually present.

Diagnosis

The condition is difficult to diagnose by patient history.

Ultrasound (US, gold standard), venography, MRI, and D-dimer assay (ELISA, latex) are valuable diagnostic tools.

Treatment

The patient's leg should be elevated about 15° to 20° and trunk should be kept horizontal.

Bed rest is recommended until local tenderness and swelling disappear. Heparin (bolus of 5,000 to 10,000 units IV followed by a continuous IV infusion of 500 units per kg every 24 hours) may be helpful.

PTT should be checked 4 to 6 hours after initial therapy and then at least every 24 hours. PTT levels should be maintained at two to three times the control value. ABGs should be monitored.

Patient should later be started on long-term anticoagulants (Coumadin); loading dose of 10 mg is given each day until PT increases.

Then, a smaller dose (5 to 7.5 mg) is given to maintain PT around 1.3 to 1.5 above the control value. Patients should be treated for 3 months for the first episode.

Lymphedema

Description

Lymphedema is characterized by the accumulation of excessive lymph fluid and swelling of subcutaneous tissue due to obstruction, destruction, or hypoplasia of lymph vessels. It may result from infection or obliteration of lymphatic tissue by excision or radiation therapy.

Signs/Symptoms

Nonpitting edema is a sign of lymphatic obstruction.

Treatment

Swelling is treated with elevation and compression; diuretics may be helpful.

Lymphangitis

Lymphangitis is the inflammation of a lymphatic vessel or vessels, usually caused by bacterial infection. The condition manifests as painful, subcutaneous, red streaks along the course of the vessel and painful, palpable, regional lymph nodes. The red streaking usually originates at the site of an infection and tracks proximal. It is often associated with fever and chills followed by nausea and malaise

Lymphadenitis

Lymphadenitis is the inflammation of one or more lymph nodes, usually caused by a primary infection elsewhere in the body.

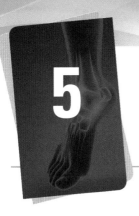

5

NEUROLOGY

NERVE ANATOMY AND TERMINOLOGY

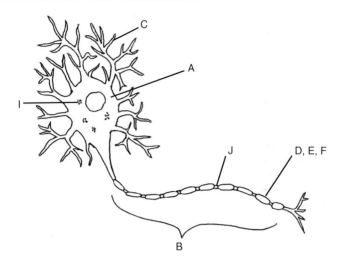

A. Perikarya—nerve cell body
B. Axon—transmits neural sig-nal to other neurons or to the organ/muscle
C. Dendrite—receives neural input from other neurons
D. Oligodendrocytes—type of glial cell (neural support cell) respon-sible for myelination of nerves within the CNS
E. Schwann cell—type of glial cell (neural support cell) responsible for myelination of nerves within the PNS
F. Myelin—a lipid-rich coating around the neural axons. Pro-duced by Schwann cells (PNS) and oligodendrocytes (CNS). Upon gross inspection, myelin is white and responsible for the "white matter" color of the brain and spinal cord.
Ganglia—a cluster of perikarya located outside the CNS
Nuclei—a cluster of perikarya located within the CNS

I. Nissl bodies—large granular bodies found in neurons. They are endoplasmic reticulum re-sponsible for protein synthesis.
J. Node of Ranvier—gaps in the myelin sheath. The action po-tential signal jumps along the axon from node to node for more rapid signal propagation.
Most nerve cell bodies (peri-karya) are found within the CNS, but sensory (afferent) and auto-nomic (visceral motor) neurons are found outside the CNS as clusters called ganglia. Sensory (afferent) perikarya are located in the dorsal root ganglia, near but not technically in the CNS. Perikarya of the autonomic ner-vous system (sympathetic para-sympathetic) are located outside the CNS. Sympathetic perikarya are found in ganglia near the spi-nal cord, and parasympathetic ganglia are found in the target organ.

Types of Neurons

Afferent	Efferent
Sensory	Motor
Direct signals toward CNS	Direct signals away from the CNS
Ganglia located in dorsal root ganglia (outside the CNS)	Ganglia located in the ventral (anterior) horn (in the CNS)

Mnemonic: SAME (*Sensory-Afferent, Motor-Efferent*)

NERVE INJURY

Sequence of nerve recovery after injury:

1. Pain
2. Temperature
3. Touch
4. Proprioception
5. Motor

Nerve Injury Classifications

Seddon Classification

Neurapraxia: Bruised nerve. Results in numbness that is reversible

Axonotmesis: Injury to axon that results in Wallerian degeneration. Nerve will regenerate over several months as long as gap is not too big.

Neurotmesis: Complete severance of the nerve, resulting in irreversible numbness

Sunderland Classification

First degree: A conduction deficit without axonal destruction

Second degree: Axon is severed without reaching the neural tube. Wallerian degeneration with regeneration. Regeneration is likely (axonotmesis).

Third degree: Degeneration of axon with destruction of fascicle with irregular regeneration

Fourth degree: Destruction of axon and fascicle and no destruction of nerve trunk, but a neuroma-in-continuity exists.

Fifth degree: Complete loss; neuroma is likely, and spontaneous recovery is rare.

Upper Motor Neuron (UMN) vs. Lower Motor Neuron (LMN) Lesions

The somatic motor nervous system is responsible for body movements. Neurons that make up this system are known as motor neurons. There are two types of motor neurons, upper motor neurons and lower motor neurons.

Upper motor neuron cell bodies are located in the cerebral cortex of the brain and the brainstem. Their axons are located in the spinal cord and brainstem and synapses with LMN. Upper motor neurons transmit impulses from the brain to LMNs.

Lower motor neuron cell bodies are located in the anterior horn of the spinal cord and the brainstem. Their axons extend to the muscles. Lower motor neurons transmit impulses from the upper motor neurons to muscles.

UMN vs. LMN LESIONS

SIGN	UMN Lesion	LMN Lesion
TONE	Increased (spasticity)	Decreased (hypotonicity)
REFLEXES	Increased	Decreased
BABINSKI	(+) Babinski	(–) Babinski
FASCICULATIONS	Absent	Present
CLONUS	Present	Absent
WEAKNESS	Present	Present

NERVE BLOCKS

Field Blocks

Ankle Block

Tibial nerve
Saphenous nerve
Medial dorsal cutaneous nerve
Deep peroneal nerve
Intermediate dorsal cutaneous nerve
Sural nerve

Digital Block (e.g., 3rd)

5th and 6th dorsal digital proper nerve
5th and 6th plantar digital proper nerve

Hallux Block

1st dorsal digital proper nerve
Deep peroneal nerve
1st plantar digital proper nerve
2nd plantar digital proper nerve

Mayo Block (for Bunions)

Saphenous nerve
Deep peroneal nerve
Medial dorsal cutaneous nerve
Medial plantar nerve

Mini-Mayo Block (for Tailor's Bunion)

Lateral dorsal cutaneous nerve

4th common dorsal digital nerve
Superficial branch of the lateral plantar nerve
4th common plantar digital nerve

Popliteal Block

Sciatic nerve (Injection is given at the posterior knee ~7 cm proximal and ~1 cm lateral to the transverse popliteal crease. At this level, it shares a neural sheath with the common peroneal nerve.)
For a complete leg block, the saphenous nerve is also injected just distal and anterior to the medial condyle of the tibia.

Local Infiltration

A localized area is flooded with anesthesia without regard to location of specific nerves. Used more commonly for ulcers, warts, and biopsies.

Bier Block (Intravenous Regional Anesthesia)

Veins, arteries, and nerves run together; so by injecting anesthetic into a vein, it diffuses out into the surrounding nerves. A tourniquet is placed around the patient's calf. An intravenous cannula is then inserted as distally as possible. The leg is then elevated for 3 to 4 minutes, or an Esmarch bandage is used to exsanguinate the extremity. The tourniquet is then inflated. The local anesthesia (usually lidocaine, plain) is then injected. The intravenous cannula is removed before preparation for operation. The block will persist as long as the cuff is inflated and disappears shortly following deflation.

Dermatomes

A dermatome is an area of skin that is supplied by a single spinal nerve. Assessing dermatomes is helpful when evaluating a patient for the presence and extent of a spinal cord injury. Dermatome innervations vary from person to person like fingerprints. Dermatomes are similar to cutaneous innervation; however, dermatomes only specify the area served by a specific spinal nerve.

Specific Points for Testing Dermatomes

L1	A point adjacent to the pubic symphysis, over the inguinal ligament
L2	Anterior superior lateral thigh
L3	Lower medial anterior thigh
L4	Over the medial malleolus or medial side of hallux
L5	Dorsum of foot
S1	Lateral heel and little toe
S2	At the midpoint of the popliteal fossa
S3	Ischial tuberosity or skin over the gluteal fold

Dermatomes

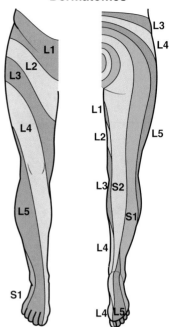

Myotomes

A myotome is a group of muscles innervated by the motor fibers of a single spinal nerve. By testing the muscle group, you can determine the integrity of that particular spinal nerve. Muscle weakness may indicate injury to the spinal cord or disk herniation at that level.

L1	Hip adduction
L2	Hip flexion
L3	Knee extension
L4	Ankle dorsiflexion
L5	Hallux dorsiflexion
S1	Ankle plantarflexion
S2	Knee flexion
S3, S4, S5	No lower extremity tests

MYOTOMES

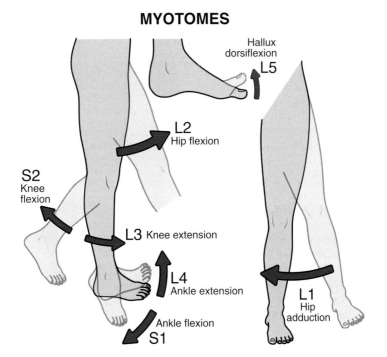

Some myotomes can be tested in an unconscious patient using tendon reflexes. A tap on the patellar ligament tests L3. A tap on the Achilles tests S1.

Cutaneous Innervation of the Lower Extremities

In addition to innervating major muscle groups, each of the major peripheral nerves originating from the lumbar and sacral plexuses carries general sensory information from patches of skin. Sensation from these areas can be used to test for peripheral nerve lesions.

Cutaneous innervation refers to the area of the skin that is supplied by a specific cutaneous nerve. Familiarity with cutaneous innervation can help diagnose damage to a specific peripheral nerve.

Cutaneous innervation

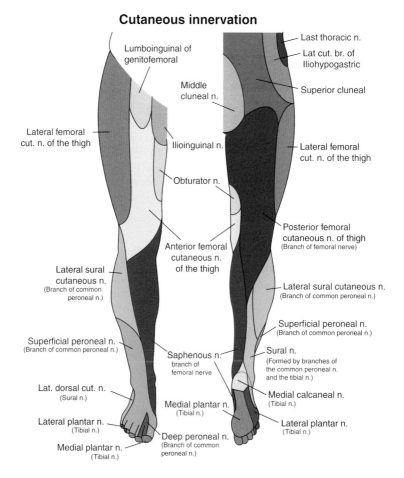

Lumboinguinal of genitofemoral

Middle cluneal n.

Last thoracic n.

Lat cut. br. of Iliohypogastric

Superior cluneal

Lateral femoral cut. n. of the thigh

Ilioinguinal n.

Lateral femoral cut. n. of the thigh

Obturator n.

Posterior femoral cutaneous n. of thigh
(Branch of femoral nerve)

Anterior femoral cutaneous n. of the thigh

Lateral sural cutaneous n.
(Branch of common peroneal n.)

Lateral sural cutaneous n.
(Branch of common peroneal n.)

Superficial peroneal n.
(Branch of common peroneal n.)

Superficial peroneal n.
(Branch of common peroneal n.)

Saphenous n.
branch of femoral nerve

Sural n.
(Formed by branches of the common peroneal n. and the tibial n.)

Lat. dorsal cut. n.
(Sural n.)

Medial calcaneal n.
(Tibial n.)

Lateral plantar n.
(Tibial n.)

Medial plantar n.
(Tibial n.)

Lateral plantar n.
(Tibial n.)

Medial plantar n.
(Tibial n.)

Deep peroneal n.
(Branch of common peroneal n.)

INNERVATION OF INTRINSIC MUSCLES

Medial Plantar Nerve (Mnemonic Laff)

1st *L*umbrical
*A*bductor hallucis muscle
*F*lexor digitorum brevis
*F*lexor hallucis brevis

Lateral Plantar Nerve

Abductor digiti minimi
Quadratus plantae

2nd lumbrical
3rd lumbrical
4th lumbrical

Deep Branch of the Lateral Plantar Nerve

Adductor hallucis muscle (both heads)
1st dorsal interosseous muscle
2nd dorsal interosseous muscle
3rd dorsal interosseous muscle
1st plantar interosseous muscle
2nd plantar interosseous muscle

Superficial Branch of the Lateral Plantar Nerve

Flexor digiti minimi quinti
4th dorsal interosseous muscle
3rd plantar interosseous muscle

Lateral Terminal Branch of the Deep Peroneal Nerve

Extensor digitorum brevis

ENTRAPMENT NEUROPATHIES

Morton Neuroma

A painful benign fibrotic enlargement of one of the common digital nerves, caused by shearing forces of adjacent metatarsal heads. This process most commonly affects the 3rd common digital nerve and less commonly the 2nd. The 3rd common digital nerve is located between and often distal to the 3rd and 4th metatarsal heads, plantar to the intermetatarsal ligament.

Signs/Symptoms

Intermetatarsal neuromas are more common in females, possibly due to shoe gear, and most common in the fourth to sixth decades of life. Pain is described as burning, cramping, or sharp and frequently radiates to the toes. Patients may also have pain radiating proximally and may notice numbness or tingling. Patients often have the sensation of walking on a wrinkle in their sock.

Pain is worse in shoes and upon dorsiflexion of MPJs (high heels). Pain is relieved by removing shoe and massaging affected area.

Lateral squeeze test—point tenderness upon palpation of the plantar aspect between the metatarsal heads while squeezing the metatarsal heads together

Mulder sign—silent palpable click that the patient feels while walking and can often be reproduced while performing the lateral squeeze test

Sullivan sign—toes adjacent to affected IS splay apart on weight bearing

Treatment

- Modification of shoe gear
- Orthotics, strapping, padding
- Corticosteroid injections
- Oral anti-inflammatory agents
- Cold therapy, stretching, and other PT modalities
- Surgery: neurectomy, EDIN, transection of the intermetatarsal ligament
- A stump neuroma can be a complication from a neurectomy surgery for a Morton neuroma. A stump neuroma occurs when the proximal nerve segment following a neurectomy attempts to regenerate and develops a bulb-shaped stump. Treatment for a stump neuroma is much the same as for a Morton neuroma.

Joplin Neuroma

A benign enlargement of the medial plantar digital proper nerve located on the plantar medial aspect of the 1st MPJ of the hallux. Signs and symptoms are similar to those of other distal focal neuropathies and include paresthesia and burning with pain at the point if compression or entrapment.

The cause is usually biomechanical (excessive pronation, hallux limitus). Treatments for a Joplin neuroma include off-weighting the nerve, orthotics, injections, NSAIDs, and neurectomy.

Tarsal Tunnel Syndrome

Entrapment or compression neuropathy within the tarsal tunnel beneath the flexor retinaculum (laciniate ligament). The tibial nerve divides into three branches beneath the flexor retinaculum: medial plantar nerve, lateral plantar nerve, and medial calcaneal nerve. Tarsal tunnel syndrome is analogous to carpal tunnel syndrome in the wrist.

Tarsal Tunnel Borders

Flexor retinaculum (laciniate ligament)—medially and posteriorly
Calcaneus and posterior aspects of talus—laterally
Distal tibia and medial malleolus—anteriorly

Cause

- Trauma (fracture, sprain, dislocation)
- Inflammatory conditions (RA, tendonitis, synovitis, diabetes)
- Space-occupying lesions (ganglion, varicosities, lipoma, neurilemoma, edema)
- Biomechanical (excessive pronation results in stretching of the tibial nerve)

Signs/Symptoms

Numbness, pins and needles, burning, or shooting pains over the entire plantar foot may occur. Symptoms are usually exacerbated by activity, such as prolonged weight bearing, walking, or running. Forced eversion of the foot may produce symptoms because this motion essentially stretches the nerve and compresses the content of the tarsal tunnel. Intrinsic muscle atrophy with hammertoe formation is a late manifestation. A positive Tinel sign, Valleix sign, or Turks test may also be present.

Treatment

Treatment should include NSAIDs, local PT nerve blocks with infiltration of corticosteroids, and orthotics to control pronation.

Surgical Treatment

Surgical treatment involves a longitudinal incision of the flexor retinaculum. Space-occupying lesions such as varicosities, cysts, or masses are removed. The tibial nerve is mobilized. Care must be taken not to damage the medial calcaneal branch of the tibial nerve as it penetrates the flexor retinaculum to provide sensory innervation to the medial heel. A tourniquet may or may not be used, however, with a vascular etiology such as varicosities; a tourniquet may hide the pathology. The flexor retinaculum is not sutured back after surgery to prevent constriction of the nerve.

MISCELLANEOUS NEUROLOGIC CONDITIONS

Multiple Sclerosis

A chronic inflammatory disease in which the immune system attacks the myelin sheath of the nerves in the CNS. Myelin damage disrupts communication between the brain and the body. Multiple sclerosis is progressive, and clinical course is highly variable and unpredictable. Generally, there is a relapsing and remitting presentation. MS can present with almost any neurologic symptom, with weakness, tingling, numbness, and blurred vision being the most common. Females are twice as likely to develop MS, and first symptoms tend to occur between ages 20 and 40. Excessive heat may accentuate symptoms, avoid hot baths and Jacuzzis. The cause is unknown but thought to be autoimmune possibly brought on by a virus or genetic defect.

Diagnosis

MRI is used to detect CNS demyelination.

Spinal tap can be useful to look for elevated levels of IgG antibodies and a specific group of proteins called oligoclonal bands.

Evoked potential (EP) tests—these tests measure the electrical activity of the brain in response to stimulation of a specific sensory nerve pathway.

Treatment

There is no cure for multiple sclerosis, and treatment is focused on speedy recovery from attacks and management of symptoms. Treatment modalities that are commonly used include corticosteroids, physical therapy, plasma exchange, and muscle relaxants.

Amyotrophic Lateral Sclerosis (ALS, Lou Gehrig DZ)

A devastating progressive degenerative disease of *both UMNs and LMNs* results in muscle weakness and atrophy throughout the body. Mental status is usually preserved. Males are twice as likely to develop the condition, and onset usually occurs when patients are in their 40s. Death usually occurs within 3 to 5 years of onset, and respiratory failure is the most common cause of death.

Signs/Symptoms

Initially, symptoms are subtle, frequent tripping or stumbling difficulty with manual dexterity, weight loss, and slurred speech. Later symptoms include difficulty swallowing (dysphagia), difficulty speaking (dysarthria), spasticity, positive Babinski sign, and hyperreflexia. Eventually, patients become completely immobile with significant muscle atrophy, contractions, and wasting. Because ALS can result in both upper and lower motor neuron lesions, symptoms can vary depending on which nerves are damaged.

Diagnosis

Diagnosis is difficult, but EMGs, NCVs, and MRIs can be helpful.

Cause

Genetic disorder

Treatment

None

Guillain–Barré Syndrome (Landry Paralysis)

An acutely progressive but self-limiting, acquired, inflammatory, demyelinating polyneuropathy resulting in rapid weakness and paralysis. The weakness spreads within several days and, in some cases, may cause life-threatening breathing difficulty. Most commonly affects those between 30 and 50 years of age. Spontaneous recovery begins 1 to 3 weeks after onset, and complete recovery usually takes place within 3 to 6 months; in more severe forms, permanent residual paralysis may occur, most notably foot drop.

Cause

Autoimmune disorder where the immune system attacks the nerves

There is often a precipitating factor such as a respiratory or digestive tract infection or a viral infection. Rarely, vaccination or recent surgery can trigger an attack.

Signs/Symptoms

Symmetrical muscle weakness usually beginning in the legs and progressing to the arms

Although sensory involvement may occur, motor weakness is always more prominent.

Decreased DTRs

Diagnosis

As with other neurologic disorders, spinal tap, EMGs, and nerve conduction studies may be helpful.

Treatment

Respiratory function must be monitored; even mild weakness may progress to life-threatening respiratory failure within hours.

Physical therapy to prevent contractures

Plasma exchange (plasmapheresis) and high-dose immunoglobulin therapy

Charcot–Marie–Tooth Disease (CMT, Peroneal Muscular Atrophy)

A group of hereditary disorders that cause damage to the *peripheral nervous system*. The main symptoms are slow progressive distal to proximal muscle weakness and atrophy. It initially affects the lower extremity and finally progresses to the upper limbs. Foot drop is often the first sign of the disease. CMT is the most common hereditary neuromuscular disorder and was named after the three physicians who first recognized the disease. There may or may not be sensory changes including peripheral neuropathy, but these are less severe than motor function deficit. Symptoms usually develop in adolescence or early adulthood, but this condition can develop in midlife too. CMT is not considered fatal, and people with most forms have a normal life expectancy.

Cause

Hereditary

Signs/Symptoms

Symptoms usually begin in the feet and legs with pes cavus, *drop foot* (slapping gait), and hammertoes.

CMT *affects the peroneus brevis while sparing the peroneus longus*; this accounts for the pes cavus deformity.

The order of muscle involvement is:

1. Plantar intrinsics
2. Tibialis anterior
3. EDL
4. EHL
5. Peroneus brevis

Loss of muscle bulk in the legs, giving the legs the classic "inverted champagne bottle" or "stork leg" appearance due to atrophy

Unsteady gait, tending to trip easily

Stocking-glove sensory loss

Decrease ankle DTRs

Diagnosis

Physical examination, EMGs, nerve conduction studies, genetic testing

Treatment

AFOs, braces and other orthopedic devices, PT, palliative foot surgery

Charcot Joint (Charcot Arthropathy)

A destructive arthropathy resulting from *peripheral neuropathy and increased bone blood flow* from reflex vasodilation. A Charcot foot results in fractures and dislocations of bones with minimal or no known trauma. Initial symptoms include swelling, redness, and increased warmth of the foot or ankle. Later, as fractures and dislocations occur, there may be significant deformity of the foot, resulting in equinus and collapse of the midfoot. Patients become weight bearing in the arch of the foot (rocker bottom foot), and plantar ulcers develop. The midfoot is the most commonly affected area, followed by the rearfoot, ankle, heel, and forefoot.

Stages

Stage 1 (acute): Red, hot, swollen foot. Radiographically, there may be signs of early bony fragmentation and joint dislocation. It is very important to off weight the foot as soon as these symptoms develop.

Stage 2 (coalescence): Redness and warmth while still present are decreased. Radiographs show early signs of bony healing.

Stage 3 (consolidation): Redness, swelling, and warmth resolve. Radiographically, bones stabilize, round off, and fuse in place. Severe deformity may be present based on the patient's weight-bearing status in stages 1 and 2.

Causes

Any condition causing neuropathy can result in a Charcot foot, most commonly diabetes.

Treatment

Non–weight bearing as soon as symptoms present

CROW boot

Accommodative footwear

Surgical intervention may be indicated based on the level of resulting deformity. Surgery may involve ORIF or excision of plantar spurs or malaligned bones that become prominent in the arch. A TAL is also very commonly required.

Friedreich Ataxia

An inherited disease that results in spinal cord and peripheral nerve degeneration and to become thinner. Most patients with Friedreich ataxia also develop scoliosis and require back surgery. The condition results in awkward unsteady movements, ataxia, and decreased sensory function, but does not affect cognitive function. Friedreich ataxia also affects the heart by causing hypertrophic cardiomyopathy, leading to decrease in the heart's pumping capacity. Symptoms typically begin between 5 and 15 years of age. Patients are usually confined to a wheelchair within 10 to 20 years after onset.

Complex Regional Pain Syndrome (CRPS)

Formerly known as reflex sympathetic dystrophy (RSD). A progressive disease of the autonomic nervous system, more specifically the sympathetic nervous system. The disease is characterized by persistent severe burning pain associated with trophic and vasomotor changes. Trophic changes may include skin and bone atrophy (Sudeck atrophy), hair loss, and joint contractures. Autonomic changes include sweating or vasomotor changes. Seventy-five percent of those affected are females. CRPS usually occurs in patients who are in their 30s and 40s. It usually occurs in one of the four extremities. The pain is initially localized to the site of injury or the distribution of the affected nerve, but with time, it spreads to involve the entire extremity. Onset can range from several days to years.

There are two types of CRPS:

CRPS Type I (RSD)

Induced by soft-tissue or bone injury. Usually caused by minor nerve injury (sprain, fracture, infection, fall). Sometimes, the nerve injury cannot immediately be identified.

CRPS Type II (Causalgia)

Induced by nerve injury

Stages

Stage 1 (Acute, 1 to 3 Months)

Constant burning pain, allodynia, hyperalgesia, hyperesthesia, hyperpathia, localized edema, joint stiffness, limitation of motion. Initially, the skin is warm, red, and dry, but near the end of this stage, it becomes cyanotic, cold, and sweaty. Bone scans with technetium (^{99}mTC) show increased uptake by the small joints. Radiographs are usually normal; changes take 5 to 6 weeks to develop.

Stage 2 (Dystrophic, 3 to 6 Months)

Continuous burning, aching pain, allodynia, hyperalgesia, hyperpathia, indurated edema. The skin takes on a cool, pale, discolored, and frequently mottled or cyanotic appearance. Dystrophic changes occur, hair growth is decreased, and nails are brittle, cracked, and ridged. Radiographs may show spotty diffuse osteopenia (Sudeck atrophy). Joints become thickened and contracted, and muscle wasting may be present. This stage is still capable of improvement.

Stage 3 (Atrophic, >6 Months)

Pain in entire limb with muscle wasting and limited movement due to contractures and ankyloses. Radiographs show marked spotty or diffuse periarticular demineralization. Prognosis at this stage is poor.

Diagnosis

Diagnosis is difficult by history and physical examination. Thermography may be helpful, decrease in temperature in either the early or late stages of the disease, possibly increased temperature localized around joints. Bone scans reveal diffuse increased uptake in the affected area using a three-phase technetium bone scan. Radiographs show spotty or diffuse osteopenia (Sudeck atrophy). Radiologic findings can take several months to develop. Doppler may be helpful in evaluating vasomotor changes. Sympathetic blocks with relief of symptoms can aid diagnosis.

Treatment

Early diagnosis and treatment are crucial for a good prognosis. Prompt diagnosis and treatment can result in remission of symptoms and complete recovery.

Treatment may include medications such as steroids, drugs used for peripheral neuropathy. Physical therapy is crucial, massage, ROM exercises, US, splinting, and contrast baths. Treatments that interfere with nerve transmission such as TENS, acupuncture, and sympathectomies are beneficial. Nerve blocks and psychotherapy are also used. Avoid surgery on these patients, if at all possible.

ELECTROMYOGRAPHY (EMG) AND NERVE CONDUCTION VELOCITY (NCV) STUDIES

Used for electrodiagnosis of neuromuscular disorders

EMG—Electromyography

Assesses the electrical activity generated by muscle fibers at rest and with activity

Results

Normal	At rest, the electrical signal should be silent, and with voluntary movement, unit potentials are roughly proportional to effort.
Denervation	In denervated muscles, there are fasciculations at rest. With voluntary movement, the number of motor units under voluntary control are decreased, and the duration and amplitude of the individual potentials are increased. The increase is due to collateral sprouting of axonal processes from surviving axons.

NCV—Nerve Conduction Velocity

Used to distinguish conditions involving the myelin sheath from those affecting the axon. They are also helpful in determining the distribution of a nerve lesion, including areas of focal nerve compression (tarsal tunnel). NCVs measure the latency of motor nerve conduction, which is the time from stimulation of a nerve to the evoked muscle response. The test is performed by stimulating one point on a nerve and measuring the time taken before the muscle responds. The test is then repeated at a second site closer to the muscle. By subtracting one time from the other, it is possible to determine the time taken for the impulse to cover the measurable distance between the two sites of stimulation. The result is a rate of meters per second (mps). Normal values vary but are almost always >40 mps.

TREATMENT FOR PERIPHERAL NEUROPATHY

Narcotic and nonnarcotic analgesics (i.e., codeine, acetaminophen, ASA)

Antidepressants (i.e., Amitriptyline-Elavil, Desipramine, Imipramine, Doxepin, Nortriptyline, Trazodone, Bupropion)

Anticonvulsants (i.e., Carbamazepine, Phenytoin, Clonazepam, Gabapentin-*Neurontin*)

Local anesthetics (i.e., Lidocaine)

Aldose reductase inhibitors (i.e., Epalrestat, Ponalresat, Alrestatin)

Topical agents (i.e., Capsaicin, Zostrix)

Vitamins (i.e., vitamin B_{12}, Biotin, Metanx)

Antiarrhythmics (i.e., Mexiletine)

Antipsychotic-phenothiazines (i.e., Prolixin)

Selective serotonin reuptake inhibitors (i.e., Paroxetine, Fluoxetine, Sertraline)

NERVE SCLEROSING INJECTIONS

Used as an alternative to surgery for Morton neuroma

Causes chemical neurolysis via Wallerian degeneration

Alcohol has a high affinity for neural tissue and causes Wallerian nerve degeneration by dehydrating the nerve.

0.5 cc of 4% alcohol sclerosing agent are injected.

Administer 3 to 7 injections 1 week apart.

Preparing solution: Aspirate 2 cc from a 50-mL vial of 0.5% Bupivacaine HCl with epinephrine. Next introduce 2 mL of absolute dehydrated alcohol into the same vial. This yields 50 cc of 4% sclerosing solution. This solution is good for about 1 month.

6 CARDIOLOGY

ANATOMY

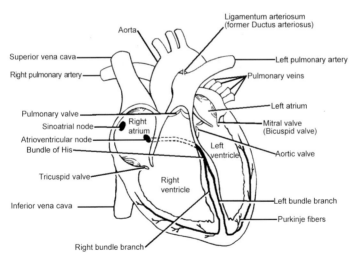

BLOOD FLOW THROUGH HEART

- Superior and inferior vena cava
- Right atrium
- Tricuspid valve
- Right ventricle
- Pulmonic valve
- Pulmonary artery
- Lungs
- Pulmonary veins
- Left atrium
- Mitral valve (bicuspid valve)
- Left ventricle
- Aortic valve
- Aorta
- Systemic circulation

HEART SOUNDS

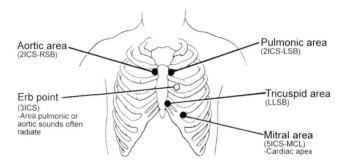

S1

- Due to closure of the atrioventricular valves (tricuspid and mitral)
- Heard loudest at mitral and tricuspid areas
- Use diaphragm of stethoscope

S2

- Due to closure of the semilunar valves (aortic and pulmonic)
- Heard loudest at aortic and pulmonic areas
- Use diaphragm of stethoscope

S3

- Caused by rapid ventricular filling
- Heard loudest at mitral area
- May be normal in young people or due to CHF or mitral regurgitation
- Use bell of stethoscope

S4

- Caused by forceful atrial ejection into a distended ventricle
- Heard loudest at mitral area
- May be normal (children, well-trained athletes) or due to HTN or aortic stenosis
- Use bell of stethoscope

MURMURS

- Use the diaphragm for high-pitched murmurs.
- Use the bell for low-pitched murmurs.
- Loudness of murmur is not proportional to the severity of disease.
- The terms *regurgitation, incompetence,* and *insufficiency* are used interchangeably.

Innocent vs. Pathologic Murmur

	Innocent	Pathologic
Timing	Systolic	Diastolic
Location	Not maximally at aortic area	Originates in heart itself
Intensity	Grade 3 or less	Can be any grade
Variation with respiration	Can vary greatly (louder on inspiration)	Usually constant
Evidence of cardiac disease	No	Yes
Age	More common in children/young adults	All ages

Murmur Loudness Scale

I—barely audible

II—faint, clearly audible

III—moderately loud with no palpable thrills

IV—loud with palpable thrill likely

V—very loud, may be audible with stethoscope partly off chest. Palpable thrill likely

VI—very loud, may be audible with stethoscope off chest. Associated with palpable thrills

NOTE: Thrills—low-frequency cutaneous vibrations associated with loud heart murmurs. The vibration can often be felt with the hand placed on the chest.

Murmur Types

Aortic Stenosis

- Loudest at aortic area
- Mid-systolic murmur
- Radiates to carotids and sometimes apex
- Crescendo–decrescendo
- Loud, harsh, medium pitched
- Ejection click and S4 often heard at apex

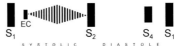

Aortic Regurgitation

- Location varies—aortic area
- Left lower sternal border
- 3rd intercostal space left
- Early-diastolic murmur
- Decrescendo
- Holosystolic
- Blowing, high pitched
- Louder sitting forward and after exhalation

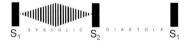

Pulmonic Stenosis

- Loudest at pulmonic area
- Mid-systolic murmur
- Crescendo–decrescendo
- Harsh, medium pitch
- Louder on inspiration
- Click often heard

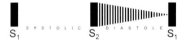

Pulmonic Regurgitation

- Loudest at pulmonic area
- Diastolic murmur
- Low pitched
- Decrescendo or crescendo–decrescendo
- Louder on inspiration

Mitral Stenosis

- Heard loudest at apex (mitral area)
- Mid-diastolic murmur
- Opening snap
- Low pitch, rumbling (use the bell)
- Decrescendo
- Accentuated by exercise
- Left lateral decubitus position

Mitral Regurgitation

- Heard loudest at mitral area or sometimes the aortic area
- Holosystolic murmur
- Radiates to left axilla
- High-pitched, blowing murmur

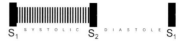

Tricuspid Regurgitation

- Loudest at tricuspid area
- Blowing, high pitched
- Holosystolic murmur
- Increases with inspiration

Atrial Septal Defect

- Loudest at pulmonic area
- Systolic murmur
- Splitting of S2

Ventricular Septal Defect

- Loudest at tricuspid area
- High pitched, harsh
- Holosystolic with mid-systolic peak

Patent Ductus Arteriosus

- Loudest at left 2nd intercostal space below left clavicle
- Continuous, "machine murmur"

READING EKGS

EKG Paper

- Little 1 mm box = 0.04 seconds
- Big 5 mm box = 0.20 seconds
- Distance between slashes at top of page = 3 seconds

Determining Heart Rate

Measure the distance between two consecutive QRS complexes

- 1 big box = 300 bpm
- 2 big boxes = 150 bpm
- 3 big boxes = 100 bpm
- 4 big boxes =75 bpm
- 5 big boxes = 60 bpm
- 6 big boxes = 50 bpm

Divide 300 by the number of big boxes between two consecutive QRS complexes.

Alternately, if the rate is slow or rhythm is irregular,

- Count the number of QRS complexes between two 3-second slash marks at the top of the page (30 big boxes) and multiply by 10.

Rhythm

Regular—a pulse with no irregularities

Regularly irregular—a pulse having an irregularity that occurs in a regular pattern

Irregularly irregular—an irregular pulse with no pattern

Components

P = depolarization of the atria
QRS = depolarization of the ventricles
T = repolarization of the ventricles

a. PR interval
  - Beginning of the P wave to the beginning of the QRS complex
  - Normal interval is between 0.12 and 0.21 seconds.
  - If >0.21 second, heart block
  - If <0.12 second, Wolff–Parkinson–White and Lown–Ganong–Levine syndromes

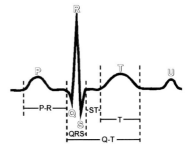

b. QRS interval
  - Beginning of Q wave to the end of S wave
  - Normal is <0.12 seconds.
  - Lengthening can occur with:
    • Beats initiated in the ventricles (i.e., PVC, VT, AIVR)
    • Bundle branch blocks
    • Pacemakers

c. Q wave
  - Hallmark of infarction
  - Q wave will appear or enlarge following an MI.
  - Most Q waves are permanent and offer valuable information when pre-oping a patient (no Sx if patient had an MI in the past 6 months) important to get old EKG for comparison.

d. ST segment
  - Between the end of QRS and the beginning of T wave
  - Elevated ST is the hallmark of myocardial injury.

e. T wave
- Inverted T wave may indicate ischemia.
- Tall, peaked T waves indicate hyperkalemia.

f. U wave
- Sometimes seen following T waves
- Associated with electrolyte disturbances (hypokalemia and hypomagnesemia)

CARDIAC RHYTHMS

1. First-degree heart block
- Delay in transmission of the electrical impulse from the atria to the ventricles
- Prolonged P-R interval beyond 0.20 seconds but constant in duration

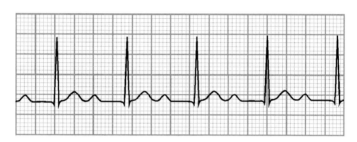

2. Second-degree heart block
- Type I (Wenckebach)
  - Not all atrial impulses reach the ventricles.
- P-R interval progressively lengthens until a QRS complex is dropped and then the cycle repeats.

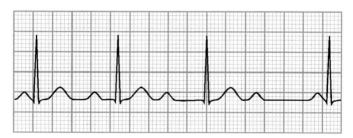

- Type II (Mobitz)
  - Not all atrial impulses reach the ventricles.

- No delay or prolongation of P-R interval

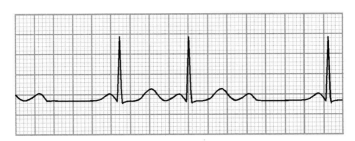

3. Third-degree heart block
   - None of the atrial impulses reach the ventricles.
   - Atrium and ventricles beat independently at their own

   regular rates (atrial rate 60 to 100 bpm, ventricular rate 40 bpm).
   - No correlation between Ps and QRSTs

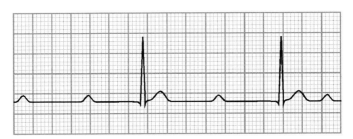

4. Sinus arrhythmia
   - NSR with varying rate depending on respiration

   - Rate increases with inspiration; rate decreases with expiration.

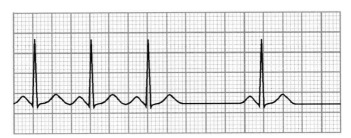

5. Asystole (sinus arrest, flatline)
- Failure of the sinus to produce an impulse, resulting in a prolonged pause

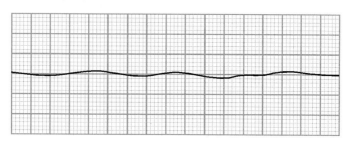

6. Sinus bradycardia
- <60 bpm

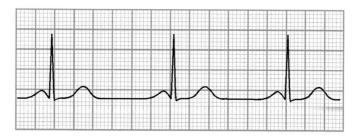

7. Sinus tachycardia
- >100 bpm

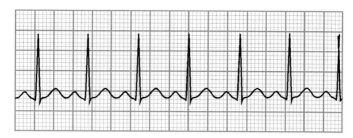

8. Premature atrial contraction (PAC)
- A focus in the atrium (other than the SA node) depolarizes prematurely.
- P wave appears early and abnormally shaped, or it may be lost in the previous T wave.
- Causes: Stimulants—coffee, tobacco, EtOH, heart disease, CHF, meds, hypoxia, low K^+ levels

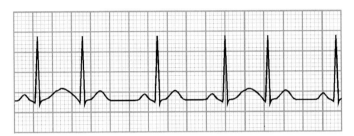

9. Paroxysmal atrial tachycardia (PAT) or paroxysmal supraventricular tachycardia (PSVT)
- A focus in the atrium (other than the SA node) depolarizes, giving rise to a series of rapid beats at a regular rate between 150 and 250 per minute.
- Begins and ends suddenly (paroxysmal)

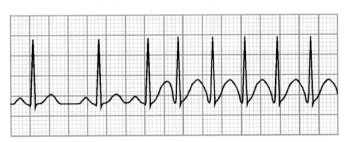

10. Atrial flutter
- Rapid firing of an ectopic atrial focus "sawtooth" pattern
- Only some beats pass to the AV node.

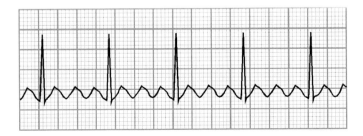

11. Atrial fibrillation
- Multiple atrial foci depolarizing in a chaotic manner
- A small number passes through the AV node.

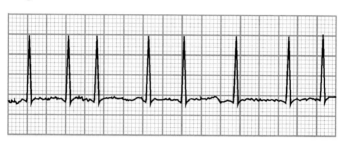

12. Premature ventricular contraction (PVC)
- Ectopic depolarization in any portion of the ventricular myocardium
- PVCs are of little concern if they arise from the same foci or if there are <5 per minute.
- If they arise from more than one foci or there are >5 per minute, it can lead to V-fib.

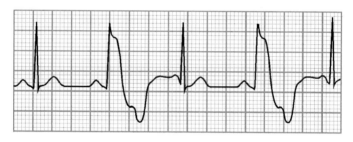

13. Ventricular tachycardia
- Ectopic depolarization of ventricles usually at a rate of 150 to 250 per minute
- Can degenerate to V-fib

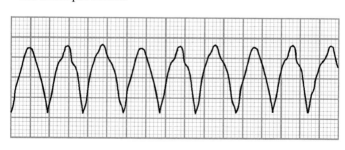

14. Ventricular fibrillation
- Rapid, irregular, disorganized ventricular rhythm
- Results in a lack of cardiac output, no pulse, no BP

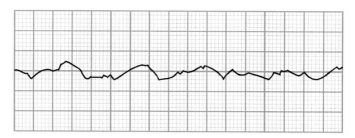

15. Normal sinus rhythm
- Rate 60 to 100
- P-R wave 0.12 to 0.2 seconds
- QRS 0.06 to 0.1 seconds
- QT 0.32 to 0.4 seconds

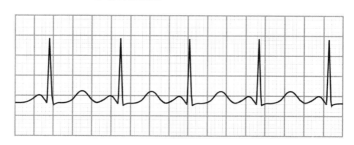

16. Wolff–Parkinson–White (WPW) syndrome
- An electrical bridge exists between the atrium and the ventricles, causing a conduction bypass of the AV node.
- Rapid impulse transmission occurs between the atrium and the ventricles, resulting in PR interval <0.12 second.

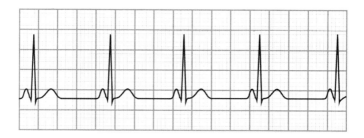

17. Junctional rhythm

- Heart beat originating in the AV junctional tissue as a safety mechanism when the higher pacemaker site (SA node) is not functioning or if the impulses are not getting through
- Inverted P wave
- The AV junctional tissue beats at 40 to 60 bpm.

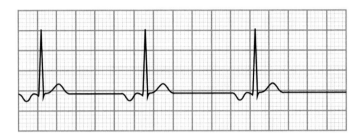

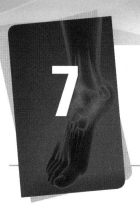

7

PHYSICAL THERAPY

THERMOTHERAPY (HEAT THERAPY)

Heat is used to reduce inflammation in subacute and chronic injuries. In the subacute and chronic stages of injury, ischemia and irritation occur from certain chemical mediators. Heat promotes drainage of these chemicals into the venous and lymphatic vessels through vasodilation. It also encourages tissue healing by increasing local circulation, which increases ROM of joints. Before heat can be beneficial, however, the active acute process of inflammation must be over.

Indications	Contraindication
Subacute or chronic inflammatory conditions	Acute injuries
Subacute or chronic muscle spasm	Impaired circulation
Decreased ROM	Poor thermal regulation
Hematoma resolution	Areas with decreased sensation
Reduction of joint contractures	Neoplasms

THERAPEUTIC SUPERFICIAL HEAT

Superficial heating modalities must be able to increase the skin temperature to between 104°F and 113°F. Transfer of heat to underlying structures is limited to <2 cm and occurs by conduction. Indicated in subacute and chronic stages of injury. Avoid heat during an active inflammatory cycle. This will increase the rate of cellular metabolism and accelerate the amount of hypoxic injury. Superficial heat modalities include heat packs, paraffin baths, and warm whirlpool.

Whirlpool

Mechanical agitation, which relaxes and massages muscles. Kinetic whirlpool combines whirlpool with ROM exercises. Can be used with ulcers that do not involve bone; Abx may be added to the water. Indications include chronic posttraumatic conditions, nerve injuries, painful stumps, decubitus ulcers, postsurgical rehabilitation, and arthritis.

Contrast Baths

Although contrast baths involve both hot and cold, the effects are that of a heat modality. Effectiveness is due to reflex hyperemia (hunting effect or response). Particularly good for stimulating circulation, reducing muscle fatigue, edema, and is useful in treating RSD.

Technique

Fill two baths, one with hot water and one with cold water (ice water).

Feet are placed alternately in each for about 1 minute.

Always start and end with cold.

Paraffin Wax

Dip foot 6 to 10 times for several seconds and then wrap in plastic and a towel and let sit for 20 to 30 minutes. Good for sprains, strains, and arthritic conditions.

DEEP HEAT

Indications	Contraindications
Chronic posttraumatic conditions	Metal implants
Nerve injuries	Pacemakers
Painful stumps	
Decubitus ulcers	
Postsurgical rehab	
Arthritis	

Ultrasound

There is an inverse relationship between frequency and depth of penetration. The higher the frequency, the more heat you can create, but the US waves do not penetrate as far.

Because of this, there must be a tradeoff between depth of penetration and therapeutic heating. A 1.0 MHz is the most popular frequency for therapeutic US as it affords a balance between depth of penetration and heating.

A 1.0 MHz can penetrate up to 5 cm. For the foot, 3.0 MHz may be used because the structures are closer to the skin. A 3.0 MHz penetrates about 1 to 2 cm.

The amount of heat generated with therapeutic US is not an exact science and patient feedback is important so tissues are not damaged.

Because of this, US is contraindicated in anesthetized areas.

Other contraindications are malignancies and acute thrombophlebitis.

THE HIGHER THE FREQUENCY, THE SHORTER THE WAVELENGTH AND THE LESS THEY PENETRATE.

Therapeutic US can be used in two ways: thermally to generate heat and mechanically as a vibration agent. Thermal US works by applying a deep heat. This is when the US machine is not being pulsed or is "continues" or 100% duty.

This is useful in patients with muscle tightness or strain. Mechanical US causes tiny vibrations in the soft tissue, which decrease swelling and inflammation and break up deep scar tissue. This modality does not create heat because it is pulsed and ~20% duty. This type is often recommended for conditions where there is built up of scar tissue (fibrosis).

Therapeutic ultrasound is a deep heating modality that uses a mechanical vibration in the form of sound waves to heat local tissues. There are other benefits to ultrasound besides deep heating, including breaking up adhesions and scars, increased tissue relaxation, and increased local blood flow.

Ultrasound machines have an option of continuous or pulsed sound waves. Continuous US produces both thermal and mechanical effects, while pulsed US produces only mechanical effects. Pulsed US is used in situations such as a fresh injury with acute inflammation where a heating effect is not desirable.

Ultrasound machines work by a process called the piezoelectric effect.

When you apply an electric field to certain crystals, they begin to vibrate, generating ultrasonic sound waves.

Ultrasound does not propagate through air; so a coupling medium is required. The coupling medium must have a low attenuation coefficient, meaning it does not absorb sound, such as US gel or water.

Indications	Contraindications
Edema	Areas with embolism
Pain	Anesthetized skin
Adhesions/scar tissue	Epiphyseal areas in children
	Bony prominences
	Vascular disease (DVT, atherosclerosis, hemorrhages)
	Acute infection
	Around metal implants, malignancies
	Patients with pacemakers

Phonophoresis

This is not a heat modality but a technique that uses ultrasound as a noninvasive way of delivering chemicals through the skin; the actual mechanism is probably via the thermal effect and acoustical streaming of the ultrasound. This technique is used for things such as topical anesthetics, anti-inflammatories, and muscle relaxants.

Shortwave Diathermy

A deep heating modality that can heat structures to a depth of 2 to 5 cm. Shortwave diathermy uses a high-frequency electromagnetic energy similar to broadcast radio waves but with shorter wavelength.

Microwave Diathermy

A less common form of electromagnetic radiation used to heat tissues.

CRYOTHERAPY

Physiologic Effects of Ice	Benefits
Vasoconstriction	Decreases swelling
Decreases cellular metabolism	Decreases inflammation
Decreases muscle spasms	Muscle relaxation
Decreases nerve activity	Analgesia

Ice Pack

Ice should be applied after an acute injury.
Ice should be alternated 10 minutes on and then 10 minutes off.
*I*ce should be accompanied by *R*est, *C*ompression, and *E*levation (RICE).

How Do You Know When to Use Hot or Cold?

There is no clear answer to this question. Some say use cold for the first 48 hours and then use heat. This response is oversimplified and often incorrect. When to use heat or cold varies from person to person and from injury to injury. It is important to evaluate the injury. The following are some general guidelines.

Question	Use Ice	Use Heat
Is the area warm to the touch?	Yes	No
Is there pain on light-to-moderate palpation of the area?	Yes	No
Does swelling increase during activity?	Yes	No
Does pain limit the joint's ROM?	Yes	No
Patient continues to show improvement with cold modalities?	Yes	No

ELECTRICAL STIMULATION

Transcutaneous Electrical Nerve Stimulator (TENS)

A pocket-sized, battery-operated device that provides mild, continuous electrical current through the skin by using two to four electrodes. TENS units can be used continuously or intermittently depending on the disease process. The intensity (output) knob is slowly turned until a slight tingling or buzzing is felt on the skin. A mild electrical current modifies and blocks the pain messages and replaces them with a buzzing, tingling sensation and can also stimulate the production of endorphins. High TENS (100 to 500 Hz) relieves pain by blocking pain fibers and is used up to 24 hours per day because when the unit is turned off, the pain cycle often returns; low TENS (1 to 50 Hz) relieves pain by endorphin release, and due to the 4-hour half-life of endorphins, it needs to only be used 15 to 30 minutes at a time.

Indications	Contraindications
Chronic pain	Pacemakers
Muscle atrophy	Pregnancy
Muscle spasms/ fatigue	
Edema	
Peripheral neuropathy	

Iontophoresis

A noninvasive way of delivering chemicals of like charge through the skin using a direct current. The compounds being delivered must be ionizable to penetrate the skin. This technique is used for things such as topical anesthetics, anti-inflammatories, and muscle relaxants.

INSTRUMENT-ASSISTED SOFT-TISSUE MOBILIZATION

Graston vs. ASTYM

These techniques were developed as a better alternative to massage for breaking up adhesions and scar tissue following injury or surgery. The techniques involve specially designed stainless steel instruments used to press or rub over injured areas and break up adhesions, scar, decrease inflammation, and promote healing. There is quite a heated debate about which is better.

Graston

Designed to break up adhesions that are formed between scar tissue and other tissues. This technique was developed before ASTYM by an athlete who injured his knee.

ASTYM

Promotes the body's natural regenerative processes to resorb and remodel tissues and break up scar tissue. Some believe that this technique tends to be less painful than Graston because it is not primarily focused on breaking up scar tissue. Instead, it promotes the body's natural regenerative processes to resorb and remodel tissues. Developed after Graston by a group of physicians and therapists.

McKenzie Method

This is spinal decompression therapy caused by a bulging or herniated disc in the cervical or lumbar spine. It consists of a series of exercises that leads to reduction of pressure on the discs of the spine.

Mulligan Concept

Mulligan manual therapy concept is a manual therapy technique where the therapist repositions a joint as the patient actively moves the joint through its range of motion.

Kinesiology Tape

Kinesiology is the study of the mechanical movements of the body. Kinesiology tape is applied on your body in specific directions to provide support to the body, without limiting the mechanics or movement of the area. Kinesio tape is different from athletic tape in that it is more flexible to allow some motion.

STRENGTHENING EXERCISES

Isometric Contraction (Static Contraction)

Muscle contraction that is not associated with joint motion or change in muscle length. Can be performed in a cast.

Isotonic Contraction (Dynamic Contraction)

Muscle contraction with associated joint motion and change in muscle length. Isotonic contractions can be either eccentric or concentric.

Eccentric Contraction

Muscle contraction in which the muscle lengthens while contracting. Contraction force of the muscle is against an overpowering weight resistance.

Concentric Contraction

Muscle contraction in which the muscle shortens as a result of the contraction. Where a weight is lifted with the force of muscle contraction.

Isokinetic Contraction

Contraction at a constant velocity at all ranges of motion by using a machine with an accommodating resistance.

DRY NEEDLING

Dry needling is similar to acupuncture in that it uses the same needles. Dry needling, however, focuses on trigger points to relax muscles as opposed to acupuncture, which focuses on meridian system and energy flow (χ). Dry needling is performed directly at the site of the knotted muscle, whereas acupuncture relieves pain by stimulating points along specific meridians that may be far away from the painful area. Dry needling is used only for orthopedic complaints, specifically muscle pain, while acupuncture is also used to treat other categories of disease such as digestive problems, high blood pressure, anxiety, flu, and many more. With dry needling, the needles are generally inserted deeper into the tissues as compared with acupuncture.

ANODYNE

Anodyne Infrared Therapy Systems are medical devices that are indicated to increase circulation and reduce pain, stiffness, and muscle spasms. The mechanism of action is, in part, due to topical heat and an increased local release of nitric oxide through infrared light or photon energy. Nitric oxide is thought to be a signaling mechanism to stimulate vasodilation.

WALKING AIDS

Crutches

Adjust the height of the crutches to allow two fingers' width between axilla and axillary pad.
The hand piece is adjusted to allow 30° of elbow flexion.

Canes

Size the cane by measuring from the greater trochanter to the ground.
Elbow should be flexed at about 30°.
The cane is held in the hand opposite the affected leg or foot.

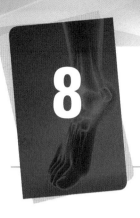

8 PLASTIC SURGERY

Skin Grafts, 127
Post-op, 130

Skin Plasties, 131
Incisions, 134

SKIN GRAFTS

Skin Graft Classification

Autograft

Skin taken from one part of the body and used to cover a wound in another part of the body. The thinner the graft, the better the "take"; the thicker the graft, the better the function. A good "take" requires absence of infection, perfect hemostasis, a good dressing, and absence of motion.

Isograft

A graft of tissue between two individuals who are genetically identical (i.e., identical twins)

Xenograft

A graft of tissue from one species used on another species

Allograft

Allograft, also called homograft, is a graft taken from one individual and placed on another individual of the same species but different genotype (not identical twins).

Amniotic Tissue Allografts

Amniotic membrane is a bilayered structure composed of both the amnion and the chorion. The amnion is the membrane directly around the embryo and in contact with the amniotic fluid. The chorion is the membrane outside the amnion and in contact with the maternal side of the placenta. Some amniotic allografts remove the chorion layer, believing this will reduce host reaction. Chorion, being on the maternal side of the placenta, has been known to contain maternal antigens. Grafts are applied stromal side down against the wound.

Amniotic Membrane Composition

Structural collagen (type I, III, IV, V, VII)

127

Extracellular matrix (ECM) proteins: Fibronectin, proteoglycans, glycosaminoglycans, laminins

Growth factors: Epidermal growth factor (EGF), transforming growth factor (TGF), fibroblast growth factor (FGF), platelet-derived growth factor (PDGF), vascular endothelial growth factors (VEGF)

Regulating proteins: Matrix metalloproteinases (MMPs) and tissue inhibitors of metalloproteinases (TIMPs), interleukins

Benefits of Amniotic Tissue Allografts

Nonimmunogenic

Antibacterial properties

Provide a matrix for cellular migration and proliferation

Reduce scar tissue

Reduced inflammation

Reduce pain at the site of application

Tissue grafts and substitutes come from many sources

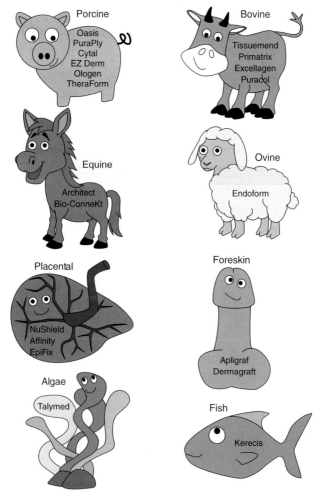

Porcine
Oasis
PuraPly
Cytal
EZ Derm
Ologen
TheraForm

Bovine
Tissuemend
Primatrix
Excellagen
Puracol

Equine
Architect
Bio-ConneKt

Ovine
Endoform

Placental
NuShield
Affinity
EpiFix

Foreskin
Apligraf
Dermagraft

Algae
Talymed

Fish
Kerecis

Autograft Types (Full Thickness vs. Partial Thickness)

Full-Thickness Skin Grafts (FTSGs)	Split-Thickness Skin Grafts (STSGs)
Contain epidermis and all of the dermis. "Take" is not as good, and infection rate is higher. Grafts do not shrink and do not change color. Hair follicles are preserved. Less susceptible to trauma.	Contain epidermis and varying amount of the dermis. The thinner the graft, the more likely it will "take," because a higher number of blood vessels are transected, and there is more opportunity for revascularization. Grafts tend to shrink (50% to 70%). Tends to pigment abnormally. More susceptible to trauma.

Meshing

Meshing is a process by which multiple full-thickness slits are placed in a graft and the graft is stretched before application to the recipient site. Meshing is performed only on partial-thickness grafts.

Advantages of Meshing	Disadvantages of Meshing
Expands tissue, allowing a smaller graft to cover a larger site. Allows drainage of hematoma/seroma through the graft. Allows the graft to drape extremely well around irregular surfaces. Increases surface area for reepithelialization.	Must heal by secondary intention. Inferior cosmetic appearance after healing. Graft becomes very delicate and easily torn.

Donor Site

Full-Thickness Graft	Split-Thickness Graft
Best donor sites are flexor surfaces, especially the groin. Pinch grafts are taken from over the sinus tarsi. The donor site is closed primarily, leaving a linear scar. Length-to-width ratio of donor graft should be at least 3:1 for adequate closure.	Common donor sites include the anterior or lateral thigh, upper inner arm, gluteal region, or the dorsum of the foot. Grafts are harvested with an instrument called a *dermatome* (e.g., Zimmer air dermatome, Padgett drum dermatome, Humby knife, Goulian knife, Brown electric dermatome), which takes thin slices of skin. After the graft is removed, control bleeding with topical thrombin and dilute epinephrine or cautery and dress with Opsite or Tegaderm.

Recipient Site

Grafts require a vascular recipient site and cannot be placed directly over cortical bone or tendon.

Control bleeding with topical thrombin, dilute epinephrine, and cauterization.

Must be free of infection, bacterial count $<10^5$ per mL

Granulation tissue must be debrided.

Graft is sutured into place leaving strategically placed long ties at various points around the graft sites for securing a stent dressing.

Stent Dressing

A type of dressing designed especially for skin grafts that functions to hold the graft in place, apply pressure, and absorb fluids. Stent dressings consist of a semipermeable nonadherent dressing (Adaptic, Owens Silk), several layers of moist saline-soaked gauze, and fluffs held in place by the tie-over sutures left in place during securing of the graft. Alternately in the case of the lower extremity, a circumferential wrap may be used.

Phases of Skin Graft Healing

Both partial- and full-thickness skin grafts heal by way of the same three phases.

Plasmatic Inhibition Phase

Occurs the first 24 to 48 hours, during which time the skin graft passively absorbs nutrients in the wound bed by diffusion. Capillary buds begin to form, but graft remains ischemic.

Inosculation Phase

By day 3, capillary buds make contact with graft.

Angiogenesis Phase

By day 5, new blood vessels grow into the graft, and the graft becomes vascularized.

POST-OP

Dressing remains on for 5 to 7 days, 2 days if unmeshed, during which time the extremity is elevated until venous circulation is established. It is important to eliminate movement/shearing so graft can "take," and this may require NWB, casting/splinting. Any fluid that accumulates under the graft must be aspirated because it creates a barrier against revascularization.

Reasons for Graft Failure

Hematoma—blood develops under graft (most common).

Infection (second most common)

Seroma—serosanguinous fluid develops under graft.

Shearing—shearing forces separate the graft from the bed.

Poor wound bed—poor vascularity, exposed tendon or bone

SKIN PLASTIES

Transpositional Flap

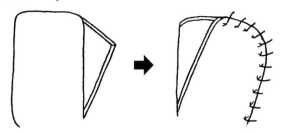

Rotational Flap

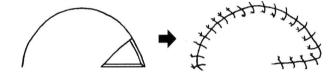

Bilobed Flap

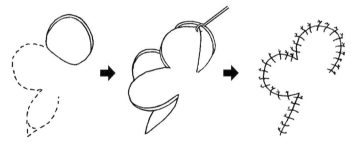

Rhomboid (Limberg) Flap

Longitudinal axis is parallel to the line of minimal skin tension.

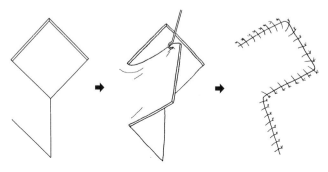

Kutler-Type Biaxial V-Y

(Advancement Flap)

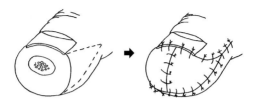

Atasoy-Type Plantar V-Y

(Advancement Flap)

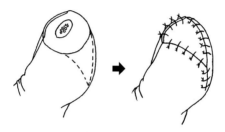

Z-Plasty

Angles that are permissible for a Z-plasty are between 45° and 60°. Angles <45° result in impaired blood flow to the flaps, and angles >60° result in severe tension. 60° result in the greatest lengthening. A Z-plasty with a 60° angle results in a 75% increase in skin length. Z-plasties are particularly useful in treating linear scar contractures.

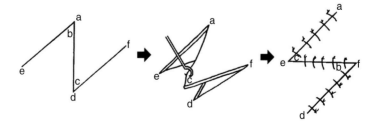

V-Y Plasty

Unidirectional skin-lengthening technique. The apex of the "V" is placed at the point of maximal skin tension.

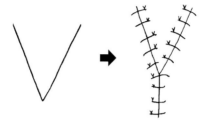

Derotational Skin Plasty for Fifth Digits

Performed in conjunction with an arthroplasty. Acts to correct for the varus (frontal) and hammering (sagittal) of the digit. The incision is made from distal-medial to proximal-lateral.

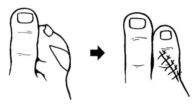

Desyndactyly Procedure

Place needles from dorsal to plantar to line up apices.

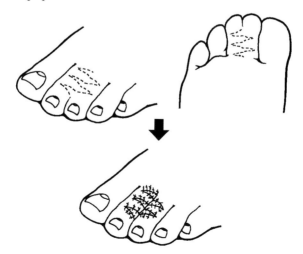

Tsuge "Inchworm" Plastic Reduction Procedure

Fishmouth incision is made around the toe just dorsal to phalange. The dorsal skin is retracted, allowing the proximal skin to buckle. The tip of the toe is excised, and the nail may be reduced in width, if desired. Six to 8 weeks after initial procedure, the dorsal redundant skin is excised.

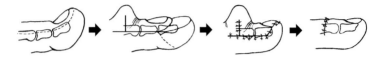

INCISIONS

Ollier Incision

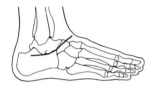

DeVries Incision

Medial longitudinal incision
Limited exposure

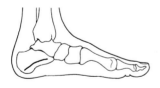
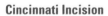

Cincinnati Incision

Transverse incision that involves extensive dissection of the posterior, medial, and lateral aspects of the foot and ankle

Do not perform in > 4 years of age.
Classic soft-tissue release for
  clubfoot

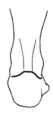

Lateral Extensile Incision

This is a full-thickness incision down to bone. Designed to outline the distribution of the peroneal artery, also protects the sural nerve, and peroneal tendons

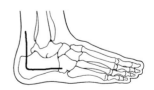

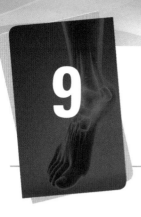

9 ARTHRITIS

SYSTEMIC FEATURES OF ARTHROPATHIES

System	Disease	Manifestation
Skin	Psoriatic arthritis	Psoriasis
	Reiter syndrome	Keratoderma blennorrhagica
	Septic arthritis (especially *Neisseria gonorrhoeae*)	Rash
	Lyme arthritis	Erythema chronicum migrans
	SLE	Butterfly rash, photosensitivity
Nasopharynx and ear	Reiter syndrome	Stomatitis
	Gout	Tophi
Eye	Reiter syndrome	Conjunctivitis
	Juvenile rheumatoid arthritis	Iridocyclitis

(*continued*)

System	Disease	Manifestation
Gastrointestinal tract	Crohn disease	Diarrhea
	Whipple disease	Diarrhea
	Ulcerative colitis	Diarrhea
Heart	Lyme arthritis	Enlarged heart, arrhythmias
	Ankylosing spondylitis	Aortic insufficiency
	SLE	Pericarditis
Nervous system	Lyme arthritis	Stiff neck, headache
Genitourinary system	SLE	Nephritis
	Gout	Kidney disease

ARTHROCENTESIS (JOINT ASPIRATION)

Joint aspiration is performed to diagnose certain conditions, including gout, various types of arthritis, and joint infection (septic arthritis). It is also used to remove excess fluid from a joint, which can cause pain and decreased ROM. Following aspiration, local anesthetic or cortisone may be injected to help with pain and inflammation.

Technique

Prep the site with antiseptic solution. Local anesthetic may be injected superficial to the aspiration site or just proximal to the site to decrease the pain from the large gauge needle (18 to 22 gauge) that will be used for aspiration.

The ankle can be approached medially, just medial to the extensor hallucis longus tendon, or laterally, just distal to the fibula. For smaller digital joints, enter the joint dorsally, just medial or lateral to the extensor tendons.

SYNOVIAL JOINT FLUID ANALYSIS

Test	Normal	Noninflammatory Arthritis	Inflammatory Arthritis	Septic
Clarity	Transparent	Transparent	Translucent	Opaque
Color	Colorless	Straw	Yellow	Variable (white)
Crystals	None	None	Possibly (gout, pseudogout)	None
Cultures	Negative	Negative	Negative	Positive
Glucose (as compared with FBS)	Equal to blood	Equal to blood	< 50 mg/dL lower than blood	> 50 mg/dL lower than blood
Mucin clot	Firm	Firm	Friable	Friable
PMN (%)	<25	<25	>50	>75
WBC	<200	200–2,000	2,000–75,000	>100,000
Viscosity	High	High	Low	Variable

DDX of Synovial Joint Fluid Analysis

Noninflammatory	Inflammatory	Sepsis
DJD	RA	Bacterial infection
Trauma	Scleroderma	
Osteochondritis dissecans	Gout	
Neuropathic arthropathies	Pseudogout	
Pigmented villonodular synovitis	Reiter syndrome	
SLE	Ankylosing spondylitis	
Scleroderma	SLE	
	Psoriatic arthritis	
	Ulcerative colitis	

RHEUMATOID ARTHRITIS

Description

Rheumatoid arthritis begins as a chronic symmetrical peripheral polysynovitis with insidious aching and morning stiffness. RA is caused by an autoimmune response that progresses to destruction of articular and periarticular structures.

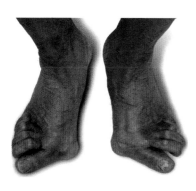

Signs and Symptoms

Symmetrical inflammatory polyarthritis (three or more joints)
Pain and swelling worse in the morning, and after rest, pain gets better with motion.

Gel phenomenon—stiffness develops after long periods of sitting or rest, and joints become painful to move.
Female-to-male ratio 3:1
Onset is 20 to 50 years of age.
Affects small joints in hands and feet (MPJs, wrists, MCJs, and PIPJ)
Possible low-grade fever, fatigue, weight loss, and malaise
Rheumatoid nodules—benign subcutaneous painless masses found at sites usually subject to trauma
Boutonnière deformity—flexion of the PIPJ of the finger with hyperextension of the DIPJ
Swan neck deformity—hyperextension of the PIPJ of the finger with flexion of the DIPJ
Baker cyst (popliteal cyst)—a synovial fluid-filled cyst, which develops in the popliteal fossa. When ruptured, symptoms mimic a DVT.
Felty syndrome—rheumatoid arthritis with associated splenomegaly and neutropenia. Patients may present with pigmented spots on the lower extremity and may have non-healing leg ulcers.

Pannus transformation—the synovium develops into a vasculature granulation tissue that produces inflammatory agents and immunoglobulin-producing lymphoreticular-like elements that destroy the articular cartilage.

Diagnosis

Blood:
- (+)RF (rheumatoid factor)
- Elevated CRP or ESR
- Normocytic MCV

X-ray:
- Fibular/ulnar deviation of phalanges
- Marginal erosions, ulnar styloid process shows early erosions
- Increased soft-tissue density
- Early increase in joint space (from pannus formation) and later decreased joint space, which can lead to ankyloses
- Juxta-articular osteopenia metatarsal heads are washed out, while the shafts may be relatively normal.

Treatment

- Rest and splints during flare-ups; ROM exercise during remission
- Anti-inflammatory drugs: NSAIDs, corticosteroids (prednisone)
- Medications
  - NSAIDs
  - Steroids
  - Disease-modifying anti-rheumatic drugs (DMARDs): hydroxychloroquine (Plaquenil), sulfasalazine (Azulfidine), methotrexate (Trexall), leflunomide (Arava)
  - Biologic agents: abatacept (Orencia), adalimumab (Humira), etanercept (Enbrel)

JUVENILE RHEUMATOID ARTHRITIS

Juvenile rheumatoid arthritis (JRA) is also called *juvenile idiopathic arthritis* (JIA). JRA is a type of arthritis that causes joint pain in children. Onset is usually before age 16. It is thought to be an autoimmune disorder. Females are affected more than males (4:1), and caution should be used during anesthesia (intubation) due to possible cervical spine problems (atlantoaxial subluxation).

Three Subtypes

1. *Polyarticular* (40%) involves many joints. This form may turn into rheumatoid arthritis. It may involve five or more large and small joints of the legs and arms, as well as the jaw and neck.
2. *Pauciarticular* (40%) involves four or less joints, most often the wrist or knees. It is also associated with eye problems (iridocyclitis).
3. *Systemic (Still disease)* (20%) involves joint swelling or pain, fever, and rash. It is also associated with systemic manifestations (splenomegaly, generalized adenopathy).

Diagnosis

Elevated ESR, C-reactive protein, ANA (NOTE: RA factor is a poor screening tool for JRA.), synovial fluid examination

Treatment

Treatment is largely the same as with RA and included ASA and other anti-inflammatory modalities.

OSTEOARTHRITIS (DEGENERATIVE JOINT DISEASE)

Description

Osteoarthritis is the most common arthritis and occurs as a result of wear and tear on joints. The cartilage that cushions the impact on the joint gradually deteriorates. As the cartilage wears down, subchondral bone is exposed, which becomes sclerotic and polished in a process called *eburnation*. Cysts may appear in the subchondral bone. Over time, the ends of the bones are also affected, with bone growing along the sides producing osteophytes. There is usually a predisposing factor, such as trauma or prior inflammatory arthritis.

Signs and Symptoms

Asymmetrical noninflammatory arthritis

Pain worse at the end of day (after use)

Pain in joint before a change in weather

Loss of flexibility

Heberden nodes (bony protuberances at the margins and dorsal surface of the DIPJs)

Bouchard nodes (bony protuberances at the margins and dorsal surface of the PIPJs)

Joints most commonly affected (neck, back, knees, hips, shoulder, 1st MPJ, and the 1st radiocarpal joint)

Diagnosis

Radiographs reveal subchondral sclerosis, loose bodies (joint mice), and asymmetrical joint space narrowing; soft tissue is normal.

Treatment

Physical therapy including ROM exercises for stiffness

Joint replacements

Synovial fluid viscosupplements—injected into joints to cushion and lubricate joint space

Synvisc (Hylan G-F 20): an elastoviscous fluid containing hylan polymers made from a chickens' comb

Hyalgan (sodium hyaluronate): a viscous solution consisting of high-molecular-weight fraction of purified sodium hyaluronate

Rheumatoid vs. Osteoarthritis

Rheumatoid Arthritis	Osteoarthritis
Inflammatory	Noninflammatory
Symmetrical	Asymmetrical
Pain worse in the morning or after rest	Pain worse at the end of the day
Osteopenia	Sclerosis
Increased soft-tissue density	Soft tissue is normal
Positive RA factor	Negative RA factor

SERONEGATIVE SPONDYLOARTHROPATHIES

Ankylosing Spondylitis (Marie–Strumpell Disease)

Description

A chronic inflammatory arthritis that affects the sacroiliac joint and, to a lesser extent, the rest of the spine. Pain and stiffness are early signs, but in advanced cases, a poker spine (very stiff, inflexible backbone) is common.

Signs and Symptoms

Onset is 15 to 35 years.
Male-to-female ratio 10:1
Lower back pain (sacroiliac joints)
Kyphosis
Recurrent acute iritis in one-third
of patients

Diagnosis

Increased sed rate, positive HLA-B27
Positive Schober test
Radiographs, abnormalities at the
sacroiliac joint, bamboo spine

Treatment

PT, NSAIDs

Reiter (Reactive) Syndrome

Description

A subacute syndrome consisting of
the tetrad:

1. Arthritis
2. Urethritis (nonbacterial)
3. Conjunctivitis
4. Mucocutaneous lesions

Most signs of the disease disappear in days to weeks; the arthritis
lasts for <6 weeks.

Types

	Sexually Transmitted	**Dysenteric**
Typical patient	Males (20–40 y)	Females and children
Cause	*Chlamydia trachomatis* (urogenital infection)	*Shigella*
		Salmonella
		Yersinia
		Campylobacter
Initial symptom	Urethritis	Enteritis (diarrhea)

Signs and Symptoms

Asymmetrical arthritis that usually
follows within 1 month of urethritis or enteritis
Much more common in males
Tetrad: arthritis, urethritis (nonbacterial), conjunctivitis, and
mucocutaneous lesions
Dysenteric form results in
diarrhea.
Usually attacks large WB joints of
LE: sacroiliac joint, knees, and
ankles
Back pain may occur with more
severe disease.
Enthesopathy: inflammation
of tendinous or ligamentous
insertions (plantar fasciitis, heel
pain)
"Sausage digits"
Radiographs: heel pain associated
with a fluffy or woolly heel spur,
periostitis
Small mucocutaneous painless
lesions, including stomatitis and
balanitis, and keratoderma blen-
norrhagica (skin lesion)
Self-limiting, most resolve in less
than a year

Diagnosis

Antibody titers
Positive HLA-B27

Treatment

NSAIDs
Tetracycline following chlamydial
infection
Relapse can occur.

Psoriatic Arthritis

Description

An inflammatory arthritis usually
involving peripheral joints. The

skin disease typically precedes the joint disease; however, arthritis can occasionally precede the psoriasis by months to years. Psoriatic arthritis is seen in ~7% of patients with dermatologic psoriasis.

Signs and Symptoms

Asymmetrical arthritis of large and small (especially the DIPJs) joints, including the sacroiliac and the spine
The prevalence of males to females affected is equal.
Peak age: 40 years
Associated with psoriatic skin and nail lesions (pitting)

Diagnosis

Positive HLA-B27, negative RA factor, negative ANA
Radiographic: "pencil-in-cup" deformity at IP joints

"Whittling" of the distal tufts of the phalanges
Ankylosis of joints

Treatment

NSAIDs, sulfasalazine, systemic steroids

INFECTIOUS ARTHRITIS
Septic Arthritis

Septic joint is an infection of a joint by a microbe. The infection usually reaches joint hematogenously; however, direct traumatic inoculation is possible. Symptoms and the severity of the condition vary depending on the pathogen. The most common joint involved is the knee, followed by the shoulder, wrist, hip, phalanges, and the elbow.

Long Bone Vasculature— Possibility of Septic Joint via Metaphysis

Infantile (0–1 y)	Childhood (1–16 y)	Adult (>16 y)
Vessels penetrate the growth plate. Joint sepsis possible.	Vessels do not penetrate the growth plate. Joint sepsis not possible.	Vessels penetrate the growth plate. Joint sepsis not possible.

Reprinted from Resnick D. *Bone and Joint Imaging*. W.B. Saunders Co; 1989:731, with permission from Elsevier.

Acute Bacterial Arthritis

Acute bacterial arthritis usually presents with fever, severe pain, and limitation of movement. The joint is swollen and tender, and the overlying skin is red and hot. Acute bacterial arthritis is a medical emergency requiring admittance to the hospital. Prognosis is good if diagnosed within 3 to 4 days.

Etiologic bacteria are generally divided into gonococcal vs. nongonococcal disease.

Nongonococcal

Tends to occur in patients with previous joint damage or immunocompromised patients. *Staphylococcus aureus* accounts for 70% of cases. Gram negatives seen in IV drug users, neutropenia, UTIs, and post-ops. In children under 2 years, the most common pathogen is *S. aureus* followed by *Haemophilus influenzae* and then Gram ($-$) bacilli.

Gonococcal

Accounts for half of all septic arthritis in the otherwise healthy sexually active young adults. Pathogen is *N. gonorrhoeae*. Usually presents as a migratory polyarticular arthritis involving several joints in rapid succession and then settling in one or two joints. There is typically a rash associated with this type of arthritis, which develops on the extremities as small, mildly painful pustules on an erythematous base, which may break down and ulcerate during healing. *N. gonorrhoeae* is seldom isolated from the synovial fluid, so all mucous membranes should be cultured, such as the throat, urethra, vagina, and rectum.

Diagnosis

Joint aspiration
Blood cultures should also be obtained.

Treatment

For acute joint sepsis, the patient should be admitted. Begin early and prompt IV antibiotic.

Antibiotic Treatment for Acute Septic Joint		
Organism	**Drug of Choice**	**Alternative Drug**
S. aureus	Nafcillin or oxacillin (150 mg/kg/d IV divided q4h)	Vancomycin (30 mg/kg/d IV divided q6h) Cephalothin (150 mg/kg/d IV divided q4h)
N. gonorrhoeae	Penicillin G (150,000 units/kg/d IV)	Cephalothin (150 mg/kg/d IV divided q4h divided q4h)
Streptococci or *pneumococci*	Penicillin G (150,000 units/kg/d IV divided q4h)	Cephalothin (150 mg/kg/d IV divided q4h)
Pseudomonas aeruginosa	Tobramycin (5–6 mg/kg/d IM/IV divided q8h) and ticarcillin	An aminoglycoside plus piperacillin, mezlocillin, or ceftazidime in full doses may be used if resistance encountered

Antibiotic Treatment for Acute Septic Joint		
Organism	Drug of Choice	Alternative Drug
MRSA	Vancomycin (30 mg/kg/d IV divided q6h)	
Other facultative Gram (−) bacilli	Gentamicin (5–6 mg/kg/d IM/ IV divided q8h) plus broad spectrum PCN (mezlocillin or piperacillin) or a third generation Ceph (cefotaxime, ceftizoxime, or ceftazidime) in doses for life-threatening infections	Tobramycin, netilmicin, amikacin plus. A third-generation Ceph, piperacillin, or mezlocillin. Each in doses for life-threatening infection

Arthrocentesis is performed daily to bid. Arthrocentesis is beneficial for many reasons:

1. Monitors response of therapy
2. Removes destructive inflammatory mediators
3. Reduces intra-articular pressure, which promotes antibiotic penetration
4. Surgical drainage may be required if the joint does not respond within 5 to 7 days of initial therapy.

Viral Arthritis

Viral arthritis presents as a self-limiting mild inflammatory nondestructive arthritis that lacks suppuration. It usually begins as a migrating polyarthralgia that rarely lasts for >6 weeks. It is most commonly caused by hepatitis B, followed by mono, rubella, or rubella vaccination; mumps; infectious mono; and parvovirus. Viral arthritis responds well to conservative regimen of rest and NSAIDs.

Tuberculosis Arthritis

Presents as a chronic, inflammatory, slowly destructive arthritis with few, if any, systemic signs. Synovial biopsies are diagnostic; joint cultures may or may not be positive for the organism. Only 50% of chest radiographs are positive. Treatment is with antituberculosis drugs (i.e., rifampin).

Fungal Arthritis

Presents as a chronic monoarticular arthritis, similar to TB. *Sporothrix schenckii* is the most common pathogen.

Lyme Dz

Presents as a migratory polyarthritis and tendonitis associated with an expanding skin rash called *erythema chronicum migrans*. The arthritis usually settles in the knee or ankle. The causative agent is the spirochete called *Borrelia burgdorferi*, and it is transmitted by a deer tick called *Ixodes dammini*.

Symptoms

Muscle aches/pains
Fatigue/lethargy
Fever/chills
Stiff neck with headache
Backache

Nausea/vomiting
Sore throat
Enlarged spleen or lymph nodes
Enlarged heart and heart-rhythm
    disturbances

Diagnosis

Specific Ab tests

Treatment

Doxycycline (100 mg bid), tetracy-
    cline (250 mg qid), or amoxicillin
    (500 mg tid) given PO × 3 weeks.

CRYSTAL-INDUCED ARTHRITIS

Gout

Description

A recurrent acute arthritis that affects peripheral joints, most notably the 1st MPJ. The arthritis stems
from a buildup of monosodium
urate crystals in and around joints
and tendons. Supersaturated hy-
peruricemic body fluids crystallize,
causing a severe red hot swollen
joint. The arthritis may become
chronic and deforming. Not all hy-
peruricemic persons develop gout.
A buildup of uric acid crystals in the
joint may be from excessive breakdown or overproduction of purines.
Gout classically begins in the evening or early morning and tends to
occur in previously damaged joints.

Signs and Symptoms

Asymmetrical monoarticular
    arthritis
Sudden onset; red hot swollen joint
Low-grade fever is sometimes
    present.
More common in men (20:1)

Joint sparing, however, chronic
    gout may be joint destructive.
Most commonly first attacks the
    1st MPJ (called *Podagra*), fol-
    lowed by Lisfranc and then the
    heel
Crunchy tophi felt in ears, olecra-
    non bursa, and Achilles tendon.

Diagnosis

Radiographs: rat bites, cloud sign,
    punched-out lesions, Martel sign
    (overhanging margins)

Gout Radiograph

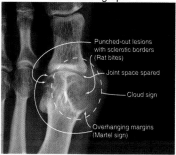

Aspiration: negatively birefringent
    yellow needle–shaped crystals,
    when parallel to axis of the lens,
    and blue when perpendicular
Blood work: hyperuricemia (>7.5
    mg per dL), not conclusively di-
    agnostic for gout

NOTE: When sending gout specimen to the lab, do not send in formalin; formalin dissolves gouty tophi.

Treatment

For effective treatment, determina-
tion must be made as to whether
the patient is an overproducer of
uric acid (metabolic gout) or an un-
derexcreter (renal gout).

	Overproducer of Uric Acid	Underexcreter of Uric Acid
Name	Metabolic gout	Renal gout (more common)
Diagnosis	Uric acid level >600 mg in a 24-h urine sample	Uric acid level <600 mg in a 24-h urine sample
Cause	Genetic enzyme defect Tumor	1° Kidney problem 2° Kidney problem (excessive acids such as lactic acid or ASA. Lead poisoning)
Treatment	Allopurinol Xanthine oxidase inhibitor 300 mg qd	Probenecid Competes with uric acid for reabsorption from kidneys 250 mg bid × 1 wk, then double the dose, then increase by 500 mg/d every 4 wk (not to exceed 2 g/d)

Effective treatment of gout should also include avoiding foods and medications that exacerbate gout.

Organ meat (liver sweetbread, kidney, heart, brains)
Lard
Anchovies and sardines
EtOH, especially red wine
Diuretics (increases osmolarity)

Pseudogout

- Also known as chondrocalcinosis, calcium pyrophosphate dihydrate (CPPD)

Description

Arthritis caused by deposition of CPPD crystals in the joint. Pseudogout most commonly affects the knee (50%), followed by the ankle, wrist, and shoulder. Symptoms are similar to those of gout, but it tends to run a longer course. Course reaches a maximum severity at 1 to 3 days and resolves in 1 week or longer. Risk of pseudogout increases with age, trauma, patients hospitalized for other medical conditions, and those with metabolic disease such as hypothyroidism, hyperthyroidism, gout, or amyloidosis. The condition is associated with a high-grade fever.

Diagnosis

Microscopic examination of joint aspiration reveals rhomboid crystals.
Radiographs reveal calcifications of the articular cartilage or meniscus.

Treatment

Immobilization, NSAID, analgesics

COLLAGEN VASCULAR DISEASES, CONNECTIVE TISSUE DZ

Systemic Lupus Erythematosus (SLE)

Definition

A chronic, remitting, relapsing, inflammatory, and often febrile, multisystemic disorder of connective tissue; acute or insidious in onset

Drug-induced lupus may be caused by procainamide, hydralazine, chlorpromazine, isoniazid, penicillamine, and griseofulvin.

Signs/Symptoms

Age of onset 15 to 35 years
Joint pain in 90% of patients (an early manifestation)
Primarily small joints of the hands and feet
Mainly in young women (10:1)
More common in blacks
Fever (90% of patients)
Abdominal pains
Butterfly rash
Skin lesions in sun-exposed areas (photosensitivity)
Fatigue, weight loss, and anorexia
Raynaud phenomenon
Alopecia
Vision problems
Proximal nail fold telangiectasis
Renal, cardiac, splenic, and pulmonary problems

Diagnosis

Increased sed rate
(+)ANA (antinuclear antibody test)
Antibodies to double-stranded DNA
Decreased hemoglobin, WBC, and platelets

Treatment

Symptomatic
  Steroids
  Antimalarials (chloroquine)
  Immunosuppressants
  Avoid sunlight

Scleroderma (Progressive Systemic Sclerosis)

Definition

A systemic disorder of the connective tissue characterized by induration, thickening, and tightening of the skin. Beginning in the hands, then face, and then other areas. There is also associated fibrotic degenerative change in various organs, especially the lungs, heart, and GI.

Signs/Symptoms

CREST (Calcinosis cutis—calcifications in the skin, Raynaud phenomenon, Esophageal dysfunction, Sclerodactyly—localized scleroderma of the digits, and Telangiectasia)
May be confined to face and hands
Onset 30s to 40s
Woman-to-men ratio 4:1
Hyperpigmentation/hypopigmentation
Dysphagia
Migratory polyarthritis
Constipation, diarrhea, abdominal bloating
Weight loss
Mask facies
Thick, hard leathery skin
Nails grow claw-like overshortened distal phalanges.
Matlike telangiectasia
Mouse-like appearance, due to skin around mouth having many furrows radiating outward

Diagnosis

Clinically
(+)ANA

Treatment

Symptomatic

Dermatomyositis/Polymyositis

Definition

Polymyositis is a chronic progressive inflammatory disease of skeletal muscle characterized by symmetrical weakness of the limb girdles, neck, and pharynx, usually associated with pain and tenderness. If associated with skin lesions, it is termed *dermatomyositis*. These skin manifestations include violaceous (heliotrope) inflammatory changes of the eyelids and periorbital area and erythema of the face, neck, and upper trunk.

Signs/Symptoms

Female-to-male ratio 2:1
Gottron sign—flat-topped violaceous papules over the dorsal aspect of the knuckles
Reddish purplish (heliotrope) facial lesions
Polyarthritis occurs in one-third of patients.
Proximal muscle weakness
Proximal nail fold telangiectasis

Diagnosis

Elevated serum CPK (creatine phosphokinase)
Muscle biopsy
Abnormal EMG
Elevated creatine (>200 mg) in a 24-hour urine specimen

Treatment

Steroids

Sjögren Syndrome

Definition

A chronic autoimmune inflammatory disorder of the exocrine glands. Resulting in decreased secretions in many areas of the body. Histologically, there is a lymphocytic infiltration of the secretory glands.

Signs/Symptoms

Women-to-men ratio 9:1
Age 40s to 60s
Often associated with rheumatic disease
Keratoconjunctivitis sicca (dry eyes)—felt as burning or itchy
Xerostomia (dry mouth)
Dry vagina
Possible loss of taste or smell
Dysphagia
Dry skin may be the only cutaneous manifestation.
Parotid gland enlargement

Diagnosis

Mild anemia, leukopenia
(+)RA factor in 70%
Schirmer test—measures quantity of tears. Litmus paper is placed in the eye for 5 minutes; if <5 mm of wetness, the test is (+).
Biopsy saliva gland

Treatment

Symptomatic

ARTHRITIS ASSOCIATED WITH INFLAMMATORY BOWEL DISEASE

Crohn Disease and Ulcerative Colitis

Rheumatologic manifestations seen in about 15% to 20% of patients
Asymmetric, nondestructive, transient arthritis
Arthritis flares tend to parallel flares of the underlying bowel disease.
Commonly involves the knees, ankles, elbows, and wrists

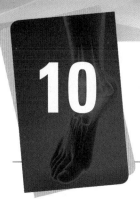

10 BIOMECHANICS

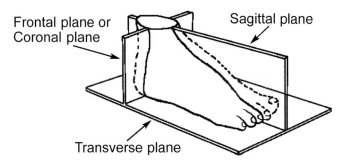

Frontal plane or Coronal plane

Sagittal plane

Transverse plane

JOINT ROM

Hip

Rotation	Int	Ext
Adults	35°–40°	35°–40°
Infants/elderly	20°–25°	45°–50°
Flexion/ extension	Flex	Ext
Straight knee	90°–100°	10°–20°
Flexed knees	120°–130°	
Abduction/ adduction		
Abduction	24°–60° (average 36°)	
Adduction	<30°	

Knee

Flexion/Extension	
Flexion	130°–150°
Extension	5°–10° (past vertical)

>10° extension is called *genu recurvatum*.

Rotation (best when knee is semiflexed at about 45°)

Med rotation	40°
Lat rotation	40°

During the last 30° of knee extension of gait, the tibia rotates laterally, with a more rapid rotation occurring at the final 5° of knee extension. When the knee is fully extended, no rotation is possible.

Genu Varum/Genu Valgum (Bow Leg/Knock Knee)

Birth	Genu varum	15°–20°
2–4 y	Straight	0°
4–6 y	Genu valgum	5°–15°
6–12 y	Straight	0°

Genu Varum/Genu Valgum

Genu varum and genu valgum "knocked knees" are frontal plane deformities that occur at the knees. They are a normal part of development, but depending on the degree and age of development, they can be pathological. Rule out rickets and Blount disease for abnormal genu valgum.

Ankle

Dorsiflexion/Plantarflexion

Dorsiflexion	20°
Plantarflexion	40°

Tibia fibular joint. The fibula rotates 12° clockwise away from the tibia during dorsiflexion.

Birth, 75°; 3 years, 20°; 10 years, 15°; 15 years, 10° to 20°

Plantarflexion	20°–40°

For normal ambulation, 10° dorsiflexion and 20° plantarflexion are required. Less than 10° of dorsiflexion is an equinus deformity. The ankle joint is most stable in the maximally dorsiflexed position.

MPJ

Flexion/Extension

	Flexion	Extension
Lesser MPJs	30°–40°	50°–60°
1st MPJ	45°	70°–90°

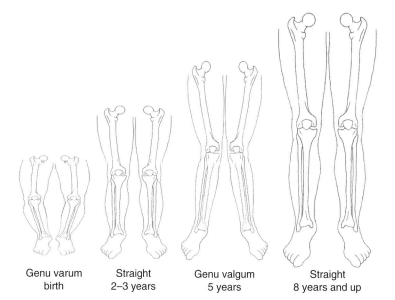

Genu varum birth   Straight 2–3 years   Genu valgum 5 years   Straight 8 years and up

Angles are measured from the long axis of the metatarsal, not the ground.

BONY ANGLES

Femur

Angle of Inclination of Femur (Mikulicz Angle)

A deformity of the hip where the angle formed between the head and neck of the femur and its shaft (*Mikulicz angle*) is decreased (coxa vara) or increased (coxa valga). Patients present with a limp and a limb length discrepancy.

Birth	140°
1 y	146°
4 y	137°
14 y	132°
Adults	120°–130° (average 127°)

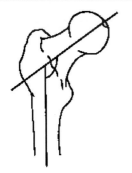

Femoral Neck Version

- Also known as angle of femoral torsion, angle of antetorsion, angle of anteversion, or angle of declination

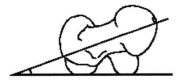

Femoral neck version is the orientation of the femoral neck in relation to the femoral condyles at the level of the knee when the femur is viewed along the axis of the shaft. In most cases, the femoral neck is anterior to the transcondylar femoral axis (called *anteversion*). When the neck axis is posterior to the condylar axis, it is termed *retroversion*.
Birth: 30°–40°
Adult: 15° (*Normal ranges are very broad.*)

Tibia

Tibial Torsion

Tibial torsion is the lateral twist of the long axis of the tibia. Tibial torsion is measured clinically by malleolar position, which is the angle between the knee axis and the medial and lateral malleoli. Note that the malleolar position is about 5° less than the tibial torsion angle.

Age	Tibial Torsion	Malleolar Position
Birth	0°	0°
1 y	6°	3°–4°
2 y	12°	6°–8°
6–8 y reaches adult value	18°–23° (average 20°)	13°–18°

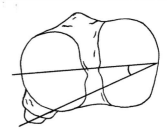

Varum/Valgum

A frontal plane deformity in which the long axis of the distal third of the tibial is angled either medially or laterally from the midsagittal plane of the more proximal two-thirds of the tibia. Tibial varum is compensated in the foot with subtalar joint pronation, and tibial valgum is compensated by supination. Tibial varum and valgum must be evaluated in conjunction with knee angles (genu varum and valgum). A genu varum of 5° plus a tibial varum of 5° mean that the subtalar joint must pronate 10° to allow the calcaneus to assume a vertical position.

Birth	5°–10° varum
>2 y	2°–3° varum (normal adult values)

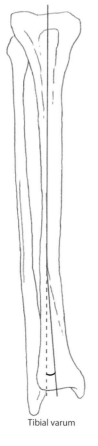

Tibial varum

Talocrural Angle

A line drawn parallel to the tibial plafond and a second line drawn connecting the tips of the medial and lateral malleoli. This measurement is useful in assessing syndesmotic injuries and ankle fractures. Normal value is 83° ± 4°.

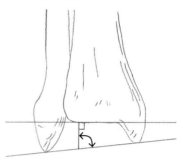

Talus

Talar Neck Angle

Long axis of the talar body and the long axis of the talar neck. There are two sets of values depending on which angle is measured.

Angle A		Angle B	
Birth	130°–140°	Birth	35°–40°
Adult	150°–155°	Adult	10°–20°

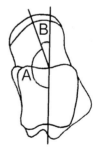

Talar Torsion (Angle of Declination of the Talus)

Lateral rotation or torsion of the talar head relative to the talar body in the frontal plane

This value increases with age and brings the supinated embryonic foot into its pronated adult position. Normal adult value is 25° to 30°.

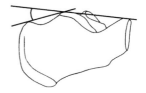

Fowler–Philip Angle

Normal 44° to 69°
Pathology >75°
Useful in evaluating retrocalcaneal bone pathology

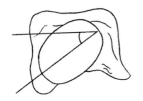

Metatarsal Declination Angle

Normal 21°

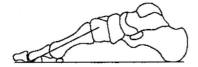

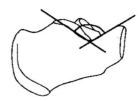

Metatarsal Length

Lengths of each individual metatarsal from base to head
Longest 2-3-5-4-1 shortest

Metatarsal Distal Protrusion

Metatarsal distal protrusion is how far distally each metatarsal extends in relation to the other metatarsals, regardless of the actual length of the bone.
Longest 2-3-1-4-5 shortest

Böhler Angle

Normal value is 20° to 40°.
Average ~30 to 35
Decreases in calcaneal fracture

Gissane Angle

Also known as critical angle, crucial angle
Normal is 120° to 145°.
Increases in calcaneal fracture

Total Angle of Ruch

Calcaneal inclination angle + Fowler–Philips angle = total angle of Ruch
Greater than 90° may be observed in a Haglund deformity.
Like Fowler–Philip angle used for retrocalcaneal bony pathology but takes the calcaneal inclination angle into account

Parallel Pitch Lines

a. Draw a line along the plantar surface of the calcaneus.
b. Draw a perpendicular line passing through the posterior aspect of the posterior facet of the STJ.
c. At the point where it passes through the posterior facet, draw another perpendicular line, parallel to the CIA.
d. If the posterior tubercle extends above the second parallel line, it is indicative of Haglund deformity.

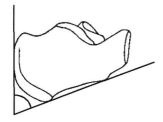

Meary Angle

Straight line through the mid axis of the talus and mid axis of the 1st metatarsal

Normal 0°

Mild flatfoot 1° to 15°

Severe flatfoot > 15°

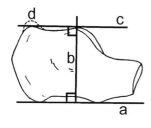

Calcaneal Inclination Angle

Average 20° to 25°

Value does not change with pronation and supination.

Decreased pes planus

Increased in pes cavus

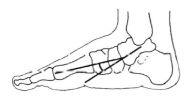

Angle of Hibbs

Long axis of the 1st metatarsal and long axis of the calcaneus on a lateral view

Less than 150° is a cavus foot.

Normal 135° to 140°

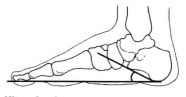

Kites Angle

Long axis of talus and long axis of calcaneus

Normal range is 20° to 40°.

Increased in pronation; decreased in supination

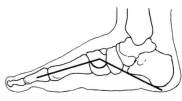

Calcaneocuboid Angle

The calcaneocuboid angle is the angle created by the lateral border of the calcaneus and lateral border of the cuboid on a weight-bearing lateral radiograph. Normal is 0° to 5°; angles >5° are found in pes planus.

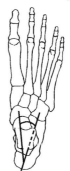

STJ

STJ axis extends anterior, dorsal medial to posterior, plantar, lateral. Axis is angled 42° dorsally in the sagittal plane and 23° medially in the transverse plane.

Subtalar joint axis

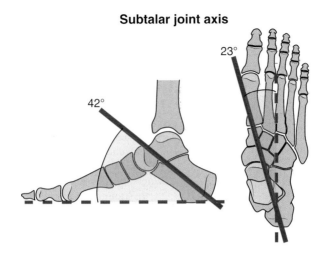

This oblique axis passes from the back of calcaneus through sinus tarsi to emerge at the superior–medial aspect of the neck of talus.

Neutral position is two-thirds the distance from the most supinated position. The average ROM is 25° to 30° (values are highly varied), and a minimum of 12° is required for normal ambulation.
PRONATION involves: dorsiflexion, eversion, abduction
SUPINATION involves: plantarflexion, inversion, adduction

Talonavicular Coverage Angle

The angle between the articular surface of the talar head and the proximal navicular
Normal < 7°

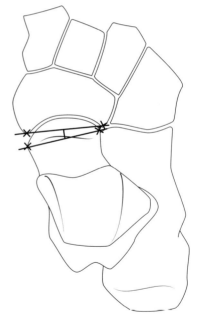

SHOE ANATOMY

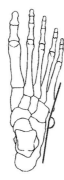

1. *Collar*
   The upper rim at the opening of the shoe
2. *Heel*
3. *Heel counter*
   The portion of the upper that surrounds the heel. Acts to reinforce the heel portion of the upper and help provide stability to calcaneus.
4. *Insole*
   The top layer of the sole that comes in direct contact with the foot. Provides traction and is made of durable material.
5. *Lace stays*
   Part of the upper on the dorsum of the shoe; often reinforced with leather and contains holes for shoe laces
6. *Midsole*
   Located between the insole and the outsole. This layer is usually responsible for absorption of the shoe.
7. *Outsole*
   Bottom layer of the sole that comes in contact with the ground.

Provides traction and is molded of durable material. Determines the flexibility of the shoe.
8. *Quarter*
   The posterior portion of the upper
9. *Shank*
   Often made of steel. Located between the insole and the outsole, the shank runs from the heel center to the ball of the shoe and acts to give support to the longitudinal arch and prevent collapse of the shoe. The shank is the section of the shoe's sole in this area.
10. *Throat*
    The area where the vamp and quarter and vamp and tongue meet
11. *Toe box* (toe cap)
    The most anterior portion of the upper that covers the toes and acts to protect the toes and help maintain the shape of the upper in the toe
12. *Tongue*
    Piece of material continuous with the vamp and covers the dorsum of the foot under the lace stays
13. *Upper*
    The section of the shoe that covers the dorsum of the foot and attaches to the sole of the shoe. The upper includes the vamp, quarter, lace stays, tongue, throat, heel counter, and toe box.
14. *Vamp*
    The anterior portion of the upper covering the forefoot and toes

Last

A last is a 3D model of the shape and cubical content of a shoe that the shoe is built around.

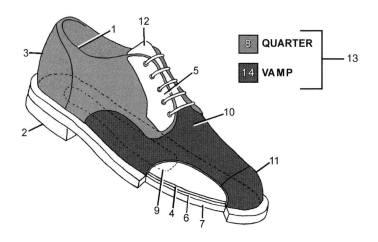

Gait Analysis

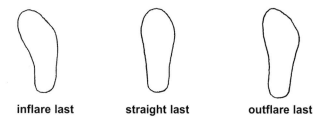

inflare last   **straight last**   **outflare last**

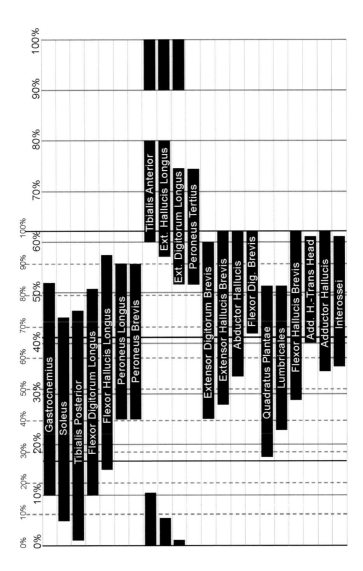

BIOMECHANICS
Limb Length Discrepancy (LLD)

A true LLD requires a 5-mm discrepancy or more to cause significant functional and structural problems. Children typically walk with a shoulder drop, but by age 13 to 14 years, compensatory scoliosis may develop. During stance, the foot of the longer leg is usually pronated and the shorter leg is supinated.

Open Kinetic Chain

Describes the movement of a body part that is NWB. Open kinetic chain pronation can be described as abduction, eversion, and dorsiflexion of the foot.

Closed Kinetic Chain

Describes the movement of a bone around a joint in a body part that is WB. Closed kinetic chain pronation can be described as talar plantarflexion and adduction in the ankle joint, and calcaneal eversion.

Flexor Stabilization

Occurs in flat feet with excessive pronation. STJ pronation allows hypermobility and unlocking of the midtarsal joint, leading to hypermobility of the forefoot. The flexors fire earlier and longer than normal in an attempt to stabilize the forefoot. The flexors overpower the interosseous muscles

and cause digital hammering or clawing. There is also a possible associated adductovarus of the 4th and 5th toes because the quadratus plantae loses its mechanical advantage.

Flexor Substitution

Occurs with weak triceps surae; the deep posterior leg and lateral leg muscles try to compensate for lack of plantarflexion. In doing so, they create a high-arched supinated foot and contract the digits. There is usually no adductovarus deformity of the digits.

Extensor Substitution

Extensor muscles normally contract to dorsiflex the ankle to allow the foot to clear the ground during swing phase. With extensor substitution, the extensors gain a mechanical advantage over the lumbricals, and the extensors will contract the MPJs. There is normally no adductovarus deformity. Causes include anything that will give the extensors a mechanical advantage over the lumbricals.

Windlass Mechanism

As the hallux is dorsiflexed, the plantar fascia is pulled under the head of the metatarsal. This brings the calcaneus toward the head of the 1st metatarsal, thereby creating an elevated medial longitudinal arch.

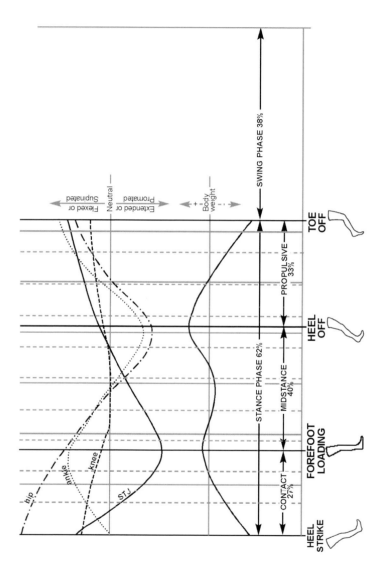

SWING PHASE 38%

STANCE PHASE 62%

PROPULSIVE 33%

MIDSTANCE 40%

CONTACT 27%

TOE OFF

HEEL OFF

FOREFOOT LOADING

HEEL STRIKE

Flexed or Supinated

Neutral

Extended or Pronated

Body weight

+ = −

hip

ankle

knee

ST J

159

Posting

Used to increase support of a part of an orthotic and tilt the contoured plate against the foot

Rearfoot posts can be used as wedges and usually have an angle between the medial and lateral planes of 4°.

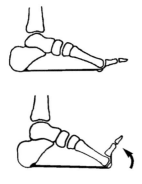

Lateral Flare

Used for lateral instability and frequent inversion sprains

Can be put on the orthotic or a shoe

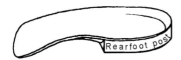

Thomas Heel

An anteromedial extension made to the heel to provide additional support to the longitudinal arch and limit late midstance pronation

A reverse Thomas heel is an anterolateral extension made to the heel to support a weak lateral longitudinal arch, rarely indicated.

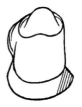

Triplane Wedge

A heel wedge thickest at its anteromedial edge

Used to supinate the foot

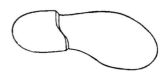

SACH Heel

A modification made to the heel of a shoe to round off the heel in a rocker-bottom manner

Allows a more cushioned fluid motion through the heel contact phase of gait

Cobra Pad

A prefabricated type of orthotic, providing arch support and off-weighting the heel

Usually constructed out of felt, it is easily fit into dress shoes.

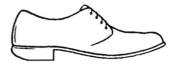

Metatarsal Bar

A pad placed just behind the metatarsal heads to reduce pressure on the 2nd, 3rd, and 4th metatarsal heads

Metatarsal bars can be incorporated into an orthotic, insole, or taped directly on the foot.

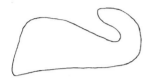

Denver Bar

Placed under the metatarsal bones to support the transverse arch extending from the metatarsal heads to the tarsometatarsal joint

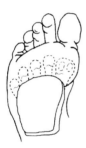

Heel Lifts

Used to treat Haglund deformity, apophysitis, LLD, and equinus

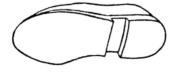

Dancer's Pad

Used to off-weight the 1st metatarsal head

Indications are sesamoiditis or fractured sesamoid.

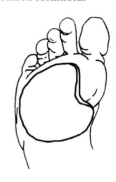

Budin Splint

Used for hammertoes to hold down the digit

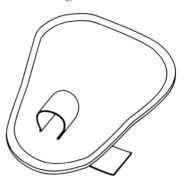

UCBL Insert

UCBL insert stands for University of California Berkeley (or Biomechanics) Laboratory where the device was developed. The UCBL insert is a custom-molded rigid device designed for maximum control of pediatric flexible flat foot. Its main distinguishing feature is a very deep heel cup with a high rigid medial, lateral, and posterior wall designed to hold the heel in neutral position.

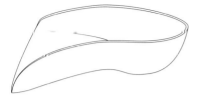

Low-Dye Strap

A strapping technique achieved with tape that alleviates the strain associated with pronation, particularly plantar fasciitis

Step 1

Apply one to three strips of 1″ adhesive tape in a *heel lock* manner.

The heel lock is applied by placing the adhesive tape on the lateral side of the foot just proximal to the 5th metatarsal head and extending around the posterior aspect of the foot to just distal to the 1st metatarsal head.

Hold the foot in the adducted (supinated) position during taping.

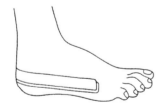

Step 2

Over the heel lock, place a *plantar rest strap* using three to four strips of 12-2″ adhesive tape.

The plantar rest strap is applied by placing the first strip on the lateral aspect of the foot just below the malleoli, across the plantar surface, and up the medial foot to the navicular.

Apply additional two or three strips distal and slightly overlapping the first

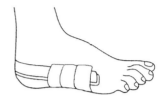

GAIT PATTERNS

Spastic Gait

Manifested by internal rotation and adduction of the entire limb with hip/knee/ankle in marked flexion. Seen with CP, familial spastic diplegia, paraplegia, and hemiplegia.

Dyskinetic Gait

A constant movement abnormality with a high degree of variability from patient to patient and gait cycle to gait cycle. It is characterized by motion involving considerable effort, often with deliberated almost concentrated steps. Seen with CP, Huntington chorea, and dystonia muscular deformities.

Ataxic Gait

Characterized by a marked instability during single-limb stance with an alternating wide/narrow base during double support. During swing phase, the limb will swing widely and cross the midline. Seen with MS, tabes dorsalis, diabetic polyneuropathy, and Friedreich ataxia.

Waddling Gait

A laboring gait exhibiting difficulty with balance proximal pelvic instability, leading to a lumbar lordosis.

May see an associated equinovarus foot type. Seen with muscular dystrophies, spinal muscular atrophy, and congenital dislocated hip.

Steppage Gait

Gait exhibits a swing-phase drop foot. Seen with Charcot–Marie–Tooth, polio, Guillain–Barré syndrome, CVA, paralytic drop foot, and facioscapulohumeral dystrophy.

Vaulting Gait

Gait changes include a high step rate, increased lateral trunk movement, scissoring, and instability from step to step, suggesting a loss of balance. Seen with myotonic dystrophy.

Equinus Gait

Gait exhibiting a swing-phase ankle plantarflexion with no heel contact.

Seen with CP, CMT, MD, spinal muscular atrophy, schizophrenia, osseous block of the ankle, and habitual toe walking.

Fenestrating Gait

Shuffling gait with loss of reciprocal arm swing, decreased velocity, decreased stride length, and increased step rate. Seen with Parkinson disease.

Trendelenburg Gait

Stance phase of each step leads to a contralateral tilt of the pelvis with a deviation of the spine to the affected side. Seen with dislocated hip or weakness of the gluteus medius muscle.

Antalgic Gait

Counteracting or avoiding pain, walking with a limp to lessen pain

11 RADIOLOGY AND IMAGING

X-rays should be taken: **WEIGHT BEARING**

ANGLE AND BASE OF GAIT

Feet abducted 15°
Medial malleoli 2″ apart

STANDARD FOOT X-RAYS

A/P, lateral, MO

EXPOSURE FACTORS

Kilovoltage peak (kVp) is the component that controls the radiographic *contrast* or *grayscale* in the film. Increasing the kilovolts produces a more penetrating x-ray, with increased *latitude*, a shorter exposure time, and less x-ray tube heat. Increasing the kVp results in less exposure to the patient.

Milliamperage (mA) controls the *quantity* or amount of x-ray emitted from the x-ray tube and is the most important component controlling radiographic *density*. To reduce radiation exposure, decrease mA.

Distance: To achieve maximum *fidelity* (true size/shape of original object), the distance of the object to the film must be kept to a minimum. A small focal spot gives better detail.

RADIOGRAPHIC TERMINOLOGY

Compton effect: The Compton effect occurs when an x-ray photon interacts with an outer shell electron. The Compton effect occurs mostly above 80 kVp. It causes less radiation to the patient and is detrimental to the image.

Grid: Composed of alternating strips of lead and aluminum spacers to control, by absorbing, scatter radiation

Collimation: A method of limiting the area of an x-ray beam, which, by law, cannot exceed the film size. A light beam from the collimator maps the area of the x-ray beam.

Photoelectric effect: Occurs at lower kVp when an x-ray photon collides with a lower shell electron. The electron is ejected, and another higher shell electron fills its space, releasing energy. The photoelectric effect is beneficial to the image but results in greater absorption of radiation by the patient.

Orthoposer: The platform that enables weight-bearing images of the foot and ankle to be obtained. X-ray film or image receptors on the orthoposer can lie flat or be placed vertically.

Hard x-rays: Hard x-rays are produced by increased kVp. They have a short wavelength, high frequency, and increased penetration and are less dangerous to the patient. Hard x-rays have higher energy, with photon energies above 5 to 10 kVp.

Soft x-rays: Soft x-rays are produced by decreased kVp. They have a long wavelength, low frequency, low penetration, and lower energy and are more dangerous to the patient.

Computed Radiography (CR) vs. Digital Radiography (DR)

CR is taken in the usual way, but uses a reusable CR-specific cassette instead of standard x-ray film. The image on the cassette is then run through a CR reader, where the image is scanned into a digital format.

DR transfers the x-ray directly into a digital signal.

Slow vs. Fast Speed Film

The larger the size of the AgBr crystals, the thicker the emulsion layer. The faster the film, the darker the image.

X-Ray Machine Requirements (Vary by State)

Dead-man–type exposure switch with a 6-ft cord

Machines <70 kVp do not need 1° or 2° barriers or special lead lined rooms. (The majority of podiatric x-rays are taken <70 kVp.)

Lead aprons, gloves, and goggles are 0.25 mm thick; gonadal shields are 0.5 mm lead equivalent.

Relative Radiographic Densities

Cortex - Cancellous - Muscle - Nerve - Tendon - Ligament - SubQ - Fat - Air

Highest density---->----Lowest density

PODIATRIC X-RAY VIEWS

Dorsoplantar (DP) or Anteroposterior (AP)

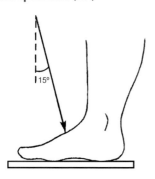

Central ray aimed at the 2nd metatarsocuneiform joint.

15° from vertical

When examining the foot for a foreign body, this view may be taken perpendicular for better spatial location.

Lateral

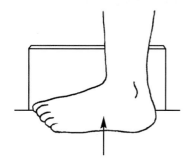

Medial side of foot against film

Central ray aimed at cuboid.

Tube is angled 90° from vertical.

Non–Weight-Bearing Medial Oblique (MO)

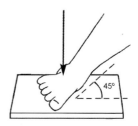

Center beam at the 3rd metatarso-cuneiform joint

Angle the foot 45° with the medial side of the foot on the image receptor.

Non–Weight-Bearing Lateral Oblique (LO)

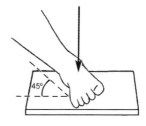

Central ray aimed at the 1st metatarsocuneiform joint.

Angle the foot 45° with the lateral side of the foot on the image receptor.

Stress Lateral or Stress Dorsiflexion

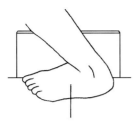

Position patient for a lateral but then have patient flex knees and maximally dorsiflex ankle.

Demonstrates any anterior ankle impingement (osseous equinus)

Plantar Axial (Sesamoidal Axial)

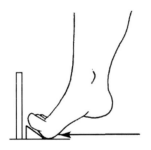

Head angled at 90° to the vertical.

Central ray aimed at the plantar aspect of the sesamoids.

Good view of sesamoids and plantar aspect of metatarsal heads

Toes dorsiflexed against film and then raise heel

Positioning device may aid in taking this projection.

Harris–Beath (SKI-Jump)

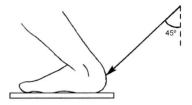

Good for posterior and middle STJ coalitions

Similar to a calcaneal axial, except ankle is dorsiflexed, giving better subtalar joint visualization.

Patient stands on film with knees and ankles flexed 15° to 20°.

First take a scout lateral film and determine the declination angle of posterior facet of STJ. Then take three views: one at the angle determined by the lateral film, one 10° above, and one 10° below.

Some advocate three arbitrary views at 35°, 40°, and 45°.

Calcaneal Axial

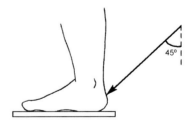

Central ray aimed at the posterior aspect of calcaneus.

Angle unit at 45°

Examines the calcaneus for fractures, abnormalities in shape, or internal fixation in major tarsal fusions

Good view for assessing the middle and posterior STJ facets

Isherwood

- Three positions to fully visualize the STJ

Medial Oblique Position

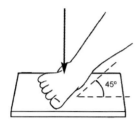

Visualizes the *anterior facet* of the STJ
Foot is positioned the same as for a non–weight-bearing medial oblique x-ray.
Central ray aimed between the fibular malleolus and the cuboid.

Medial Oblique Axial Position

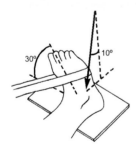

Visualizes the *middle facet* of the STJ
Foot adducted 30° from image receptor.
Dorsiflex and invert the foot using a sling.
Central ray aimed between the fibular malleolus and the cuboid.
Tube head angled 10° cephalad.

Lateral Oblique Axial Position

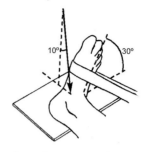

Visualizes the *posterior facet* of the STJ
Foot abducted 30° from image receptor.
Dorsiflex and evert the foot using a sling
Central ray between the tibial malleolus and navicular tuberosity
Tube head angled 10° cephalad

Stress Inversion (Talar Tilt)

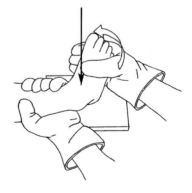

Position the stress inversion view the same as an ankle AP view.
Examiner wears lead gloves.
Stabilize lower leg with one hand while forcefully inverting foot with other hand.
Performed following ankle inversion sprains, may need to anesthetize foot (common peroneal block) for pain relief and to relax foot

Assess lateral ligamentous injury, specifically the ATF and CFL.

Positive is a test >10° or if the talar tilt is 5° greater than the unaffected ankle.

Anterior Drawer or Push–Pull Stress

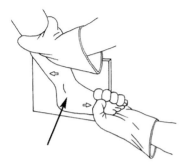

Patient supine or sitting with leg in lateral position. Stabilize leg with one hand and place an anterior dislocating force on the foot with the other hand.

Central ray aimed at the medial malleoli.

Taken following ankle trauma to assess the ATF

Good visualization of the tibial plafond and medial space between the medial malleolus and body of the talus

Lateral space between the lateral malleolus and the talus cannot be visualized.

A positive test is a 6 mm or greater.

Anterior translation of the talus is measured by the distance from the posterior lip of the tibial joint surface to the nearest point of the talar dome.

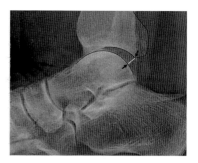

Ankle-AP

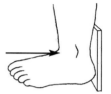

Foot positioned straight ahead.

Central beam parallel to the floor and aimed between malleoli.

Good visualization of the tibial plafond and medial space between the medial malleolus and the body of the talus. The space between the lateral malleolus and talus may not be visualized.

Ankle-Lateral

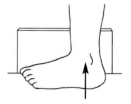

Medial side of foot against film

Central beam parallel to floor and aimed at the center of the ankle

Good for trochlear surface of talus and its articulation with the tibia and fibula

Ankle-Medial Oblique

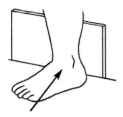

Leg internally rotated 45° from the central beam.
Central beam parallel to floor and aimed at the center of the ankle.
Good view of tibiofibular syndesmosis

Ankle-Lateral Oblique

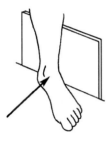

Leg externally rotated 45° from the central beam.
Central beam parallel to floor and aimed at the center of the ankle.

Mortise View

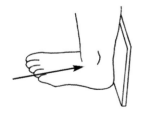

Leg internally rotated ~15° from central beam, and attempt to place the malleoli on a plane parallel to the film.

Central beam parallel to floor and aimed at the center of the ankle.
The arch formed by the tibial plafond and the two malleoli is referred to as the *ankle mortise*. This view is intended to adequately visualize the mortise.

Canale View

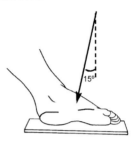

This view is the same as the AP view, but the foot is fully plantar-flexed and pronated 15°.
This view provides a good view of the talar neck for fractures in this area.

Broden I View

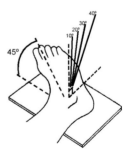

Broden views are special calcaneal radiographs to show the congruency of the subtalar joint. Often taken intraoperatively to assess calcaneal fracture reduction.
The ankle is at 90° and the foot is adducted 45°, and the central beam aimed at the lateral malleoli.

Four cephalad views at 10° intervals off the perpendicular (40°, 30°, 20°, and 10° cephalad)

Allows visualization of the middle and posterior STJ facet, useful in comminuted fractures of the calcaneus

The 40° projection shows the anterior portion of the posterior facet, the 10° projection shows the posterior portion of the posterior facet, and the middle facet can usually best be seen at one of the intermediate projections.

Broden II View

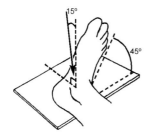

X-ray beam is tilted 15° caudally.
Three projections are taken at 3° to 4° intervals.
This view allows visualization of depressions in the posterior facet of the STJ.

ACCESSORY BONES

1. Os vesalianum
2. Os trigonum
3. Os peroneum
4. Os sustentaculum tali
5. Os calcaneus secundarius
6. Os tibiale externum
7. Dorsal 1/2 of bipartite medial cuneiform
8. Plantar 1/2 of bipartite medial cuneiform
9. Os intercuneiform
10. Os intermetatarseum I
11. Os talonavicular dorsale
12. Fabella—accessory sesamoid bone found behind the knee in the lateral head of the gastrocnemius muscle *(not shown)*

Accessory ossicles

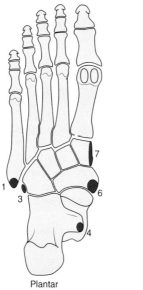

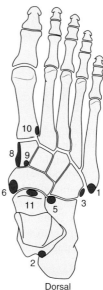

Plantar   Dorsal

OSSIFICATIONS

Ossification centers

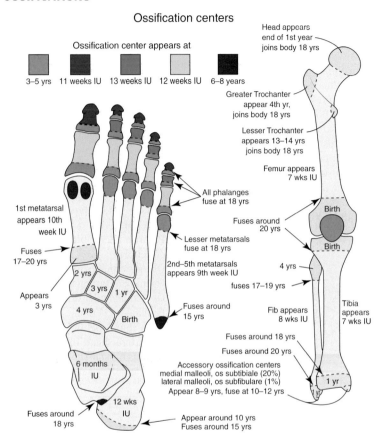

Ossification center appears at

3–5 yrs   11 weeks IU   13 weeks IU   12 weeks IU   6–8 years

Head appears
end of 1st year
joins body 18 yrs

Greater Trochanter
appear 4th yr,
joins body 18 yrs

Lesser Trochanter
appears 13–14 yrs
joins body 18 yrs

Femur appears
7 wks IU

Birth

Fuses around
20 yrs

Birth

4 yrs

fuses 17–19 yrs

Tibia
appears
7 wks IU

Fib appears
8 wks IU

1st metatarsal
appears 10th
week IU

All phalanges
fuse at 18 yrs

Fuses
17–20 yrs

Lesser metatarsals
fuse at 18 yrs

2nd–5th metatarsals
appears 9th week IU

2 yrs

3 yrs   1 yr

Appears
3 yrs

4 yrs   Birth

Fuses around
15 yrs

6 months
IU

Fuses around 18 yrs

Fuses around 20 yrs

Accessory ossification centers
medial malleoli, os subtibiale (20%)
lateral malleoli, os subfibulare (1%)
Appear 8–9 yrs, fuse at 10–12 yrs

1 yr

Fuses around
18 yrs

12 wks
IU

Appear around 10 yrs
Fuses around 15 yrs

MAGNETIC RESONANCE IMAGING

MRI is an imaging modality that uses the body's natural magnetic properties to generate detailed images. MRI is noninvasive and uses no ionizing radiation. Average magnetic field strength is between 0.2 and 3 T (Tesla). Open MRIs are available for patients who are claustrophobic; these units have less field strength.

How It Works

MRI works by using the body's natural hydrogen molecules. Hydrogen is a good choice because it is the simplest element with an atomic number of 1 and an atomic weight of 1. Hydrogen is also abundant in both water and fat, making it a good choice.

When hydrogen is in its ionic state (H^+), it is essentially just a proton. A proton is positively charged and has a magnetic spin or wobble. All the protons (hydrogen ions) wobble in a chaotic manner and cancel out any magnetism. By applying an external magnet, the protons (hydrogen) in the body align with the MRI's magnetic field.

Once the protons (hydrogen ions) are aligned, a radio frequency pulse is applied, which pushes the protons (hydrogen) into a higher energy level. The radio is then turned off, and the higher energy gained by the protons (nuclear magnetic resonance signal) dissipates and is transmitted to the receiver coils. The radio frequency coils act as both transmitter and receiver. The protons (hydrogen) in different types of tissues realign at different speeds and produce different signals. The computer then converts these NMR signals into images.

MRI Commonly Used in Podiatry

T1

T1 images are produced by measuring the time taken for the magnetic vector to return to its resting state. T1-weighted images produce hyperintense signal with fat, bone marrow, nerves, and lipomas. T1 images are sometimes referred to as anatomic images.

T2

T2 images are produced by measuring the time needed for the axial spin to return to its rest state. T2-weighted images produce hyperintense signal with water (inflammation), blood, edema, and fluid-filled tumors. Most diseases manifest themselves by an increase in water content (inflammation); so, T2 images are referred to as pathologic image.

Weight	Fat	Water	Muscle	Ligament	Bone
T1	*Bright*	Dark	Intermediate	Dark	Dark
T2	Intermediate	*Bright*	Intermediate	Dark	Dark

Short-T1 Inversion Recovery (STIR)

STIR is a type of fat suppression. The high signal produced by fat can mask subtle contrast differences, which can mask pathology. STIR is used to nullify the signal from fat to allow greater visualization of other tissues.

MR Arthrography

Used primarily in the shoulder and hip. Involves injecting a contrast material into the joint and then performing an MRI.

MRI Contraindications

Pacemakers
Metal clips
Metal valves
Metal stints
Slivers of metal embedded in the eye
Cochlear implants
Stents
Internal fixation is not a contraindication, although it is recommended that the hardware be in at least 6 weeks. This gives it enough time for adequate bone incorporation.

COMPUTED AXIAL TOMOGRAPHY (CAT) SCAN

A CAT scan is an x-ray that uses computed axial tomography to generate cross-sectional images. CAT scans are less expensive and quicker than MRIs but have a high radiation exposure. CAT scans are used in podiatry for coalitions, complex fractures, and Charcot foot.

BONE SCANS (SCINTIGRAPHY)

Bone scans have good sensitivity and poor specificity.

Radioactive compounds (radiopharmaceuticals) are slowly injected into the patient and localized in specific organs.

A scintillation probe or detector is positioned over the target, and emitted γ-photons are converted to visible light and counted.

Hot spot: Area of high radiopharmaceutical uptake

Cold spot: Area of low radiopharmaceutical uptake

Identifies areas of increased bone turnover or osteoblastic activity (i.e., fractures, bone tumors)

Bone scanning allows early diagnosis of a stress fracture (as early as 7 hours postinjury).

Podiatric Indications

Osteomyelitis, trauma/inflammatory arthritis, stress fracture, tumors, nonspecific pain

Technetium-99 (Tc-99m)

Highly selective for bone metabolism (osteoblastic activity)

Normal uptake seen at tendon insertion, site of bone growth in children, epiphyseal plates, areas of constant stress, or osseous remodeling

Will pick up in any areas of focal inflammation or bone turnover

Used to identify fractures, tumors, infections

Technetium is combined with an appropriate bone-imaging agent:
Tc-99MDP (methylene diphosphate)
Tc-99MAA (macroaggregated albumin)

Tc-99m Macroaggregated Albumin (Tc-99MAA)

Assesses capillary bed perfusion in diabetics

Assesses healing potential in ischemic ulcers

Tc-99m Methylene Diphosphate (Tc-99MDP)

Used to identify areas of increased bone metabolism (fractures) and increased blood flow

A stress fracture will show up as early as 7 hours after injury.

Normal uptake is found in tendon insertions and epiphyseal plates, and areas of constant stresses or osseous remodeling.

Images are obtained at 2 to 4 hours.

Osteoblastic-mediated chemo-absorption onto the surface of hydroxyapatite crystals

Physical half-life of 6 hours

Useful 140-keV γ-photon

50% is excreted by the kidney; so, adequate hydration/voiding is important to reduce the radiation exposure to bladder wall.

Four-Phase Bone Scan (Tc-99 MDP)

First phase—radionuclide angio-
gram (blood flow phase)
Images are taken 1 to 3 seconds
apart immediately following
injection.
Shows dynamic visualization of
blood flow
Provides information about the
relative blood supply to the
extremity
Second phase—blood pooling
images
Images are taken 5 to 10 minutes following injection.
Quantifies relative hyperemia or
ischemia
Third phase—delayed image
(bone-imaging phase)
Images are taken 3 to 4 hours
following injection.
Visualizes regional rates of bone
metabolism
This phase is useful to determine cellulitis vs.
osteomyelitis.
By the third phase with cellulitis, there should be a flushing and cleaning returning
toward normal density. With
osteomyelitis, Tc-99 will incorporate into the bone and
show increased density.

Fourth phase
Images are taken at 24 hours.
Used in the diagnosis of osteomyelitis; at this phase, it
shows greater bone activity
and less soft-tissue activity. If
the ratio at 24 hours has increased more than one whole
number compared with the
third phase, it is positive for
osteomyelitis. If the ratio at
24 hours is decreased more
than one whole number
compared with the third
phase, it is negative for osteomyelitis. If the ratio at 24
hours is less than a whole
number different compared
with the third phase, it is
inconclusive.

Gallium-67 Citrate (Ga-67)

Gallium binds to WBC, plasma
proteins, siderophores, and
iron-binding proteins (transfer-
rin, ferritin, lactoferrin).
Identifies neoplasms and inflammatory disorders
Imaging is performed at 6 to 24
hours for infections.
Imaging is performed at 24 to 72
hours for tumors.
Excreted by the kidneys
Half-life is 78 hours; thus, radiation
dose is high.

Indium-111 (In-111)

Binds to cytoplasmic components
of the WBC membrane
Spleen and liver light up because
of WBC destruction at these
locations.
Used for leukocyte-mediated
pathology—inflammatory
disorders
Images are taken at 18 to 24 hours.
More accurate at assessing acute
infection, while Ga-67 is more
sensitive for subacute and
chronic infection
Half-life is 67 hours.
Rather than simply injecting the
radiopharmaceutical, In-111
bone scans involve drawing
blood from the patient, isolat-
ing WBCs, labeling them (with
In-111), and then reintroducing
them back into the bloodstream.

Indium is more accurate at assessing infection if gallium studies are inconclusive.

Thallium-201 (Ti-201)

Used to assess foot perfusion

Combined Tc and Ga Bone Scan

Combining technetium (bone-imaging radionuclide) and gallium (inflammatory-imaging nuclide) gives more information than either scan alone. Technetium should be given first, because it has a shorter half-life, followed by gallium at 24 to 48 hours. When referring to Tc as either (+) or (−), they are referring to phase 3 (bone-imaging phase). Tc reveals if bone is involved, and Ga reveals if WBCs are involved.

Results	Diagnosis	Explanation
Ga(+) Tc(+)	OM	Ga(+) indicates that infection is present, and Tc(+) indicates that bone is involved.
Ga(+) Tc(−)	Cellulitis	Ga(+) indicates that soft-tissue infection is present, and Tc(−) indicates that bone is not involved.
Ga(−) Tc(+)	Osteoarthropathy Stress fraction Chronic OM	Ga(−) indicates that there is no infection, and Tc(+) indicates that bone is involved.

FLUOROSCOPY

Fluoroscopy is a type of x-ray machine that allows real-time moving images. It is also referred to as a *C-arm* because the unit is the shape of a "C," with the x-ray beam at one end and the image receptor at the other. It is a mobile unit that can be easily manipulated in surgery to assess joint motion and internal fixation or to locate foreign bodies.

DIAGNOSTIC ULTRASOUND

Picture of the Ultrasound Spectrum

Ultrasound is a term to describe sounds of frequencies above 20,000 Hz, beyond the range of human hearing. Diagnostic ultrasound produces sound waves that bounce off body tissues and makes an echo. The ultrasound machine receives the echoes and sends them to a computer that uses them to create an image called a sonogram. Diagnostic US uses sound waves to visualize structures. Unlike US used in physical therapy, diagnostic US produces very little heat. This is accomplished by limiting the intensity (temporal average intensity). Diagnostic US can be used in the presence of pacemakers and metallic implants.

How Ultrasound Work

Ultrasound waves are produced by vibrating a quartz crystal. Quartz crystal is piezoelectric, meaning they vibrate when stimulated by electricity. When just the right amount of electricity is applied, the crystal will resonate, producing US waves. The piezoelectric crystal is located in the transducer or probe that is directly applied to the skin with a coupling agent such as ultrasound gel. Ultrasound does not travel through air.

Ultrasound

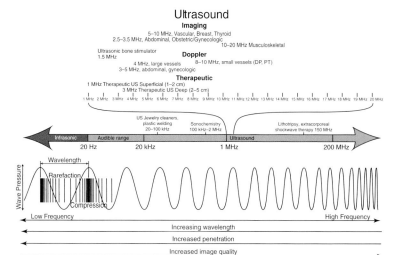

Imaging
5–10 MHz, Vascular, Breast, Thyroid
2.5–3.5 MHz, Abdominal, Obstetric/Gynecologic
10–20 MHz Musculoskeletal

Ultrasonic bone stimulator
1.5 MHz

Doppler
4 MHz, large vessels   8–10 MHz, small vessels (DP, PT)
3–5 MHz, gynecologic

Therapeutic
1 MHz Therapeutic US Superficial (1–2 cm)
3 MHz Therapeutic US Deep (2–5 cm)

1 MHz 2 MHz 3 MHz 4 MHz 5 MHz 6 MHz 7 MHz 8 MHz 9 MHz 10 MHz 11 MHz 12 MHz 13 MHz 14 MHz 15 MHz 16 MHz 17 MHz 18 MHz 19 MHz 20 MHz

US Jewelry cleaners,
plastic welding   Sonochemistry
20–100 kHz   100 kHz–2 MHz

Lithotripsy, extracorporeal
shockwave therapy 150 MHz

Infrasonic | Audible range | Ultrasound

20 Hz   20 kHz   1 MHz   200 MHz

Wavelength

Wave Pressure
Rarefaction
Compression

Low Frequency   High Frequency

Increasing wavelength
Increased penetration
Increased image quality
Increasing energy

Types of Transducers

Linear transducers: Crystal arrangement is linear, shape of beam is rectangular, near-field resolution is good. This is a high-frequency probe ideal for musculoskeletal and superficial vessels.

Convex (Curved) transducers: Crystal arrangement is curvilinear. Good for deeper structures; abdominal, transvaginal, transrectal.

Phased-array transducer: Crystal arrangement is phased array or "stacked" construction, shape of beam is triangular, near-field resolution is poor. Used for cardiac examinations, abdomen, and brain.

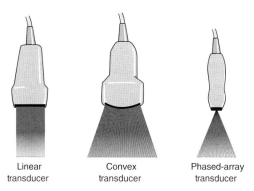

Linear
transducer

Convex
transducer

Phased-array
transducer

Types of Diagnostic Ultrasound

B-mode-(B)rightness mode. This is a traditional US scan. It is the most commonly used and displays as fluorescent dots. The more intense the reflection, the brighter the dots. It scans a plane through the body that is viewed as a two-dimensional image in grey scale. This type of ultrasound is good for visualizing musculoskeletal structures.

B-mode

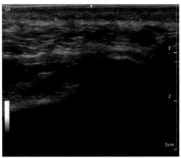

M-mode-(M)ovement mode. A single scan line is emitted over time and displayed graphically. This allows fast moving tissues to be studied in a still frame displayed graphically over time. Most useful in echocardiography where the fast moving valve leaflets are difficult to see on conventional B-mode. M-mode is of no value in the foot.

M-mode

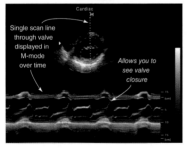

Single scan line through valve displayed in M-mode over time

Allows you to see valve closure

DOPPLERS

Spectral Doppler: Spectral Doppler is a mode of ultrasound that gives information on direction and velocity of flow that is gathered either audibly, graphically, or both. There are two types of spectral Doppler, pulsed and continuous. These are usually portable hand-held devices. The ideal angle to hold the Doppler is at a 45° angle or less to the blood flow, but not >60°.

Pulsed-wave (PW) Doppler: With PW Doppler, there is one transducer crystal, and it alternates between sending and receiving. A pulsed signal is emitted to a specific depth, where you want to measure blood flow velocity. With PW, there is better range resolution and specificity but a lower spectrum of velocities. PW Dopplers are more useful in cardiology because you are able to determine the velocity of blood in a specific location in the heart (range resolution). It is also useful when you have multiple vessels on top of each other. Pulsed-wave Doppler has a limit on the maximum velocity it can test. Nyquist limit is the upper limit of blood velocity that can be detected by pulsed-wave Doppler.

Continuous-wave (CW) Doppler: With CW Doppler, there are two transducer crystals. One is constantly transmitting, and one is constantly receiving. CW has higher sensitivity, but there is range ambiguity. Requirement for a Doppler is to have a continuous wave (CW) Doppler, direction sensitivity and bidirectional flow capabilities, audible output, and recording. A complete color spectral analysis is preferred as it allows us to distinguish between forward and reverse flow. CW Doppler is able to detect the presence and direction of flow but unable to distinguish signals arising from vessels at different depths. Therefore, it lacks range resolution. These are the simple hand-held Dopplers; they are portable and inexpensive. They are used at bedside to ascertain flow in superficial vessels such as the DP or PT.

Pulsed wave vs. Continuous wave

Sample volume

Pulsed-wave Doppler
One crystal.
Unable to measure high velocities.
Range resolution.

Continuous-wave Doppler
Two crystals.
Able to measure high velocities.
Range ambiguity.

Color Doppler: Color Doppler is not considered a type of spectral Doppler but operates on the same principles as pulsed wave. Color Doppler detects blood velocity as a Doppler shift and displays a positive Doppler shift (blood moving toward to probe) in red and negative Doppler shift (blood moving away from the probe) in blue.

This color display is overlayed onto a grayscale B-mode ultrasound image. When possible, the probe should be positioned in the direction of the heart at a 45° angle. By doing so, arterial blood will display red and venous blood will display blue.

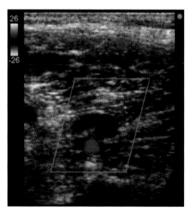

Duplex US Machine

Called a duplex Doppler because it combines both traditional ultrasound (B-mode) with Doppler ultrasound

The top is a color image with directional flow overlayed onto a two-dimensional grayscale B-mode ultrasound image (basically a color Doppler).

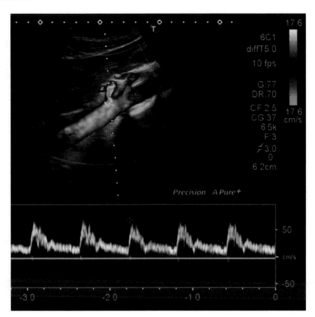

The bottom of the screen depicts the waveform using spectral Doppler.

When you order an US to rule out a DVT, this is the type of scan performed.

DOPPLER WAVEFORMS

Normal peripheral arterial blood flow has a triphasic waveform. Keep in mind the terms *monophasic*, *biphasic*, and *triphasic* were developed for nondirectional audio Doppler and often do not correspond well with digital waveform readouts.

First phase: Initial high-velocity systolic flow due to left ventricular contraction

Second phase: Early diastolic reversal of flow due to peripheral resistance. The absence of the second reverse flow phase does not necessarily mean there is vascular disease. The second phase may be absent if there is low peripheral resistance, such as during exercise or reactive hyperemia. This phase also decreases as blood moves further from the heart and blood flow smooths out.

Third phase: Late diastole flow in which there is elastic recoil that pushed blood forward after the aortic valve closes. The loss of the third phase may occur due to arterial wall calcifications, which comes with age but is worsened by conditions such as atherosclerosis and diabetes.

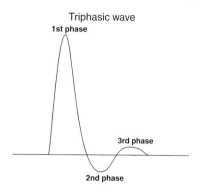

Triphasic wave

Biphasic Waveform

Arteries with biphasic waveforms may have normal blood flow or represent arterial insufficiency depending on the specific aspects of the waveform.

Normal biphasic waveform

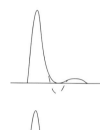

No 2nd phase
This occurs with low peripheral resistance where there is no reverse flow. This may occur with hyperemia or during exercise. Blood flow to extremity may be normal.

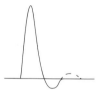

No 3rd phase
Due to calcified vessel walls. There is no third phase due to lack of elastic recoil of the artery. Blood flow to extremity may be normal.

Abnormal biphasic waveform

Widened and blunted 1st phase
A biphasic waveform with a widened or blunted 1st phase would indicates poor blood flow.

Monophasic

Arteries with monophasic waveforms indicate arterial insufficiency and are associated with an abnormal blunted elongated single wave.

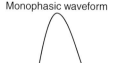

Monophasic waveform

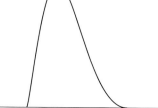

Tardus Parvus

A Doppler waveform pattern shown downstream from severe arterial stenosis (stenosis > 80%). Usually caused by aortic valve stenosis, which is most commonly caused by aging.

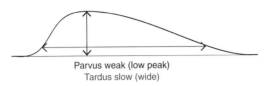

Parvus weak (low peak)
Tardus slow (wide)

Diagnostic Ultrasound Terminology

Near Field

Structures in the upper half of the monitor

Far Field

Structures that appear in the bottom half of the monitor

Echogenic

When the US wave encounters a very dense object, such as bone, the sound wave bounces back, allowing very little sound wave to pass through the tissue. The result is a bright white image.

Anechoic

When the US wave passes through an object without any echo, the image is black. Examples of this would be a fluid-filled cyst (ganglion cyst).

Hyperechoic

Brighter echo showing up as white. Examples of hyperechoic structures include bone, scar tissue, tendon (hyperechoic relative to muscle), ligament, nerves (hyperechoic relative to muscle), and ulcer sinus tract (relative to surrounding ulceration).

Hypoechoic

Less echo showing up dark on monitor. Examples of hypoechoic structures include fluid-filled cyst, muscle, ulcerations, inflammation, and tendon tears.

Homogeneous

Uniform in pattern

Heterogeneous

Irregular in pattern

Identifying Foot Pathology With Ultrasound

Plantar Fasciitis

Normal plantar fascia is <4 mm in thickness, and hyperechoic with multiple parallel lines on longitudinal scan. Abnormal plantar fascia measures >4 mm thick and decreased echogenicity indicative of inflammation.

Plantar Fibromas

Fusiform-shaped heterogeneous hypo-echoic mass adjacent to the plantar surface of the plantar fascia

Morton Neuroma

A discrete well-defined round hy-poechoic mass just proximal to the metatarsal head in the interspace

Ganglion

Presents as a well-defined anechoic (black) lesion

Tendinosis and Tendon Tears

Present as hypoechoic thicken-ing (inflammation); may also be hypoechoic area surrounding the tendon, indicative of fluid and in-flammation. The torn fusiform portion of tendon is heterogeneous as compared with the rest of the tendon.

US-Guided Injections

During US-guided injections, the needles will be hyperechoic and the bolus of anesthetic or cortisone will appear as hypoechoic infiltration.

Indications for Diagnostic Ultrasound

Plantar fasciitis, tears
Muscle injury
Capsulitis

Heel spurs
Morton neuroma
Stress fractures
Achilles injury
Tendonitis/tendon tears
Ligament tears
Soft-tissues masses (fibromas)
Cysts/ganglions
Bursitis
Foreign bodies
US-guided injections, aspirations, and biopsies

Arthrogram

Dye is injected into a joint, and the joint is x-rayed.
Ankle:
If dye leaks around the tip of the fibula. Leaks anterior to the lateral malleolus and laterally alongside it = tear in the ATF.
If dye leaks into the peroneal sheath = tear in the calcaneofib-ular ligament
If contrast leaks into the tibio-fibular syndesmosis = tear in the distal anterior tibiofibular ligament
If contrast leaks into the posterior facet of the STJ = tear in the posterior talofibular ligament. (In 10% of cases, this may repre-sent a normal variant.)
A normal arthrogram should coat the entire joint and extend into the syndesmotic recess, which normally should not exceed 2.5 cm.

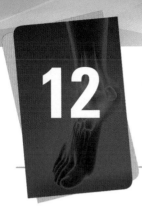

12 BONE TUMORS

Bone tumors are either primary or metastatic. Primary bone tumors can be either benign or malignant. Radioisotope scans (Tc-99MDP) can estimate the local intramedullary extent of the tumor and screen for other skeletal areas of involvement. For potentially active and aggressive lesions, an MRI is useful. Definitive diagnosis requires a biopsy.

In general, less aggressive lesions have a narrow zone of transition, a geographic pattern of destruction, and no periostitis of adjacent soft-tissue involvement. Sclerosis of the surrounding normal bone also indicates a slow-growing lesion.

TYPES OF PERIOSTEAL RESPONSE

These periosteal reactions are not pathognomonic for any particular tumor but indicate the aggressiveness of the lesion.

Buttressing (Thick Periostitis)

Slow-growing tumor presses against the periosteum and thickens the cortex. Usually indicates a benign lesion, but can be malignant.

Buttressing

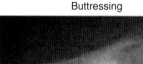

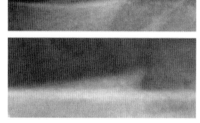

Codman Triangle

A triangular elevation of periosteum from an aggressive, usually malignant, bone tumor, most notably Ewing sarcoma and osteosarcoma. As a tumor enlarges, it pulls the periosteum away from the bone, forming a triangle. The periosteum may then begin to ossify before being pulled away again. This can result in a multi-layered triangle.

Codman triangle

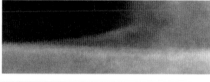

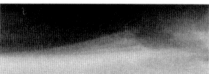

Sunburst

Delicate linear divergent spic-
   ulations of periosteum bone
   formation separated by spaces
   containing blood vessels.
   Spiculated periosteal reaction
radiating from the point-source
lesion. They develop from the
growth of the tumor into the
soft tissue with subsequent
ossification. Seen in malignant aggressive lesions such as
osteosarcoma.

Sunburst

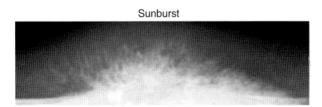

Onion Skin

Multiple layers of new periosteal
   bone in a lamellated pattern.
   Seen in aggressive lesions such
   as Ewing sarcoma.

Onion skin

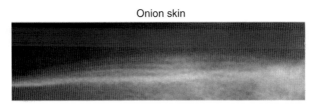

Hair-on-End

Delicate parallel spiculated rays
   of periosteum bone formation
   separated by spaces containing
blood vessels, similar to
sunburst pattern, but rays are
all parallel. Seen in Ewing
sarcoma.

Hair-on-end

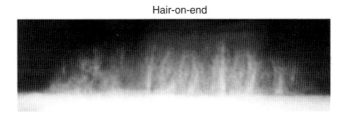

PATTERNS OF BONE DESTRUCTION

Geographic

Well-defined margins with a narrow zone of transition from normal to abnormal bone. Indicative of a slow-growing, less aggressive lesion.

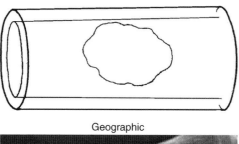

Geographic

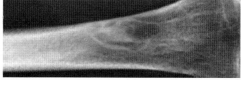

Moth-Eaten

Less well-defined lesion margins with ragged borders and a wider zone of transition between normal and abnormal bone

- More aggressive pattern than geographic and indicates a faster growing lesion, but less aggressive than permeative
- Appears as multiple small holes in the bone

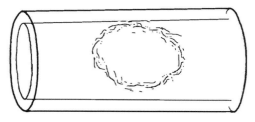

Moth-eaten

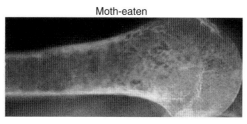

Permeative

Poorly defined lesion margins with a wide zone of transition; the lesion boundaries are not easily discerned from normal bone. Aggressive, rapidly growing lesion seen in malignant bone tumors. Typically presents as multiple small streaks running through the cortical bone.

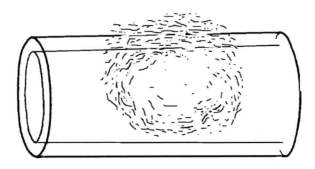

Permeative

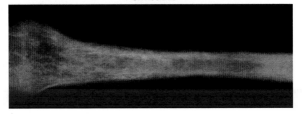

MOST COMMON SOURCES OF METASTATIC BONE TUMORS

Breast, lung, prostate, kidney, and thyroid

MOST COMMON BENIGN PRIMARY BONE TUMOR

Osteochondroma

MOST COMMON MALIGNANT PRIMARY BONE TUMOR

Osteosarcoma

NOTE: Multiple myeloma is more common than osteosarcoma but is often considered a marrow cell tumor versus a bone tumor.

Age of tumor development

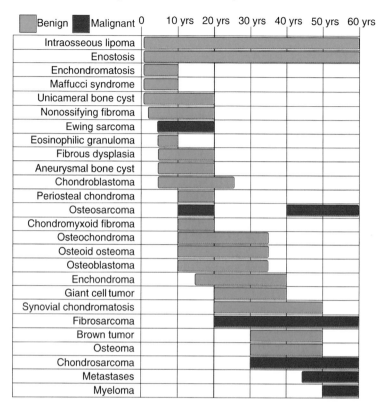

BONE TUMORS AT A GLANCE

	MALIGNANT	BENIGN		
<20 years	**Ewing Sarcoma** -Onion skin	**Chondroblastoma** -ephyseal	**Enchondromatosis** -multiple enchondromas -Ollier dz -Maffucci syndrome	**Eosinophilic granuloma** -immune system reaction
	Osteosarcoma -sunburst	**Aneurysmal bone cyst** -soap bubble appearance -metaphyseal -blood-filled cyst		**Chondromyxoid fibroma**
			Interosseous lipoma -neutral triangle -central calcifications	**Osteochondroma** -cartilage covered bony protuberance
		Enchondroma		
		Periosteal chondroma -chondroma on surface of bone	**Osteoid osteoma** -nocturnal pain relieved by ASA & NSAIDs	**Nonossifying fibroma** -multilocular bubble like appearance
		Enostosis -bony island -thorny radiation	**Fibrous dysplasia** -ground glass -shepherds crook	**Unicameral bone cyst** -simple bone cyst fallen fragment
			Osteoblastoma -a large osteoid osteoma (>1.5 cm)	
>20 years	**Osteosarcoma** -sunburst	**Giant cell tumor** -soap bubble appearance -epiphyseal	**Enostosis** -bony island -thorny radiation	
	Chondrosarcoma -endosteal scalloping	**Osteoma** -surface of bone	**Synovial chondromatosis** -rice bodies in joint	
	Fibrosarcoma -no periosteal reaction	**Interosseous lipoma** -neutral triangle -central calcifications	**Enchondroma**	
	Myeloma		**Brown tumor** -hyperparathyroidism	

- ▢ EPIPHYSIS
- ▢ METAPHYSIS
- ▢ DIAPHYSIS

GENERAL REPRESENTATION OF THE LOCATION OF BONE TUMORS

BONE TUMORS BY LOCATION

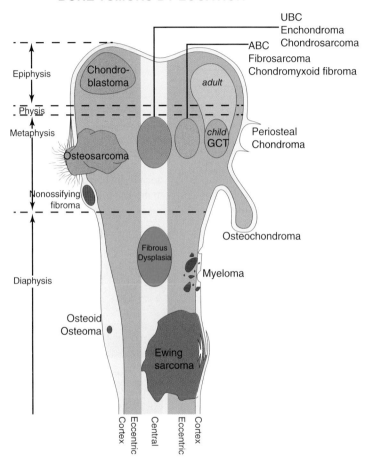

BONE-FORMING TUMORS

NOTE	
1st decade	(age 0–9)
2nd decade	(age 10–19)
3rd decade	(age 20–29)
4th decade	(age 30–39)
5th decade	(age 40–49)
6th decade	(age 50–59)

Osteoma

Relatively rare benign bone-forming tumor. Similar to an enostosis but occurs on the surface of bone. Most common in the fourth to fifth decades of life and are more common in females (3:1).

Osteomas are technically not neoplasms but hamartomas. Hamartomas are developmental or genetic abnormalities versus as neoplasm where one cell mutates and becomes a tumor.

Most commonly seen in the skull, specifically the sinuses and mandible. They can rarely occur in long bones.

Lesions are usually asymptomatic incidental finding and remain unchanged on serial x-rays.

Radiographic appearance: Homogeneous, smooth, dense bony protrusion from the intramembranous bone on the surface of bone

Osteomas may be associated with Gardner syndrome.

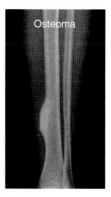

Osteoma

Osteoid Osteoma

Benign bone-forming tumor occurring in the first and second decades of life, more common in males (2:1)

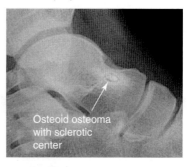

Osteoid osteoma with sclerotic center

Osteoid osteoma

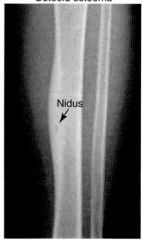

Nidus

Usually located intracortically in the _diaphysis_ of long bones, proximal femur is the most common location, followed by the tibia. In the foot, the talus and calcaneus are most commonly involved.

Symptoms are pain, worse at night, _relieved by aspirin or NSAIDs._

Radiographic appearance: Oval or round well-demarcated radiolucent area (nidus), surrounded by a zone of uniform bone sclerosis. The nidus growth is self-limited and usually does not exceed 1.5 cm in diameter. The nidus may be purely radiolucent or has a sclerotic center.

Osteoid osteomas usually become asymptomatic over time and spontaneously heal. This process can take about 2 years, so most patients opt for surgery. Surgical resection with curettage or radiofrequency ablation of the nidus is curative.

Osteoid osteomas are hot on a bone scan.

DDx includes Brodie abscess. Differentiation can be made by the fact that Brodie abscess is located in the medullary canal in cancellous bone and osteoid osteomas are in the cortex. Osteoblastomas also look similar to osteoid osteomas, but they are >1.5 cm.

Enostosis (Bone Island)

A benign bone tumor mostly seen as an incidental and asymptomatic finding on x-ray. Occurs in all age groups. Can occur anywhere but is most common in the ribs, spine, and pelvis.

Enostosis is technically not neoplasm but hamartoma. Hamartomas are developmental or genetic abnormalities versus as neoplasm where one cell mutates and becomes a tumor.

Enostosis

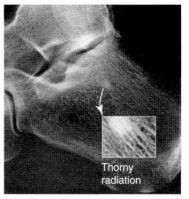

Thorny radiation

Radiographic appearance: Intramedullary sclerotic area with discrete margins and radiating spicules "_thorny radiation._" Lesions do not distort the shape of the bone or protrude from the cortical surface.

Bone scan will be cold. This can help differentiate them from a sclerotic bone metastasis, which will have an intense amount of uptake. Serial x-rays should be taken at 1, 3, 6, and 12 months to assure they are not growing, which could indicate a metastasis. The most common causes of osteoblastic metastasis are breast cancer and prostate cancer.

Osteoblastoma (Giant Osteoid Osteoma, Osteogenic Fibroma)

Rapidly growing, benign, bone-forming tumor; rarely becomes malignant

Occurs in the second and third decades of life and is more common in males

Most commonly seen in the spine, skull, and the diaphysis of long bones

Symptoms include mild pain not relieved by aspirin.

Radiographic appearance: Well-circumscribed, expansile, osteolytic lesion (>1.5 cm) with areas of calcifications and cortical thinning. Characterized by osteolysis and osteosclerosis with cortical thinning and osseous expansion.

DDx: Histologically and radiographically similar to osteoid osteoma, and differentiation is primarily made by its size; osteoblastomas are >1.5 cm. Larger lesions may resemble giant cell tumor or aneurysmal bone cysts.

Osteoblastomas are hot on a bone scan.

Treatment is excision.

Osteosarcoma (Osteogenic Sarcoma)

Malignant bone-forming tumor

Age 10 to 25 years and >40 years

Male-to-female distribution is equal.

Most commonly found in the metaphyseal region around the knee (distal femur or proximal tibia)

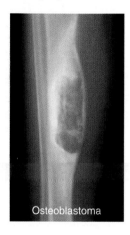

Osteoblastoma

Osteoblastoma

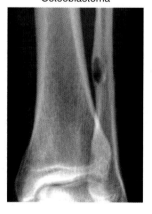

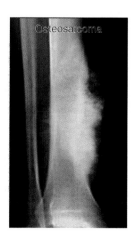

Osteosarcoma

Usually occurs in teenagers during rapid growth spurts or in patients over 40 years who have a preexisting condition, most notably Paget disease

Symptoms: Pain, swelling, and fever (R/O osteomyelitis); the osteoid-producing nature of the tumor often yields an elevated alkaline phosphatase level.

Radiographic appearance: Appearance is variable depending on osteolytic or sclerotic nature of lesion. A mixed pattern of osteolysis and osteosclerosis is most typical. Penetration of cortical bone usually occurs with a Codman triangle or "sunburst" appearance.

Prognosis is poor.

Radiographic appearance: Osteosclerosis inside the lesion with periosteal reaction. Aggressive periosteal reactions such as sun ray spicules, sunburst appearance, or Codman triangle may be present. Cortical breach is common, and there may be an adjacent soft-tissue mass. Associated with Paget disease.

Variable with combination of bone destruction and bone formation. Sun ray spicules/sunburst appearance and Codman triangle may be evident. Cortical breach common, adjacent soft-tissue mass. Joint space rarely involved (25% lytic, 35% sclerotic, 40% mixed). Telangiectatic type purely lytic.

Synovial Chondromatosis (Synovial Osteochondromatosis)

A rare benign condition involving the synovium

Multiple loose cartilaginous bodies in the joint "rice bodies," which may or may not be ossified

The knee is most common, but any joint can be involved.

Symptoms include pain, swelling, decreased range of motions, and locking of the joint.

Synovial chondromatosis

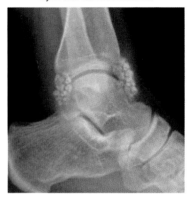

Brown Tumor (Osteitis Fibrosa Cystica)

Diffuse osteopenia with multiple osteolytic lesions dispersed throughout skeleton.

Brown tumors are more likely the result of a preparative process than a neoplastic process. Where bone loss is rapid, there may be bleeding with reparative granulation tissue and proliferating fibrous tissue replacing normal marrow. The hemosiderin deposited during this process is what makes the tumor brown.

Brown tumors arise in an environment of excess osteoclastic activity, specifically hyperparathyroidism.

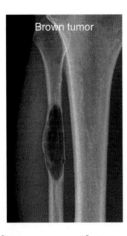
Brown tumor

The disease can manifest at any age but is most common among persons older than 50 years. Highest incident between the third and sixth decades.

Male-to-female ratio 1:3

One of the manifestations of hyperparathyroidism

Histologically, they are identical to giant cell tumors; blood work can distinguish the two. Patients with Brown tumors have PTH > 2000, and serum Ca^{2+} raised.

Most commonly seen in the maxilla and mandible, clavicle, ribs, and pelvic bones. Most commonly in the diaphysis of tubular bones and maxillary bones. Radiographically, they are well-defined, lytic lesions. The cortex may be thin and expanded.

Enchondroma (Chondroma)

Slow-growing, benign tumors that arise from hyaline cartilage. They are usually asymptomatic unless they are pressing on other structures or there is a pathologic fracture. Radiographically,

they vary widely and may present with calcifications. Chondral-type calcifications have unique descriptors, including; punctate, stippling, flocculent, rings, arcs, or popcorn. When they are located centrally in the bone, they are termed *enchondromas*; if they originate on the surface of bone, they are called *periosteal chondromas, juxtacortical chondromas*, or *chondromas*. There are also conditions that develop multiple chondromas termed *enchondromatosis*. Enchondromatosis includes Ollier disease and Maffucci syndrome.

Chondroma
(Enchondroma)

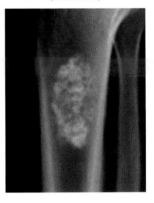

Enchondroma

An enchondroma is a chondroma that forms in the medullary canal. They tend to occur in the third and fourth decades of life, and male-to-female distribution is equal. Enchondromas are often asymptomatic, and painless swelling may be the only symptom.

Enchondroma

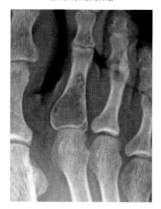

They are mostly found in the metaphysis and diaphysis of the tubular bones, especially the hands and feet. The proximal phalanx is the most common site. They can also be found in the pelvis.

Radiographic appearance: Well-defined central medullary lobular lesion in the metaphysis of long bones with some calcification and endosteal scalloping. Cortical expansion and pathologic fracture are possible.

Bone scan is hot.

Endosteal scalloping is the focal erosion of the inner layer of the cortex (endosteum) by an intraosseous process. Generally associated with slow-growing medullary lesions, although low-grade chondrosarcomas also present with scalloping.

Endosteal scalloping

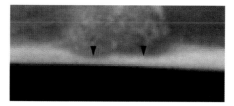

Enchondromatosis, also known as Ollier disease, is a nonhereditary condition characterized by multiple enchondromas. The condition occurs during the first decade of life and is most commonly seen in the hands. Patients have shortened, bowed affected limbs, and it has a high incidence of malignancy (up to 25%).

Maffucci syndrome, like Ollier disease, presents with multiple enchondromas; is found mostly in the hands; and occurs during the first decade of life. Maffucci syndrome is distinguished from Ollier disease by the presence of soft-tissue hemangiomas. These hemangiomas often form phleboliths, which can be seen on x-ray. A phlebolith is a small blood clot in a vein that hardens and calcifies over time. Malignant transformation into chondrosarcoma and angiosarcoma occurs in 30% of cases.

Maffucci syndrome

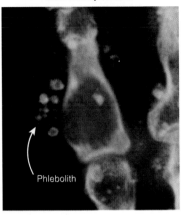

Phlebolith

Periosteal chondroma

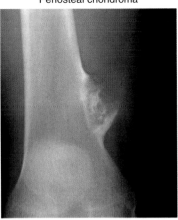

Periosteal Chondroma (Juxtacortical Chondroma)

A chondroma that forms on the surface of bone

May occur in any age group, but mostly during the second decade of life, and male-to-female distribution is equal.

Humerus and femur are usually affected and, to a lesser extent, the hands and feet.

Symptoms may include swelling and mild pain.

Radiographic appearance:
The lesion is located on the surface of the bone. The tumor caused sclerosing of the underlying bone with buttressing of the peripheral walls that may take on a dished-out appearance. Calcifications may be present.

Chondroblastoma (Codman Tumor)

Benign cartilage-forming tumor that occurs during the second and third decades of life. They are more common in males (2:1), and symptoms include local pain and swelling.

Located in the epiphysis of long tubular bones, especially around the knee (distal femur or proximal tibia), also seen in the proximal humerus. When found in the foot, it is usually in the talus or calcaneus.

Radiographic appearance:
Well-defined round or oval osteolytic lesion classically located eccentrically in the epiphysis. May have a thin sclerotic border, and up to 50% of lesions may have calcific foci within the lesion.

Although benign, chondroblastomas will continue to grow if left alone, so treatment usually involves surgical excision.

Chondroblastoma

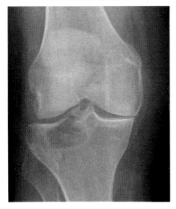

Chondromyxoid Fibroma

Rare, benign cartilage-forming tumor. Occurs during the second and third decades of life. Occurs in the metaphysis of long tubular bones (especially tibia) and is more common in males (2:1).

Symptoms include slowly progressing local pain, tenderness, and swelling.

Classic location is the upper 1/3 of the tibia, 25% of cases. Other relatively common sites are the small tubular bones in the foot, distal femur, and pelvis.

Radiographic appearance: Lobulated or oval, eccentrically located, expansile, lytic lesions with well-defined sclerotic borders. They tend to be elongated in shape, and unlike many other tumors of cartilaginous origin, there are no matrix calcifications. Endosteum is usually sclerotic and scalloped. Intralesional trabeculae tend to be coarse and thick. This distinguished them from giant cell tumors and nonossifying fibromas,

which have thin trabeculae. Large lesions may penetrate the cortex, resulting in an osseous defect. In spite of this cortical erosion, the lesion is benign, and soft-tissue involvement is rare. Might easily be misdiagnosed as a fibrosarcoma.

Chondromyxoid fibroma

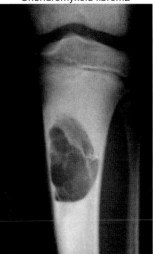

Chondromyxoid fibroma

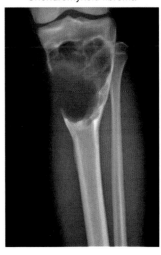

Osteochondroma

Benign cartilage-covered osseous protuberance

Occurs during the first, second, and third decades of life

More common in males (1.5:1)

Occurs in the metaphysis of long tubular bones (especially femur, humerus, and tibia)

Radiographic appearance: Cartilage-covered osseous protuberance (exostosis) with normal trabeculation <u>pointing away from the joint</u>. Lesions can be sessile (wide base) or pedunculated (mushroom shaped). Most commonly seen subungually in the foot and may contribute to the formation of a pincer nail.

Symptoms include a painless slow-growing mass.

Most common benign tumor; however, there is a 1% change of malignant degeneration.

Osteochondroma

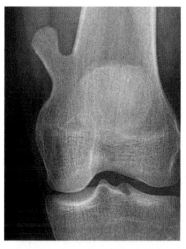

Chondrosarcoma

Malignant cartilage-forming tumor

More common over age 60

Males are affected more often than females (1.5:1).

Lesions can occur almost anywhere, the most commonly affected bone being the femur.

In long bones, it is generally found in the metaphysis. Chondrosarcomas arising near the surface of the bone (peripheral chondrosarcomas) usually arise from preexisting osteochondroma.

Symptoms include a slowly progressing pain.

Chondrosarcoma occurs more in the pelvis and scapula and is uncommon in the hands and feet.

Chondrosarcoma

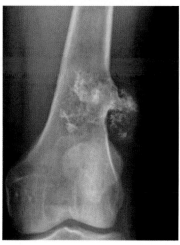

Radiographic appearance: The diagnostic distinction between a benign enchondroma and low-grade chondrosarcoma is difficult because they can look the same. Chondrosarcoma tends to be larger with significant endosteal scalloping and cortical destruction. Also, of great clinical value, chondrosarcomas tend to be painful, while chondromas are not.

Nonossifying Fibroma

Benign lesion of bone composed of connective tissue

Occurs during the first and second decades of life

Occurs in cortical bone in the metaphysis region of long tubular bones, often around the knee (distal femur proximal tibia)

Lesions are usually asymptomatic, self-limiting, and heal over time being replace by normal bone.

Radiographic appearance: Well-circumscribed, subcortical, eccentric, multiloculated lesion with scalloped margins. Geographic well-marginated, multilocular appearance. Intercortical osteolysis single or multiple bubble like areas.

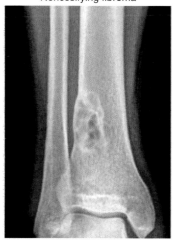

Nonossifying fibroma

Fibrous Dysplasia

An uncommon genetic bone disorder where normal bone is replaced by fibrous (scar-like) tissue. It may affect one bone (monostotic) or multiple bones (polyostotic). When it is associated with endocrine dysfunction, specifically precocious puberty in girls, and cutaneous pigmentation, café-au-lait spots with irregular, ragged, or "coast-of Maine" boarders, it is known as McCune–Albright syndrome.

Shepherd Crook

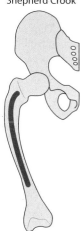

Fibrous dysplasia

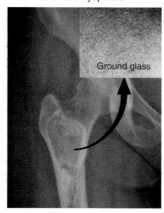

Ground glass

Most commonly involves the bones in the skull and face. Patients present with asymmetry of face. Also can affect the long bones in the arms and legs, the pelvis, and ribs. Fibrous dysplasia may be asymptomatic or painful and may result in abnormally shaped bones or pathologic fractures.

Lesions in long bones are usually intramedullary and predominantly diaphyseal in location.

Lesions are usually painless and have a hazy quality classically described as a "ground-glass" appearance. They are well-defined often with a border of reactive sclerosis. Lesions in the proximal femur may result in a pronounced varus curvature referred to as a "Shepherd crook" deformity.

Fibrosarcoma

Malignant tumor of fibroblasts that has a tendency to recur

Occurs during the third, fourth, fifth, and sixth decades of life, and males and females are affected equally.

Usually found in the metaphysis of long tubular bones (especially femur, tibia). 80% are found around the knee. Symptoms can include pain, swelling, and limited motion with possible pathologic fracture.

Fibrosarcoma

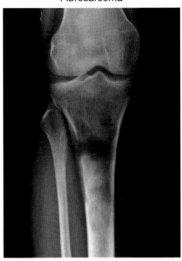

Radiographic appearance: Osteolytic lesion with a geographic, moth-eaten, or permeative pattern of bone destruction. In spite of the cortical destruction, there is relatively little periosteal reaction (no onion peel, sunburst, etc.). Extension into soft tissue is also common. Invasive or well-defined margins depending on differentiation of tumor. May look like osteosarcoma.

Bone scan is hot.

Call occur primarily or secondary to Paget disease, osteonecrosis, chronic osteomyelitis, or an area of previous irradiation

Patients with neurofibromatosis are at increased risk. Certain preexisting lesions such as fibrous dysplasia, chronic osteomyelitis, bone infarcts, and Paget disease. Also, previous irradiated areas of bone have a greater chance of developing a fibrosarcoma.

Giant Cell Tumor

Aggressive benign tumors composed of connective tissue, stromal cells, and giant cells

Occurs during the third and fourth decades of life

More common in females

Usually <u>originates in the metaphysis, but quickly extends into the epiphysis</u> and subchondral bone. These tumors cannot extend into the epiphysis until skeletal maturity because the tumor cannot cross the growth plate.

Giant cell tumor

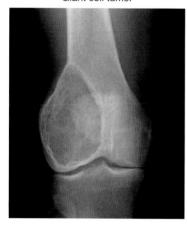

Seen in long tubular bones, especially around the knee (distal femur or proximal tibia)

Symptoms include pain, with possible swelling and limitation of motion.

May be associated with Paget disease

Radiographic appearance: Eccentric, osteolytic (cystic), multilocular lesion extending to the subchondral bone. Large extensive periostitis is generally not present; the cortex can be eggshell thin. Well-defined geographic lesions in the epiphysis/metaphysis. Junction with normal bone often poorly defined. Cortex thinned and sometimes ballooned. Delicate and thin "<u>soap-bubble</u>" appearance. Lytic lesion with geographic nonsclerotic margins.

Have a tendency to recur

Unicameral Bone Cyst (Solitary Bone Cyst, Simple Bone Cyst)

Benign fluid-filled tumors of unknown origin that occurs during the first and second decades of life

More common in males (2:1)

In patients younger than 20 years of age, these lesions generally occur in the metaphysis of tubular bones (especially proximal humerus and the femur). Lesions in patients over 20 years of age generally occur in the pelvis or calcaneus.

Unicameral bone cyst

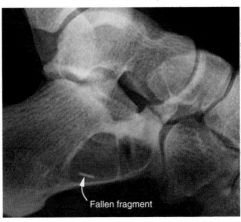

Fallen fragment

Usually asymptomatic but may result in a pathologic fracture

Radiographic appearance: Centrally located, radiolucent, possibly multilocular lesion with cortical thinning and very mild osseous expansion. Calcaneal lesions are well-defined, radiolucent lesions usually occurring at the neutral triangle. There may be a fractured piece of bone in the lesion, "fallen fragment" sign, which is a classic UBC finding. UBCs differ from ABC and GCT in that there is no or minimal ballooning of the cortex.

Fallen fragment sign: Pathologic fractures cause bone fragments to fall into the cyst and migrate to the dependent position. The fragment will not migrate to the bottom of the cyst unless the cyst contains fluid with low viscosity, which makes them pathognomonic for UBCs.

Recurrence rate is high in children.

Treatment is surgical evacuation of cyst and curettage. UBC aspirate is clear straw colored.

Aneurysmal Bone Cyst (ABC)

Benign blood-filled cyst that occurs during the first, second, and third decades of life. They are unusual, in that they are rapidly growing painful lesions, but are benign. They are not a true neoplasm.

Although often primary, they do occur secondarily from vascular injury. They may be seen alongside of other bone lesions, such as nonossifying fibroma, chondroblastoma, giant cell tumor, fibrous dysplasia, osteoblastoma, and osteosarcoma.

Aneurysmal bone cyst

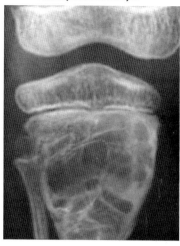

Usually found in long tubular bone, most notably the fibula, femur, and tibia. 15% of cases are found in the calcaneus.

Can be asymptomatic, but the majority experience pain and soft-tissue swelling

Intraosseous lipoma

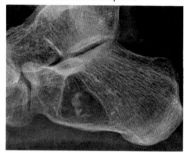

More common in females (2:1)

Symptoms include pain and swelling, with possible pathologic fracture.

Radiographic evaluation: An eccentric, osteolytic (possibly trabeculated) expansive (ballooning) lesion, which may extend out into the soft tissue. Lesions are usually located in the metaphysis of long tubular bones and the spine. In cross-sectional imaging, we will see multiple, delicate, fluid-filled sacs with a "soap-bubble" appearance. Appearance is similar to giant cell tumors, but unlike GCTs, they do not extend into the epiphysis. A thin "eggshell" covering of expanded cortex is often seen.

Intraosseous Lipoma

Benign tumors of fatty tissue

Can present at any age and are distributed equally between males and females

Radiographic evaluation: Osteolytic lesion surrounded by a thin, well-defined sclerotic border. Internal osseous ridges are frequently present, and bone expansion may be seen. When the calcaneus is involved, lesions are usually in the neutral triangle (as with unicameral bone cysts) and there is often a central calcification (unlike unicameral bone cysts).

Ewing Sarcoma

Aggressive malignant tumors occurring in children. Ewing sarcomas originate in bone marrow cells and have a poor prognosis. They usually occur between the ages of 7 and 20 years and are more common in males (3:2).

Most commonly located in the diaphysis of the femur, pelvic bones, tibia, and humerus. Tubular bone (tibia, fibula, clavicle). Usually originates in the legs bones or pelvis.

Symptoms mimic an infection and include pain, swelling, fever, weight loss, and leukocytosis.

Ewing sarcoma

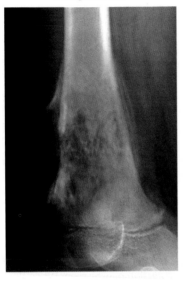

Ewing sarcoma also known as a round cell tumor

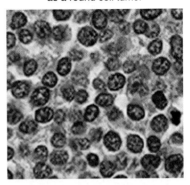

Radiographic evaluation: Aggressive, permeative or moth-eaten, osteolytic lesion with cortical erosions, periostitis (onion skin, Codman triangle), and a soft-tissue mass.

Prevalent in Caucasians, but rarely seen in the Afro-Caribbean races

Trauma often precedes the development of this tumor.

Ewing sarcomas are the most common type of small round cell tumor of bone. The tumor is composed of masses of small undifferentiated round cells. Nuclei are prominent with minimal cytoplasm and very little stroma between cells.

Eosinophilic Granuloma

Eosinophilic granulomas are a form of Langerhans cell histiocytosis. It involves the overproduction of Langerhans cells, which is a component of the immune system. A condition of both human and veterinary pathology. It is more of a disorder of immune regulation rather than neoplasm and occurs more in males (2:1). Eosinophilic granulomas are most common in flat bones (skull, pelvis) but may originate in any location of any bone (diaphyseal, metaphyseal, or epiphyseal). Symptoms include pain and soft-tissue swelling.

Radiographically variable and may appear benign (geographic) or malignant (permeative/moth-eaten). Skull lesions have sharp punched-out borders that are uneven across the inner and outer border, causing a beveled-edge appearance.

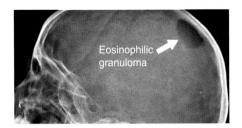

Eosinophilic granuloma

Myeloma (Multiple Myeloma)

Most common malignant bone tumor and affects people in their fifth to seventh decades of life. Multiple myeloma is often referred to as the most common type of malignant bone tumor, although technically myeloma is not a bone tumor, it is a malignant proliferation of bone marrow plasma cells. Myeloma begins with the B cells, which then differentiate into plasma cells. The function of the plasma cells is to secrete antibodies (IgM, IgG, IgA, etc.). These abnormal plasma cells are ineffective at producing antibodies.

The malignant plasma cells secrete a monoclonal immunoglobulin called M-protein. These monoclonal immunoglobulins produce an abundance of Bence Jones proteins that are excreted in urine. Bence Jones proteins are toxic to the kidneys.

Radiographic appearance: Multiple sharply circumscribed punched-out lytic lesions. The lytic lesions in the bones are caused by calcium coming out of the bones. This excess calcium causes hypercalcemia, which further damages the kidneys.

Multiple myeloma

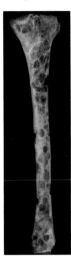

Symptoms: Symptoms are often ignored because they are mistaken for general body aches from age and arthritis. Myeloma symptoms include bone pain, renal failure, pathologic fractures, and reoccurring bacterial infections.

Diagnosis: Increases in serum calcium and Bence Jones protein found in the urine.

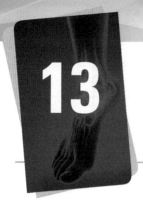

BONE HEALING

BONE HEALING

Requires immobilization (fixation) and compression (optimal is 12 to 18 lb per in^2)

Bone can regenerate back to 100% of its strength following a fracture.

The body has a difficult time healing bone ends that are >1 cm apart or fractures where the gap is greater than the radius of the bone at that level.

Osteoblasts deposit bone, and osteoclasts resorb bone.

Four Overlapping Stages of Bone Healing

Inflammation

Peaks at 48 hours and subsides at about a week

Inflammation, in addition to its normal role, also acts as an immobilizer by causing:
  Pain—patient protects the area
  Edema—acts as a hydrostatic splint

Soft Callus

Begins several days after injury and persists for about 1 to 2 months

Fibrous and cartilaginous tissue develops at each end of the fracture

If the soft callus fails to unite the two sides of the fracture (as with an amputation), it will cease to grow and be resorbed.

Hard Callus

If a soft callus is successful in connecting the fracture, it begins to ossify.

Occurs at around 3 to 4 months

Remodeling

Lasts for several years

Excess callus is resorbed.

Final bone morphology is determined by Wolff law. Wolff law states that bone will adapt to the loads under which it is placed.

Two Types of Bone Healing

Bones heal by either primary (intramembranous) or secondary (endochondral) ossification. Fracture stability dictates which type of healing will occur. Primary bone healing requires absolute stability, while secondary bone healing requires relative stability. In reality, bones usually heal by a combination of both processes. Different fixation modalities can dictate which type of bone healing will occur.

Relative vs. absolute stability spectrum

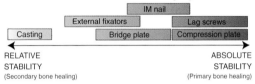

Primary Bone Healing	Secondary Bone Healing
Bone heals by haversian remodeling (simultaneous remodeling and direct formation of new bone)	Involves the formation of callus/cartilaginous and fibrous tissue intermediates that are later replaced by bone
Little to no callus formation	Callus formation (irritation callus)
Requires absolute stability (good bone opposition and no interfragmentary motion)	Occurs when there is motion at the fracture or osteotomy site
Preferred method of bone healing	Less desirable method of bone healing
Intermembranous	Endochondral
Requires absolute stability	Requires relative stability
Requires low strain	Requires high strain

Bone Healing Complications

Type	Definition	Treatment
Delayed union	Healing has not advanced at the average rate for the location and type of fracture/osteotomy. Time frame cannot be arbitrarily set, but most doctors consider a delayed union at around 4 to 6 months.	Delayed unions can often be healed by strict immobilization alone.

(*continued*)

Type	Definition	Treatment
Nonunion	A fracture or osteotomy that is a minimum of 9 months old and has not shown radiographic progress for 3 months.	Generally, intervention including a bone stimulator or operative means is required to heal a nonunion. Atrophic nonunions often require a bone graft.
Pseudoarthrosis	End stage of a nonunion. A fibrocartilaginous surface develops at the bone fracture site, and a joint space develops that may contain synovial fluid.	Operative intervention is the only reliable method of forming a union involving a pseudoarthrosis.

NOTE: A malunion is a fracture that heals in an anatomically incorrect position.

NONUNION CLASSIFICATION (WEBER AND CECH)

Hypertrophic (Hypervascular) Nonunions

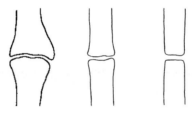

Elephant Foot	Horse Hoof	Oligotrophic
Hypertrophic	Mildly hypertrophic	Not hypertrophic
Large callus	Poor callus	Minimal or no callus
Greatest chance of healing		Vascularization is present on bone scan

Hypertrophic nonunions are vascularized and have a callus present on radiograph. They can typically be treated by stable fixation alone.

Atrophic (Avascular) Nonunions

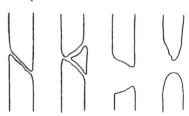

Torsion Wedge	Comminuted	Defect	Atrophic
Intermediate fragment that has healed to one of the main fragments, but not the other	Intermediate fragment that has become necrotic	Characterized by the loss of a fragment such that the two ends are too far apart to unite	End result of a defect nonunion, ends of the fragments become osteoporotic and atrophic

Atrophic nonunions show no evidence of callus formation on radiograph and are ischemic or cold on bone scan. Atrophic nonunions require decortication and bone grafts to heal.

Pseudojoint

Typically, pseudojoint has adequate vascularity but excessive motion/instability. They form a fibrocartilaginous surface over the fractured ends of the bone and require surgery to fuse.

Factors Contributing to Nonunions

Local Factors	General/Systemic Factors
Infection	Smoking
Poor fixation	Diabetes
Insufficient immobilization	Endocrinopathies (thyroid, parathyroid, testosterone deficiency, vitamin D deficiency)
Distracted fracture	Malnutrition
Vascular status	Medications (steroids, chemotherapy, bisphosphonates)
Severity of injury (comminution, local tissue damage)	Bone quality

BONE GROWTH STIMULATORS

Work by using the bioelectrical principles of bone healing. Endogenous bioelectric potentials have been found to have an electronegative reaction at the fracture site.

Compression = electronegative potentials = osteoblasts = bone formation

Tension = electropositive potentials = osteoclasts = bone resorption

Types of Bone Growth Stimulators

Electrical Bone Stimulators

Direct Current (Invasive)

Direct current bone stimulators are surgically implanted devices with a cathode being placed directly on the bone and an anode on the skin. DC stimulators provide constant uniform current at the fracture site. The advantage of DC bone stimulators is compliance because they cannot take it off. The disadvantages are that it requires a surgical procedure to implant, potential for short circuits from the leads touching hardware, and limited battery life (6 to 8 months).

Electromagnetic Field Bone Stimulators (Noninvasive)

Capacitive Coupling (CC)

Electrodes are placed on the skin on either side of the fractures site.

An alternating current is then used to create an electric field within the fracture site. These units are small and light weight but may cause irritation of the skin from the electrodes.

Inductive Coupling (IC)

Uses wire coils through which a current is passed and a magnetic field is generated. The magnetic field, in turn, generates an electrical current at the fracture site. These units are large and heavy, which affect compliance, but they are the least invasive type of bone stimulator. They can be applied over a shoe or cast. There are two types:

Pulsed Electromagnetic Field (PEMF)

A time-varying magnetic field producing an induced electric field

Combined Magnetic Field (CMF)

A time-varying magnetic field superimposed on a static magnetic field. There is improved compliance with these units because they need only be worn 30 minutes a day.

Ultrasound Bone Stimulators (Noninvasive)

Ultrasonic bone stimulators cause micromotion at the fracture site; this encourages a soft callus formation. Bone is formed by endochondral ossification. The US used for bone healing is low-intensity pulsed ultrasound (LIPUS). The US used for physical therapy modalities is a much higher intensity and is contraindicated in fractures.

BONE GRAFTS

Graft Type

Autograft

A bone graft from one's own body or identical twin. Short-term storage of graft is best accomplished by wrapping the graft with a moistened saline sponge. Immersing the graft in saline solution is detrimental to the graft.

Allograft (Homograft)

Bone from same species, usually freeze-dried (lyophilized) bone bank bone. Some brands require reconstitution with sterile saline infusion before use.

Xenograft (Heterograft)

Bone from different species

Synthetic Grafts

Hydroxyapatite, tricalcium phosphate, type I collagen, marine coral

Autograft vs. Allograft

Allograft (Lyophilized)	Autograft
Freeze dried/ devoid of water	Freshwater is present
Noncellular bony matrix	Cellular bony matrix
No osteoinductive properties	Osteoinductive properties
Allows creeping substitution	Allows creeping substitution
Unlimited amount	Limited amount
Slower healing	Faster healing
Bone bank bone	Requires a donor site

Cortical vs. Cancellous Graft

Cortical Bone	Cancellous Bone
Dense	Porous
Used to provide stability (can be fixated)	Used to fill defects
Few viable cells	Many viable cells
Incorporation is slow	Incorporation is faster
Does not revascularize	Does revascularize
Does not facilitate osteogenesis	Facilitates osteogenesis
Allows creeping substitution	Allows creeping substitution
Not completely replaced by new bone	Completely replaced by new bone
Radiolucent when healing	Radiodense when healing
Haversian system	No haversian system
Graft is weakest at 8 weeks	Graft becomes stronger each week

Harvesting Sites for Autograft

Iliac crest
  Best source of cancellous bone
  Proximal anteromedial tibia
Fibula
  The middle third to half of the bone may be removed without any ill effects.
  Rarely, the entire proximal ¾ may be removed.
  The distal ¼ should always be left to maintain ankle joint integrity.
  The fibula graft is removed by a Henry approach.
  Good source of cortical bone

Calcaneus
Proximal tibia
Distal tibia
Greater trochanter
Rib

Harvesting a Medullary Calcaneal Autogenous Bone Graft

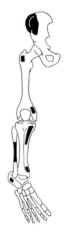

Lateral incision over the calcaneus (avoid the neutral triangle, the sural nerve, and the calcaneofibular ligament attachment). Drill holes to outline a cortical window and cut window with a power saw. The cortical window is then pried from its bed. Curette out cancellous bone as needed through the window. If cortical bone is not needed, replace the window after packing the defect with lyophilized bone.

Papineau Bone Graft

An open cancellous bone graft for the management of large defects resulting from radical debridement of infected bone and soft tissue. Infected nonunions of long bones are debrided, and cancellous bone graft chips are packed at the site. No coverage of soft tissue is performed; instead, the graft is left exposed beneath a nonadherent dressing. Granulation tissue forms over the bone graft, and later, a tissue flap or skin graft can be applied.

Graft Healing

Osteogenic

Contains viable osteoblasts

Creeping Substitution

The process by which most cellular elements in the graft die and are slowly replaced by viable bone. Transplanted bone is invaded by vascular granulation tissue, causing the old bone to be resorbed and subsequently replaced by the host with new bone.

Osteoconduction

The scaffolding effect of the bone graft that acts as a conduit for migration of viable cells. This scaffolding is the matrix that allows creeping substitution to occur.

Osteoinduction

The presence of a bone morphogenetic protein inductor substance that induces pluripotential primitive mesenchymal cells to differentiate into osteoblasts

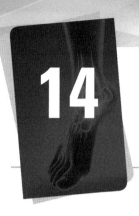

14 DERMATOLOGY

SKIN LAYERS

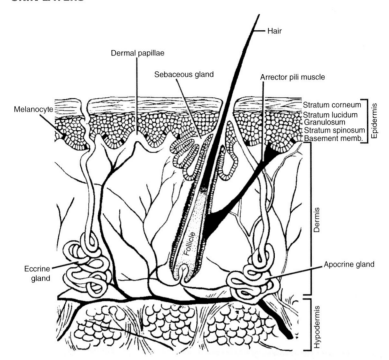

Epidermis

- About 0.04 mm thick

Stratum Corneum (Horny Layer)

The outer most layer of the epidermis composed of dry, flattened, anuclear, dead, keratinized cells that ultimately flake from the body

Stratum Lucidum

A clear translucent layer of the epidermis

Granulosum Layer

Several layers thick; the cell's cytoplasm contains keratohyalin granules.

Stratum Spinosum

Several cell layers thick; contains intercellular bridges, giving the cells a spiny appearance

Basement Membrane (Stratum Germinativum, Basal Layer)

Deepest layer of the epidermis composed of a single layer of rapidly proliferating cells that slowly migrate upward to ultimately become the stratum corneum. It takes 4 weeks for basal cells to reach the surface and be shed.

Dermis

- About 0.5 mm thick

The dermis is the dense connective tissue stroma forming the bulk of the skin. It contains blood vessels, lymphatics, nerve ending, and hair follicles. The dermis is connected to the epidermis by finger-like projections called *dermal papillae*. These dermal papillae form ridges (fingerprints) at the surface of the skin.

Papillary Layer

Upper 1/3 of the dermis, contains Meissner corpuscles (light touch)

Reticular Layer

Lower 2/3 of the dermis, contains Pacinian corpuscles (vibration and pressure)

Subcutaneous Tissue (Panniculus, Hypodermis)

Composed of fatty connective tissue

ADDITIONAL CELLS

Melanocytes

Melanocytes produce melanin, which absorbs ultraviolet light and protects the tissue; they are intermingled among the basal cells. Ultraviolet radiation activates melanocytes (tanning).

Langerhans Cells

Langerhans cells are dendritic cells (antigen-presenting immune cells) involved with the immune system. They are found throughout the epidermis, especially the stratum spinosum.

GLANDS

Sweat Glands

Eccrine Sweat Glands

Distributed all over the body, most numerous in the palms and soles. They produce an odor-free watery substance and are involved in cooling the body. They open out onto the skin, not in the hair follicle.

Apocrine Sweat Glands

Found abundant in the axillae and anogenital region, their ducts open into the hair follicles. They are adrenergic mediated and produce a viscous sticky odorous substance.

Present at birth but do not become active until puberty

Sebaceous Glands

Secrete sebum into the hair follicle and are located all over the body, except the palms and soles. Oil glands found mostly on the face, neck, and upper body. Secrete sebum, which is an oily, wax-like mixture of triglycerides and cholesterol. Secrete sebum by holocrine secretion whereby the entire cell content becomes excreted due to autolysis.

DERMATOLOGIC LESIONS

Primary Lesions

Bulla: Fluid-filled, elevated lesions over 0.5 cm in diameter

Burrow: An intraepidermal tunnel usually caused by insects or parasites

Cyst: Noninfected, deep-set collection of material surrounded by a histologically definable wall

Macule: Flat, circumscribed lesions measuring up to 1 cm in diameter. Cannot be felt, but can be seen.

Nodule: Circumscribed, solid, elevated lesion measuring up to 1 cm in diameter. Differs from a papule in that it has the added dimension of depth in the underlying tissue.

Papule: Circumscribed, solid, elevated lesions measuring up to 1 cm in diameter

Patch: Flat lesion measuring over 1 cm in diameter

Plaque: Circumscribed, thickened, elevated lesion over 1 cm in diameter

Pustule: A vesicle or bulla containing pus

Tumor: Circumscribed, solid, elevated lesion measuring >1 cm in diameter. Differs from a papule in that it has the added dimension of depth in the underlying tissue.

Vesicle: Fluid-filled elevated lesions <0.5 cm in diameter

Wheal (hives): A well-circumscribed, elevated lesion that appears and disappears rapidly (minutes to hours)

Secondary Lesions

- Changes due to evolution of the primary lesion

  Crust: Dried masses of serum, pus, or blood, generally mixed with debris—"scabs"

  Erosion: Deep excoriations in the epidermis, but the dermis is not breached, leaves no scars.

  Excoriation: Scratch marks usually seen where there is pruritus

  Fissure: Linear, deep, epidermal cracks, commonly found in areas of dry or thick skin that may extend into the dermis

  Lichenification: Thickening of the skin with exaggeration of skin lines, giving a leathery appearance, often associated with hyperpigmentation. May be due to excessive scratching or rubbing.

  Maceration: Epidermis becomes overly hydrated and turns white.

  Scales: An exfoliative condition marked by flaking laminations of the epidermis

  Scar: "Cicatrix," the formation of fibrous connective tissue, which has replaced dermis or deeper layer, lost as a result of trauma or disease

  Ulcer: Loss of the epidermis and a portion of the dermis

  Xerosis: Dry skin

DERMATOLOGIC TESTS

Auspitz Sign

Pinpoint bleeding that occurs when the scales of a psoriatic lesion are removed

Diascopy (Glass Slide Test)

Press a clear glass slide against the lesion and look for blanching. Dilated capillaries (erythema) will blanch, hemorrhagic lesions (purpura) will not.

Excisional Biopsy

Method of choice for diagnosis and removal of dermal and subcutaneous cysts and tumors (epidermal cysts and lipomas) and also for malignant melanoma

Can be used for lesions too big to punch biopsy

Fungal Culture

Dermatophyte test medium (DTM) is used to grow dermatophyte cultures. Cultures require about 10 days to grow; medium will turn red if dermatophytes are present. If the DTM turns red, it is diagnostic for dermatophytes; however, a false (+) may be seen with saprophytes and so the colonies must be examined. Dermatophytes have powdery white colonies. Saprophytes have shiny colonies, which may be white, brown, black, or green in color.

KOH Test

A KOH test can be performed on hair, skin, or nail to diagnose dermatophytes.

Technique

Scrape the scales from a lesion onto a slide with a blade.

Apply a drop of 10% to 20% potassium hydroxide (KOH). KOH dissolves keratin so that the skin, nail, or hair shaft becomes clear.

KOH will dissolve keratin alone, but the process may be speeded up by adding gentle heat or DMSO.

Examine under microscope for the presence of fungus; if present, the septated fungal hyphae can be seen growing through the epithelial cells.

Nikolsky Sign

A skin finding in which the top layer of skin slips away from the lower layer when slightly rubbed. An epidermal detachment produced by lack of skin cohesion, seen in bullous diabeticorum.

PAS

Periodic acid–Schiff stain test is a staining method for diagnosing fungus. PAS stains polysaccharides such as the carbohydrates found in the cell wall of the fungal hyphae. The cell walls of fungi stain magenta.

Punch Biopsy

Method of choice for most inflammatory or infiltrative diseases. Yields a full-thickness specimen of the skin.

Shave Biopsy

Particularly suited to lesions confined to the epidermis such as seborrheic keratoses or molluscum contagiosum

Small Nerve Fiber Biopsy

Tests the small unmyelinated nerve fibers (C fibers) in the skin. With small fiber neuropathy, neurologic examination, EMG, and nerve conduction studies may be normal because they test the large nerve fibers. The ideal biopsy site is the calf at 10 cm proximal to the lateral malleolus. Two standard tests are available:

Epidermal nerve fiber density (ENFD) test: Measures the density of the small nerve fibers in the skin

Sweat gland nerve fiber density (SGNFD) test: Measures the density of the small autonomic nerve fibers in the sweat glands. SGNFD test is a more sensitive test for small fiber neuropathy than ENFD.

Tzanck Test

Used to diagnose viral disease (herpes simplex, herpes zoster, and molluscum contagiosum)

Technique involves scraping a fluid and base of vesicle or bullae onto a glass slide. The slide is fixed with methanol and stained with Wright stain. The presence of multinucleate giant cells suggests herpes infection.

Wood's Light Examination

A black light with a 360-nm wavelength (UV) filtered through glass, used to diagnose certain infections by causing different colors to fluoresce

Erythrasma *(Corynebacterium minutissimum)* fluoresces coral red.

Tinea capitis *(Microsporum canis)* fluoresces light, bright green.

Pseudomonas aeruginosa fluoresces green.

Tinea versicolor fluoresces yellow gold.

Ash leaf macule (tuberous sclerosis): accentuated hypopigmentation

DERMATITIS/ECZEMA

Contact Dermatitis

Dermatitis caused by contact with certain substances found in the environment, causing inflammation of the epidermis and dermis. The most common and classic example of this is poison ivy. Another common cause is nickel, which is widely used in jewelry and in metal clasps on women's underclothes. In podiatry, contact dermatitis is commonly due to the rubber found in the toe box of most shoes or the cement used to bind shoes together.

Classification

a. Irritation contact dermatitis
   Nonimmunologic mechanisms, whereby a single exposure causes a reaction (i.e., detergents, fiberglass)
b. Allergic contact dermatitis
   Acquired immunologic response. The first contact causes no reaction, but the exposure sensitizes the skin to future exposures (i.e., poison ivy).

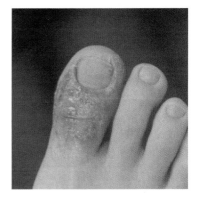

Presentation

Irregular poorly demarcated patches of erythema and edema, on which there are superimposed closely spaced vesicles, punctate erosions exuding serum, and crust. May be seen with a subchronic or chronic lesion lichenification.

Treatment

Avoid contact with the offending agent.

Increase aeration: Avoid shoes with plastic uppers, wear cotton or wool socks instead of synthetic ones, apply drying powders.

Topical hydrocortisone cream for pruritus. In moderate-to-severe cases, treat pruritus with oral meds (Benadryl, Atarax, Vistaril).

Astringent soaks (Burow solution, Epsom salt). This will decrease inflammation and reduce weeping.

Moisturizing lotions may also be soothing and help with lichenification and fissuring.

Topical Abx for secondary bacterial infections

Atopic Dermatitis

Dermatitis resulting from a hereditary predisposition to a lowered cutaneous threshold to pruritus. This leads to scratching and rubbing that turn into eczematous lesion. There is usually a positive family history of allergic rhinitis, hay fever, asthma, or migraine headaches. Atopic dermatitis is often exacerbated by sudden changes in temperature, humidity, and stress/anxiety, and females may have eruption just before their menstrual period.

Classification

a. Infantile atopic dermatitis
    Usually starts at about 2 to 6 months and mostly seen on the face. In about half the infants, it clears up by age 2 and never returns; in the other half, it clears up and then reappears in late childhood or early teens (childhood atopic dermatitis).

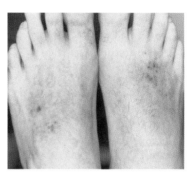

b. Childhood atopic dermatitis
    Starts in late childhood/early teens. Most commonly seen on the antecubital and popliteal fossae. In about half of these individuals, the condition clears up in adolescence; in the remaining half, it persists into adulthood (adult atopic dermatitis).

c. Adult atopic dermatitis
    As the person grows older, the rash usually seems to shrink and become localized. It can be found anywhere on the body but has a predilection for the flexures, front and sides of the neck, eyelids, forehead, face, wrists, and dorsum of the hands and feet.

Presentation

Irregular, often asymmetrical, poorly demarcated patches of erythema and edema, on which there are superimposed closely spaced vesicles, punctate erosions exuding serum, and crust. With a subchronic or chronic lesion, lichenification may be seen.

Treatment

Increase aeration: Avoid shoes with plastic uppers, wear cotton or wool socks instead of synthetic ones, apply drying powders.
Topical hydrocortisone cream for pruritus. In moderate-to-severe cases, treat pruritus with oral meds (Benadryl, Atarax, Vistaril).
Astringent soaks (Burow solution, Epsom salt) will decrease inflammation and reduce weeping.
Moisturizing lotions may also be soothing and help with lichenification and fissuring.
Topical Abx for secondary bacterial infections

Urticaria

An allergic reaction resulting in transient pruritic wheals or small erythematous papules that erupt in minutes to hours and disappear usually within 24 hours or less. Patients often have a history of atopic dermatitis. In severe reactions, anaphylaxis may occur.

Causes

Food (milk, eggs, shellfish, nuts)
Drugs (PCN)
Parasites

Treatment

Antihistamines (hydroxyzine, terfenadine)

Nummular (Discoid) Eczema

Pruritic dermatitis occurring in the form of coin-shaped plaques composed of grouped small papules/vesicles on an erythematous base. Especially common on the lower legs of older males during the winter. Lesions often have an associated bacterial infection, and treatment should include oral dicloxacillin or erythromycin in addition to topical corticosteroids.

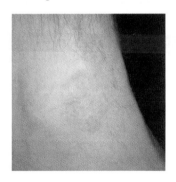

Lichen Simplex Chronicum (Neurodermatitis)

A circumscribed area of lichenification resulting from repeated physical trauma (rubbing/scratching)

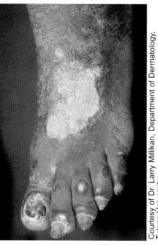
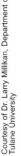

Courtesy of Dr. Larry Millikan, Department of Dermatology, Tulane University

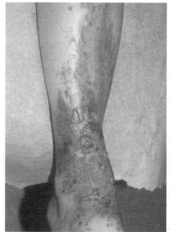

Courtesy of Dr. Larry Millikan, Department of Dermatology, Tulane University

Stasis Dermatitis

Dermatitis of the lower leg related to PVD. Presents as erythematous scaling plaques with exudation, crusts, and superficial ulcers. Usually found just proximal to medial malleolus.

Symptoms include mild pruritus, pain, edema, and nocturnal cramps, and a painful ulcer may be present. Often associated with brown reticulated hemosiderin hyperpigmentation.

Treatment

Saline or Burow wet dressing, later topical corticosteroids

Unna boot

Reduce edema (elevate leg, supportive stockings, leg muscle pumps)

If an ulcer is present, use wet to dry compressive bandages.

Systemic antibiotics are necessary if cellulitis is present.

Dyshidrotic Eczematous Dermatitis (Dyshidrosis)

A special vesicular type of hand and foot eczema associated with pruritus. There is a predilection for the sides of the fingers, palms, and soles of the feet. Presents as small vesicles deep seated (appearing like "tapioca") in clusters, occasionally bullae. Later stages present with scaling, lichenification, painful fissures, and erosions. Despite the name, sweating plays no role in the pathogenesis. There is a bullous form called *pompholyx*. Emotional stress and ingestion of certain metals (nickel, cobalt, or chromium) have been suggested as possible precipitating factors.

Treatment

Vesicular stage—saline or Burow wet dressing/soaks

Eczematous stage—topical corticosteroids

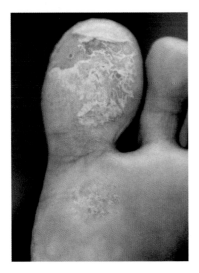

(T/Gell). Hydrocortisone creams and lotions may also be used.

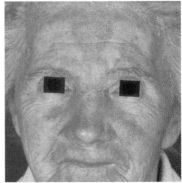

From Fitzpatrick TB. *Color Atlas and Synopsis of Clinical Dermatology*. 2nd ed. McGraw-Hill Inc; 1992:55.

Seborrheic Dermatitis

A common chronic inflammatory disorder characterized by scaling and redness, usually worse in the winter. It does not cause hair loss.

Presentation

Flaky, white scales over erythematous patches. Most commonly seen in those 20 to 50 years; in children, it is called "cradle cap."

Location of Lesions

Scalp, eyebrows, malar area, nasolabial folds, retroauricular creases, beard, presternal area, and central back. Less commonly seen in the axillae, groin, submammary area, and umbilicus.

Treatment

Antiseborrheic shampoos are the standard therapy for the scalp—1% selenium sulfate suspension (Selsun Blue), zinc pyrithione (Head and Shoulders, Zebulon), and tar derivatives

Pyoderma Gangrenosum

A rare disease frequently associated with GI diseases (ulcerative colitis, Crohn dz). Consists of large ulcers with characteristic purple overhanging edges, which develop rapidly from pustules and tender nodules. Exact etiology is unknown; lesions occur particularly on lower legs, abdominal, and face. Responds to systemic steroids.

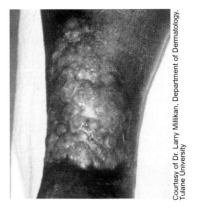

Courtesy of Dr. Larry Millikan, Department of Dermatology, Tulane University

BACTERIAL INFECTIONS

Impetigo

A common contagious superficial skin infection seen in preschool children and young adults

Cause

Usually *Staphylococcus aureus*

Location of Lesions

Most often presents on the face, arms, legs, or buttock

Presentation

Initially presents as a red rash with many small blisters; the blisters later break, forming a crusted stage. In the crusted stage, there are golden yellow crusts that appear "stuck on" on an erythematous base.

Bullous impetigo presents as scattered thin-walled bullae arising in normal skin and containing clear yellow fluid without later becoming crusted.

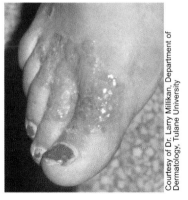

Courtesy of Dr. Larry Millikan, Department of Dermatology, Tulane University

Treatment

Curable in 7 to 10 days with 2% mupirocin (Bactroban) ointment and oral antistaphylococcus penicillins or erythromycin × 10 days

Pitted Keratolysis

Superficial pitting in the stratum corneum on the soles of the feet, giving rise to a "moth-eaten" appearance. It is the result of a keratolytic enzymes produced by bacteria. Often associated with hyperhidrosis and bromhidrosis.

Cause

Corynebacterium or *Micrococcus sedentarius*

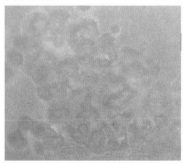

Treatment

Topical and/or oral erythromycin
Measures should also be taken to reduce foot perspiration.

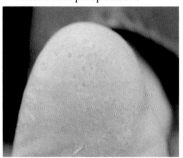

Erythrasma

A bacterial infection affecting the intertriginous areas of the body (between toes, groin, and axillae). There is a higher incidence in warm, humid climates and in diabetics. It often results as a secondary infection as a result of tinea.

Cause

C. minutissimum

Diagnosis

Wood's lamp will cause the area to fluoresce "coral red."

Presentation

Lesions are scaling, fissuring, and slightly macerated. In the feet, it most commonly occurs between the third and fourth toes, resembling tinea.

Treatment

Oral erythromycin or tetracycline Relapses are common within 6 to 12 months.

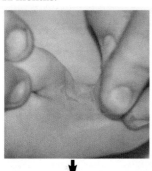

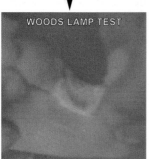

WOODS LAMP TEST

Cellulitis

An acute, severe, rapidly spreading skin infection (more specifically an infection of the connective tissue just beneath the skin). Any break in the skin can potentially result in cellulitis. Erysipelas—acute superficial form of cellulitis involving the dermal lymphatics.

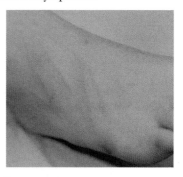

Cause

Staph or Strep (most common pathogens are group A *Streptococcus pyogenes* and *S. aureus*)

Location of Lesions

Most common on the lower leg

Presentation

Sudden onset of tender, edematous erythema in an area of the skin that is warm to the touch as compared with the contralateral side. Spreads rapidly, and red streaking may be seen from the cellulitis toward the heart with swollen lymph glands nearest the cellulitis. If left untreated, sepsis can occur.

Treatment

Oral antibiotics
Warm water soaks over the area of cellulitis to relieve pain/inflammation and hasten healing

Elevation and restricted movement of affected area

Folliculitis

A superficial contagious bacterial infection of a hair folliculitis usually caused by *S. aureus*. Most common on the neck, face, buttocks, and breast. Treatment involves applying moist heat to allow the lesion to come to a head and drain.

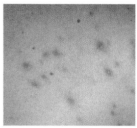

Republished with permission of Elsevier, from Goldstein BG. *Practical Dermatology*. Mosby; 1997:76, Fig. 7-6; permission conveyed through Copyright Clearance Center, Inc.

Furuncle

A contagious deep bacterial infection of a hair follicle usually caused by *S. aureus*. A furuncle, also known as a *boil*, is the result of a worsening case of folliculitis. Lymphadenopathy may be present. Most common on the neck, face, buttocks, and breast. Treatment involves applying moist heat to allow the lesion to come to a head and drain. Incision and drainage and oral antibiotics may be required.

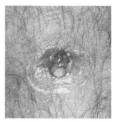

From Dockery GL. *Color Atlas of Foot & Ankle Dermatology*. Lippincott-Raven; 1999:143, Fig. 8.9.

Carbuncle

A cluster of furuncles that coalesce when the infection spreads through small tunnels underneath the skin. If associated with cellulitis or fever, systemic antibiotics are required.

FUNGAL INFECTION

Dermatophytosis (Cutaneous Mycoses)

Dermatophytosis is a superficial fungal infections caused by one of three genera of fungi: *Trichophyton*, *Microsporum*, and *Epidermophyton*. Dermatophytes only live on dead cells, and they do not become systemic, although they can elicit an immune response.

Dermatophyte infections, regardless of fungal species, are usually named for the body part affected.

Tinea pedis—athlete's foot
Tinea unguium—nail fungus
Tinea corporis—skin (ringworm)
Tinea barbae—beard hair
Tinea capitis—scalp hair
Tinea cruris—groin

Three Main Dermatophyte Genera

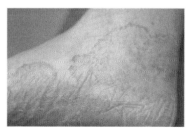

a. *Microsporum*

Microsporum	*Canis*	Animal source
	Audouinii	Human source
	Gypseum	Soil source
	Infects skin and hair.	
	Responsible for childhood tinea capitis. Rarely cause tinea pedis.	
	Microsporum species fluoresces green under UV light.	

b. *Epidermophyton*
Epidermophyton floccosum
  - Third most common cause of tinea pedis (5% to 10%)
  - Infects skin and nail
c. *Trichophyton*
  - Responsible for most tinea pedis and tinea capitis
Trichophyton mentagrophytes
  - Second most common cause of tinea pedis (45%)
  - Most acute type
  - Inflammation with vesicles or bullae
  - Occurs on the plantar skin and may resolve into a keratosis
  - There is also an intertriginous form, which is most common.
  - Occurs at the IS, especially the third and fourth
  - Characterized by maceration, scaling, and fissuring with pruritus and malodor
Trichophyton rubrum
  - Most common cause of tinea pedis (50%) and accounts for 75% of all superficial fungal infections
  - Infects skin, nail, or hair
  - Squamous form
  - Moccasin distribution—affects the plantar surface and sides of the foot

  - May be accompanied by keratosis
  - May coexist with intertriginous form
Trichophyton tonsurans and *Trichophyton schoenleinii*
  - Most common causes of tinea capitis

Dermatophytid

Dermatophytid is a secondary eczematous eruption that develops at a distant site as a result of a fungal infection of the feet. Most commonly seen on the hands and wrists or fingers, but can also present on the face or trunk. Dermatophytid is not infected with the fungus but rather a secondary allergic reaction. The lesions are pruritic and usually appear as fluid-filled bumps or red spots. Dermatophytid goes away after the original fungal infection is treated.

VIRAL INFECTIONS
Verruca (Plantar Wart)

Plantar warts are common contagious benign tumors caused by a virus. They are caused by human papillomavirus and are more common in older children. They are painful only when under a weight-bearing surface of the foot. Commonly confused with a callus (see the following table).

Warts vs. Callus	
Wart	**Callus**
Skin lines go around lesion	Skin lines go through lesion
WB or NWB surfaces	WB surfaces
Pain on lateral pressure	Pain on direct pressure
Center—pale/spongy punctate bleeding	Center—hard
Affects children and young adults	Affects middle aged and adults

Treatment

Surgical excision, liquid nitrogen, various topical acids, laser
Spontaneous remission occurs in about 60% of cases with or without treatment and may reoccur at the same or a different site.

and may be a single isolated lesion or multiple scattered lesions. Often disappear spontaneously within 1 to 2 years.

Treatment

Same treatment as warts

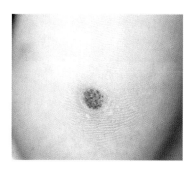

Molluscum Contagiosum

Contagious viral infection of the skin. Common in children. In adults, it is often sexually transmitted.

Cause

Poxvirus

Presentation

Discrete, round, smooth, umbilicated, pearl white, or skin-colored papules measuring 1 to 3 mm in diameter. Lesions are asymptomatic

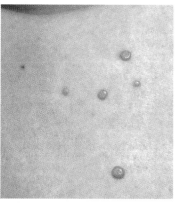

From Fitzpatrick TB. *Color Atlas and Synopsis of Clinical Dermatology.* 2nd ed. McGraw-Hill Inc; 1992:69.

Herpes Simplex

Recurrent herpetic eruptions can occur due to overexposure to the sun, febrile illnesses, physical or emotional stress, immunosuppressive drugs, or menstruation. The virus remains dormant in the nerve ganglia. Incubation is 2 to 20 days (average 6 days).

Herpetic whitlow is a painful herpetic eruption that occurs on the distal phalanx through a cutaneous break.

Cause

HSV-1 (herpes simplex virus 1): Found on the mouth, on the lips, conjunctiva, or cornea

HSV-2 (herpes simplex virus 2): Found on the genitalia (STD)

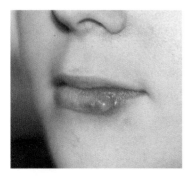

Presentation

Associated with a prodromal period of tingling discomfort or itching in the area where the eruption will occur. Initially presents as single or multiple clusters of small vesicles, filled with clear fluid on an erythematous base. After several days, the blisters rupture and leave painful, shallow ulcers that heal in 2 to 4 weeks.

Diagnosis

Tzanck smear (requires fluid from one of the vesicles)

Treatment

Acyclovir (oral or topical)

Herpes Zoster (Shingles)

An acute CNS infection involving the dorsal root ganglia. Triggered by systemic disease, particularly Hodgkin disease or immunosuppressive therapy. Occurs at any age but most common after age 50 years; reoccurrence is rare, 4%.

Ramsay Hunt syndrome—herpes zoster involving the face and auditory nerve. Involves pain in the ear and facial paralysis.

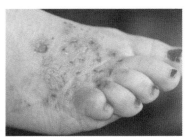

Causes

Varicella-zoster virus

This is the same virus that causes chicken pox. Arises from a reactivation of the virus that has lain dormant in the sensory root ganglia for many years. During a shingles outbreak, these individuals can spread chicken pox.

Presentation

Prodromal symptoms occur 3 to 4 days before an outbreak and include chills, fever, malaise, and GI disturbances. Presents as crops of clear fluid-filled vesicles on an erythematous base; erupts along the cutaneous area (dermatomes)

supplied by a peripheral sensory nerve. After several days, the blisters rupture and leave painful, shallow ulcers that heal in 2 to 4 weeks. Postherpetic neuralgic pain in the cutaneous area supplied by a peripheral sensory nerve may linger long after skin lesions are gone.

	Herpes Simplex	Herpes Zoster
Common name	Cold sores, genital herpes	Shingles
Causative agent	HSV-1, HSV-2	Varicella-zoster virus
Presentation	Single or multiple vesicles	Crops of vesicles
Location	Mouth, eyes, genitalia	Along dermatomes
Prodrome	Itching and tingling in the area of eruption	Chills, fever, malaise, GI problems
Pain	Moderate to severe	Severe
Reoccurrence	Common	Rare

Diagnosis

Tzanck smear (requires fluid from one of the vesicles)

Treatment

Locally applied wet compresses are soothing, pain meds, acyclovir.

Varicella (Chicken Pox)

Highly contagious primary infection caused by the zoster virus, varicella. Transmitted by airborne droplets as well as direct contact. Patients are contagious from several days before vesicles appear until the last crop of vesicles crusts over. Incubation period is 2 weeks.

Signs/Symptoms

Successive crops of pruritic vesicles, which progress to pustules, crusts, and sometimes scar. Mild headache, fever, and malaise may be present.

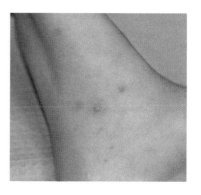

Diagnosis

Tzanck test

Treatment

Symptoms in children are usually mild, and antiviral treatment is not indicated. In adults, oral acyclovir 1,000 mg q6h × 5 days is used.

In 1995, the chicken pox vaccine (varicella vaccine) became part of the standard childhood immunizations. The vaccine is a live but weakened (attenuated) virus.

SCALING PAPULAR DISEASE

Psoriasis

A common, chronic, inflammatory dermatitis that affects 2% of the population. Affects whites more than blacks. Onset is usually between 10 and 40 years, and there is often a positive family history. Typical course is chronic remission and recurrence. Mostly a cosmetic problem unless associated with joint pain (psoriatic arthritis). Stress and cold weather may exacerbate flare-ups.

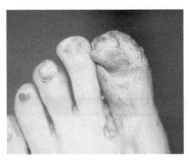

Location of Lesions

Usually involves the scalp, extensor surfaces of the extremities (especially knees and elbows), the back, and the buttock

Presentation

Lesions are well-circumscribed, erythematous, "salmon pink" papules or plaques covered with silvery shiny scales. Lesions are not pruritic and heal without scaring. Pitting of the fingernails and toenails is seen in 25% of patients.

Auspitz phenomenon—removal of silvery scales results in pinpoint bleeding.

Treatment

Keratolytics
Topical corticosteroids
Exposure to sunlight generally helps heal lesions; however, occasionally, sunburn can exacerbate the condition.
Methotrexate is used to treat severe resistant cases.

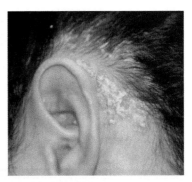

Pityriasis Rosea

A self-limited, mild inflammatory skin disease characterized by scaly lesions. Occurs most often in young adults (between age 10 and 35 years). Spontaneous remission usually occurs in 1 to 4 months; recurrences are rare.

Cause

Unknown, probably by an infectious agent

Presentation

Lesions are round or oval and slightly erythematous with fine scales and have a slightly raised border.

A "herald" or "mother" patch found on the trunk usually precedes the generalized eruption by 5 to 10 days and is usually larger than the rest of the lesions. The generalized eruption consists of many lesions 2 to 5 cm in diameter and continues to develop for weeks. Patches on the back typically radiating from the spinal column in a "Christmas tree" pattern. Pruritus may or may not be present.

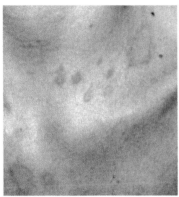

Republished with permission of Elsevier, from Goldstein BG. *Practical Dermatology*. Mosby; 1997:177, Fig. 14-13; permission conveyed through Copyright Clearance Center, Inc.

Treatment

Usually, none is needed.
Pruritus can be controlled symptomatically.

Lichen Planus

A recurrent, benign, pruritic, inflammatory eruption of the skin. Lesions may disappear in weeks or persist for years. Most common in people over 40 years of age. Associated with oral lesions in about half of patients. May result in sudden hair loss in patches on the head; 10% of patients develop pterygium. Moderate-to-severe pruritus is common.

Cause

Unknown; may be caused by certain drugs; stress can precipitate an attack.

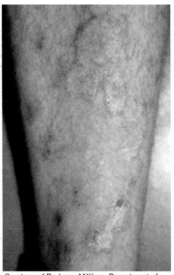

Courtesy of Dr. Larry Millikan, Department of Dermatology, Tulane University

Location of Lesions

Seen symmetrical in the flexor surfaces of the wrists, forearm, lower abdomen, back, and mucous membrane

Presentation

Skin
Flat, topped, violaceous, shiny, polygonal-shaped papules measuring 2 to 4 mm in diameter with a network of fine white lines (Wickham striae)

Mucous Membrane (Buccal Mucosa, Tongue, Lips)
Milky white papules with a fine white lacework (Wickham striae)
On rare occasion, long-standing oral lesions may develop carcinoma.

Treatment

Treatment consists of topical corticosteroids with occlusion. Erosions usually resolve in weeks to months; however, lesions may persist for years, especially on the shins or in the mouth.

BENIGN TUMORS

Common Moles

Common benign growths derived from altered melanocytes. Classification system is based on the location of cells.

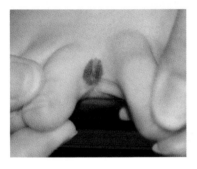

Junctional Nevi

Flat and hyperpigmented. Nevus cells are found at the epidermal layer above the basement membrane.

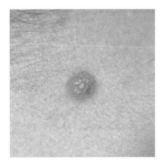

Dermal Nevi (Intradermal Nevi)

Raised and flesh colored (sometimes pigmented). Nevus cells are entirely within the dermis. Common on the face, rarely malignant.

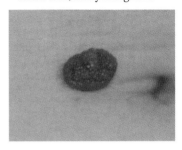

Compound Nevi

Raised and hyperpigmented. A combination of a junctional nevi and dermal nevi—they contain cells found in both the dermis and the epidermis.

Skin Tag

Common, soft, small, flesh-colored, or hyperpigmented pedunculated lesions that may occur anywhere, but most common at intertriginous sites. They are asymptomatic and only a cosmetic concern. They are more common in obese people. Tend to become longer and more numerous over time. Removal is most often for cosmetic reasons (liquid nitrogen or excision).

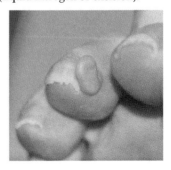

VASCULAR TUMORS

Angioma/Hemangioma

Capillary Hemangioma (Strawberry Mark)

Soft, bright red, vascular nodule plaques that develop at birth or soon after birth. They disappear spontaneously by age 5 years. Treatment is rarely necessary.

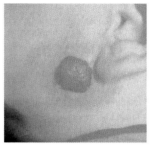

Republished with permission of Elsevier, from Goldstein BG. *Practical Dermatology*. Mosby; 1997:278, Fig. 20-13; permission conveyed through Copyright Clearance Center, Inc.

Port-Wine Stain (Nevus Flammeus)

An irregularly shaped red or violaceous macular vascular formation, which is present at birth and does not disappear spontaneously. Treatment may be with skin-colored dyes or copper vapor laser. Occasionally associated with two syndromes: Sturge–Weber syndrome and Klippel–Trenaunay–Weber syndrome.

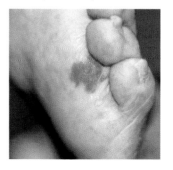

Spider Angioma

A focal telangiectatic network of dilated capillaries radiating from a central papular punctum. Associated with pregnancy or hepatic disease.

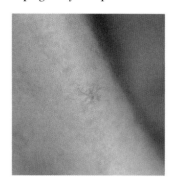

Cavernous Hemangioma

Edematous vascular lesion characterized by soft compressible tissue. May be associated with surface varicosities or nevus flammeus–like changes. Lesions are not apparent at birth but become visible during childhood. Lesions are asymptomatic.

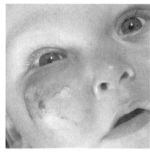

From Fitzpatrick TB. *Color Atlas and Synopsis of Clinical Dermatology*. 2nd ed. McGraw-Hill Inc; 1992:163.

Pyogenic Granuloma

A benign skin lesion composed of small blood vessels, usually occurring before age 30. There is an increased incidence during pregnancy.

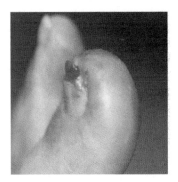

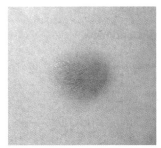

From Fitzpatrick TB. *Color Atlas and Synopsis of Clinical Dermatology.* 2nd ed. McGraw-Hill Inc; 1992:175.

Presentation

Rapidly developing, bright red, or violaceous or brown-black nodule with a slightly constricted base. Lesions generally do not hurt and bleed easily when only slightly touched.

Location of Lesions

Commonly occurs at nail margins and grooves, especially in conjunction with ingrown toenails

Treatment

Excision

Dermatofibroma

Common button-like dermal fibroma usually occurs on the extremities, most commonly the leg

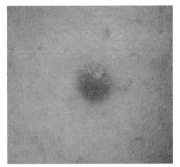

Reproduced with permission from Dockery GL, Crawford ME. *Color Atlas of Foot and Ankle Dermatology.* Lippincott Williams & Wilkins; 1999: Fig. 6.24.

Diagnosis

Dimple sign—lateral compression with thumb and index finger yields a depression or "dimple"

Presentation

Lesions are firm papules or nodules usually between 3 and 10 mm. They can be skin color, pink, tan, or brown.

Location of Lesions

Extremities, most commonly the leg

Treatment

Lesions are benign and require no treatment unless they pose a cosmetic problem or are subject to repeated trauma.

Keloid

A hypertrophic scar that extends beyond the site of injury often with claw-like extensions. More common in blacks, and there may be a familial predisposition.

Treatment

Controversial but may include surgical excision and steroid injections

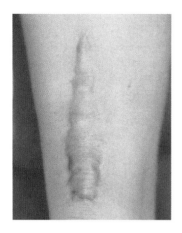

Glomus Tumor

A benign, extremely painful, vascular tumor arising from a glomus body. Glomus bodies consist of an arteriovenous shunt surrounded by a capsule and are involved in body temperature regulation. Glomus tumors are most commonly found subungually.

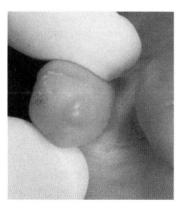

From Dockery GL. *Color Atlas of Foot & Ankle Dermatology*. Lippincott-Raven; 1999:114, Fig. 6.56.

Cause

Unknown

Presentation

Painful, blue-red, moderately firm papule usually <1.0 cm in diameter. Rarely ulcerate or bleed. Characterized by paroxysmal pain

Location of Lesions

Commonly found subungual

Treatment

Surgical excision is curative.

Kaposi Sarcoma

A multicentric systemic vascular tumor characterized by violaceous nodules and edema secondary to lymphatic obstruction. Before HIV was uncommon and seen in greatest frequency in Eastern Europe and Jewish and Italian immigrants over 60 years of age. Now occurs mainly in homosexual males with HIV.

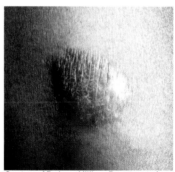

Courtesy of Dr. Larry Millikan, Department of Dermatology, Tulane University

Presentation

Bluish red, purple to violaceous, or dark brown macules, nodules, and patches that spread and may coalesce to form large plaques or nodules. Lesions are asymptomatic.

Location of Lesions

Most frequently found on the feet or legs

Treatment

In HIV patients, treatment is not often indicated since infection usually dominates the clinical cause.

MALIGNANT TUMORS

Basal Cell Carcinoma

Most common type of skin cancer, sometimes called *rodent ulcer.* More common in fair-skinned individuals, metastasis is rare.

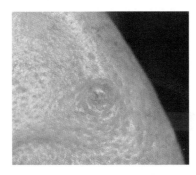

Causes

Excessive sunlight or radiation exposure

Location of Lesions

Occurs on sun-exposed areas, especially the face

Presentation

Highly variable, most commonly begin as a small, asymptomatic, smooth, hemispherical, translucent, shiny papule with a pearly border. Later, dilated blood vessels and, occasionally, specks of brown or black pigment can be seen. The lesion gradually enlarges into a mass of pearly nodules or a papular plaque that maybe darkly pigmented. Later still, it may develop into an ulcerated, crusted, or bleeding lesion surrounded by a nodular rim (rodent ulcer).

Treatment

Excision, curettage, cautery, or cryotherapy and, in severe cases, radiation therapy

Squamous Cell Carcinoma

A malignant tumor of epithelial keratinocytes (skin and mucous membrane) with a high incidence of metastasis. Bowen disease is a superficial variant of squamous cell carcinoma that resembles a localized patch of psoriasis, dermatitis, or tinea.

Marjolin ulcer is a squamous cell carcinoma that develops in an area of previous trauma, chronic inflammation, or scarred skin. Marjolin ulcer is the carcinoma most frequently associated with chronic venous ulcers.

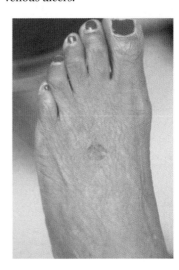

Cause

Exogenous carcinogens (i.e., sunlight exposure, ingestion of arsenic, radiation, smoking)

More common on fair-skinned people and people over 55 years old. Males are more affected than females; however, on the legs, females predominate.

Location of Lesions

Occur on sun-exposed areas, specifically the face or back of the hands. On the foot, often arise in previous damaged skin, especially scars.

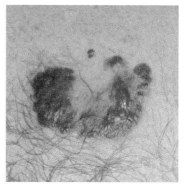

From DeVita VT. *Cancer, Principles and Practice of Oncology.* Lippincott; 1982:1131, Fig. 31-9.

Presentation

Clinical presentation is highly variable. They may begin as a small erythematous scaly nodule that ulcerates. Superficial, discrete, hard lesions resembling a verruca arise from an indurated elevated base, dull red color with telangiectasias.

Treatment

Excision, curettage, cautery, or cryotherapy and, in severe cases, radiation therapy

Melanoma

Description

Malignant tumor of the melanocytes arising from preexisting nevi or de novo. Found primarily on sun-exposed areas of fair-skinned individuals. Predilection for the backs of men and the legs of women. When it occurs in blacks, it is often found on the palms, soles, or nail beds. Majority present between 30 and 60 years of age. Any pigmented skin lesion with recent change in appearance should be suspect.

Types

a. *Superficial spreading melanoma*
   Most common (70%)
   Occurs in younger patients
   Spreads radially before invading deep
   Pigmented macular/papular lesion with irregular borders

b. *Nodular melanoma*
   15% of cases
   Worst prognosis (becomes invasive early)
   Uniformly pigmented, bizarrely colored nodule
   Commonly ulcerates

c. *Lentigo maligna melanoma* (malignant freckle)
   5% of melanomas
   Slowest growing, least likely to metastasize
   Macular patch of mottled pigmentation
   Enlarged radially before spreading deep
   Occurs on sun-exposed areas
   More common in older patients older than 60 years

d. *Acral lentiginous melanoma*
10% of melanomas
Aggressive, invades early
Occurs chiefly on the palms
and soles, often on the digits
or subungula (melanotic
whitlow)
Usually found on nonwhite
individuals

Signs and Symptoms

a. ABCDEs
*A*symmetrical
*B*orders—irregular, notched
*C*olor—multicolored (pink,
white, purple, gray, tan,
black, blue, or brown)
*D*iameter—>6 mm in diameter
(approximately the diameter
of a pencil eraser)

Amelanotic Melanoma

Occurs when a melanoma arises
from a melanocyte devoid of pigment. May occur in any of the four
clinicopathologic variants. Presents as erythematous papules or
nodules lacking significant pigmentation. Often misdiagnosed as
basal cell carcinoma, squamous
cell carcinoma, and other nonpig-
mented skin tumors.

*E*levation—lesions are usually
elevated.
b. Any pigmented skin lesion with
recent change in appearance
should be suspect.
c. Palpable regional lymph nodes
(late manifestation)
d. Hutchinson sign—seen in subungual melanoma. Pigment changes
in the eponychium secondary to
leaching of the pigment from a
subungual melanoma.

Pathologic Staging

Clark Classification (Depth of Invasion)

Stage I	Limited to the epidermis
	No basement membrane involvement
Stage II	Through basement membrane into papillary dermis
Stage III	Filling the papillary dermis
Stage IV	Into the reticular dermis
Stage V	Into the subcutaneous fat

Breslow Classification (Thickness of Tumor)

Depth of Lesion (mm)	Survival Rate at 10 Years (%)
<0.75	97
0.76–1.50	87
1.51–3.00	67
>4.00	40

Treatment

Excision

Breslow Thickness	Margins/Depth of Excision
In situ (earliest stage)	0.5–1 cm of normal skin and extend down to subQ
≤1 mm	1 cm of normal margins and extend to fascia
1.01–2 mm	1–2 cm of normal margins
≥2.01 mm	2 cm of normal margins

CUTANEOUS MANIFESTATIONS OF DIABETES

Necrobiosis Lipoidica Diabeticorum

May be an important clinical finding as it precedes the onset of diabetes mellitus in 15% to 20% of patients

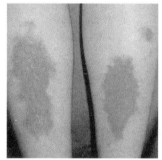

Reproduced with permission from Goodheart HP. *Goodheart's Photoguide of Common Skin Disorders.* 2nd ed. Lippincott Williams & Wilkins; 2003: Fig. 25.2.

Cause

Caused by an obliterative endarteritis, characteristic of diabetic microangiopathy

Presentation

Begins as a red or red-brown, flat, well-circumscribed lesion that slowly expands. The active border remains erythematous and sharply demarcated, but the center appears atrophic, yellow, waxy, shiny, and telangiectatic as lipids are deposited. Dermal vessels become telangiectatic, and the subcutaneous vessels become visible. These lesions may persist for years and ulcerate from minor trauma. Lesions can be anywhere from 0.5 to 25 cm in diameter.

Location of Lesions

90% of lesions are found on the shins.

Treatment

Unless ulcerated, lesions do not have to be treated. A high-potency topical corticosteroid applied to the active margin may arrest the progression. Resolution and/or prognosis are not related to the patients' glycemic control.

Xanthoma Diabeticorum

Sudden onset of crops of asymptomatic yellow papules each with an erythematous rim. Located mostly over the extensor surfaces (knees, elbows, back, buttocks, and truck). Usually arises during the hypertriglyceridemic phase of uncontrolled diabetes. Spontaneously disappears over several weeks after the serum lipid level has returned to normal.

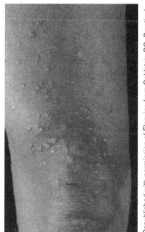

Republished with permission of Elsevier, from Goldstein BG. *Practical Dermatology.* Mosby; 1997:278, Fig. 20-13; permission conveyed though Copyright Clearance Center, Inc.

Bullous Diabeticorum

Occurs as spontaneous asymptomatic blisters on the extremities, especially the feet. The blisters are sterile and filled with clear fluid, which range from a few millimeters to several centimeters in diameter. Lesions begin as tense lesions, but as it enlarges, it becomes flaccid. The exact cause of the blisters is unknown, although photosensitivity has been suggested as initiating factor. Blisters heal over a 6-week period without scarring. Lesions require no treatment; however, the blisters may be incised and drained if they are in a precarious position.

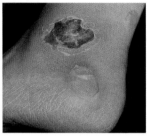

Reprinted from Habif TP. *Clinical Dermatology*. Mosby; 1990:411, Fig. 16-4, with permission from Elsevier.

Diabetic Dermopathy

Atrophic, hyperpigmented, circumscribed skin lesions found bilaterally on the shins or feet. Occur in 30% to 60% of diabetics. The pigmentation is due to hemosiderin deposits. Lesions are asymptomatic and require no treatment.

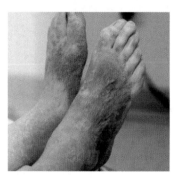

MISCELLANEOUS

Scabies

A contagious intensely pruritic parasitic infection of the skin. Impregnated female mites tunnel into the stratum corneum and deposit eggs along the burrow. Larvae hatch within a few days and congregate around the hair follicle. Transmitted mostly by person-to-person contact, also by towels, cloths, and bedding. The mite can only survive 2 days off the skin.

Scabies is the basis for the colloquial term *the seven-year itch* as it tends to occur in communities in a 7-year cycle.

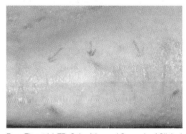

From Fitzpatrick TB. *Color Atlas and Synopsis of Clinical Dermatology*. 2nd ed. McGraw-Hill Inc; 1992:133.

Cause

Skin infestation by a mite *Sarcoptes scabiei*

Presentation

Characteristic initial lesions are gray or skin-colored burrows, seen as a fine waxy dark line a few millimeters to 1 cm long with a minute papule at the open end.

Location of Lesions

Lesions occur predominately on the finger and toe webs, the flexor surfaces of the wrists, around the elbows and axillary folds, around the areolae of the breasts in females and on the genitals in males, along the belt line, and on the lower buttocks. Scalp and face are usually spared.

Diagnosis

Diagnosis is confirmed by scrapings taken from the burrows, which will demonstrate the parasite.

Treatment

5% permethrin cream (cover entire body from neck down for a minimum of 12 hours)

Single-dose PO ivermectin (Stromectol)

Syphilis

STD

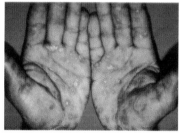

Republished with permission of Elsevier, from Goldstein BG. *Practical Dermatology*. Mosby; 1997:197, Fig. 15-6; permission conveyed through Copyright Clearance Center, Inc.

Cause

Spirochete, *Treponema pallidum*

Stages

Primary syphilis
  Incubation period is 3 weeks.
  Painless ulcers or canker develop at the site of inoculation.

There is often regional lymphadenopathy.

Secondary syphilis
  Appears 2 to 6 months after initial infection
  Lesions are asymptomatic, round or oval, brown-red, or pink, dry macules and papules measuring 0.5 to 1 cm in diameter.
  Lesions may be generalized to the trunk or localized on the head, neck, palms, or soles.
  Usually associated with a flulike syndrome (headache, sore throat, generalized arthralgia, malaise, fever)

Tertiary syphilis
  Lesions begin as nodules that ulcerate, resulting in "punched-out" lesions called a *gumma*. Twenty-five percent of patients will have neurosyphilis (peripheral neuropathy, mental deterioration) or cardiovascular syphilis.

Diagnosis

VDRL (venereal disease research laboratory) test. This blood test tests for the antibodies to the bacteria that cause syphilis.

Treatment

PCN

Rosacea

A chronic acneform inflammation of the pilosebaceous units of the face (usually cheeks and nose). Also known as *adult acne*. Occurs predominately in females between 30 and 50 years of age. Recurrences are common, but the disease tends to disappear after a few years.

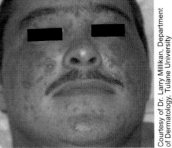

Courtesy of Dr. Larry Millikan, Department of Dermatology, Tulane University

Cause

- Unknown, but reactions have been triggered by alcohol, hot or spicy foods, stress, and heat stimuli in the mouth (hot liquids)

Presentation

Patients have periodic reddening of the face (flushing) with increase in skin temperature. Lesions are characterized by telangiectasias, erythema, papules, and pustules appearing especially in the central area of the face. Lesions last days to weeks.

Treatment

Reduce stress level, eliminate food, or drink that exacerbates condition.
Topical 0.75% metronidazole
Oral tetracycline
Corticosteroids are contraindicated; they have been known to worsen the condition.

Acanthosis Nigricans

A diffuse velvety thickening and hyperpigmentation of the skin that may precede other symptoms of malignancy by 5 years. Underlying endocrine disorder and malignancies must be ruled out.

Location of Lesions

Lesions are most common in the axillae and on the neck, also the groin, antecubital fossa, knuckles, submammary, and umbilicus. In the feet, there may be hyperpigmentation over the knuckles of the toes.

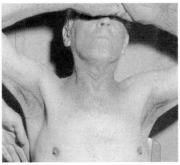

From Fitzpatrick TB. *Color Atlas and Synopsis of Clinical Dermatology*. 2nd ed. McGraw-Hill Inc; 1992:733.

Classifications

Type 1: Hereditary, benign
Type 2: Benign, associated with endocrine disorders (diabetes)
Type 3: Pseudo, complication of obesity
Type 4: Drug induced
Type 5: Malignant

Granuloma Annulare

Benign, confluent, firm, pearly, white papules or nodules that spread peripherally to form rings with normal skin in their center. Recurrences are common, and lesions are usually asymptomatic and self-limiting. In 75% of cases, lesions disappear spontaneously in 2 years. May also present as a subcutaneous nodule appearing much like a rheumatoid nodule. Possible higher incidence in diabetics.

Location of Lesions

Lesions are usually present on the feet, legs, hands, or fingers.

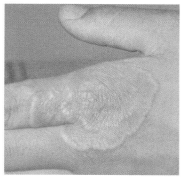

From Fitzpatrick TB. *Color Atlas and Synopsis of Clinical Dermatology*. 2nd ed. McGraw-Hill Inc; 1992:247.

Treatment

Intralesional triamcinolone acetonide injections

Topical corticosteroids with occlusion

Porokeratosis Plantaris Discreta

Benign, slow-growing, hyperkeratotic, exquisitely tender papules. Lesions are caused by hypertrophy of the stratum corneum around the duct of a sweat gland (eccrine sweat duct).

Generally a solitary lesion found on the sole of the foot, which is often misdiagnosed as warts or callus

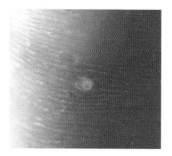

Callus/Corns

Heloma Molle

A soft interdigital callus often white from maceration. When found at the fourth IS, it is usually caused by pressure from the head of the proximal phalanx 5th toe against the base of the proximal phalanx 4th toe.

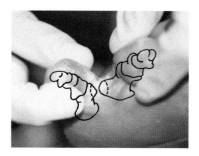

Heloma Dura

A hard callus on the dorsum of the toe or on the tip of the toe. Caused by a bony prominence such as hammertoes, mallet toes, or claw toes.

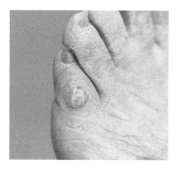

Intractable Plantar Keratoma (IPK)

Nucleated callus plantar to a metatarsal head

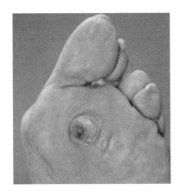

percent of normal individuals have one to three café-au-lait spots. Extensive café-au-lait macules with a "coast-of-Maine," or irregular, edge may indicate McCune–Albright syndrome. The spots are due to heavily pigmented melanocytes of neural crest origin.

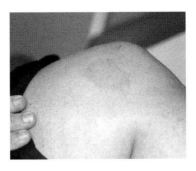

Café-Au-Lait Spots

Hyperpigmented macules on the trunk and legs. They are associated with several genetic disorders, most commonly neurofibromatosis (von Recklinghausen disease). Ten

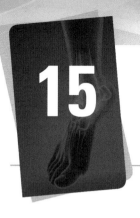

15 WOUND CARE/DIABETES

DIABETES

Diabetes is a metabolic disease that causes high blood glucose. This occurs either because insulin production is inadequate or because the body's cells do not respond properly to insulin. Insulin is a hormone produced by the pancreas that moves glucose from the blood into the cells. Nine percent of Americans (30 million people) have diabetes. When monitoring diabetes, it is better to err on the side of hyperglycemia; hypoglycemia can result in permanent neuron destruction.

Three Types of Diabetes

Type 1

IDDM
The body does not produce insulin.
Usually develops before age 40, juvenile onset
Accounts for only 10% of diabetics
Requires insulin injections

Type 2

NIDDM
The body does not produce enough insulin for proper function, or the cells in the body do not react to insulin.
Can sometimes be controlled with diet, exercise, and weight loss
Overweight people are at greater risk, and the risk also increases with age.

Type 3

Gestational diabetes

A type of hyperglycemia that occurs during pregnancy
Occurs in 1% to 3% of women
Disappears in 97% of cases at the end of pregnancy

Type 1 vs. Type 2 Diabetes

Type 1	Type 2
IDDM	NIDDM
Juvenile onset	Adult onset
Prone to ketosis	Ketosis resistant
Onset <30 years of age	Onset usually over 40 years of age
Accounts for 10% of diabetic	Accounts for 90% of diabetic
Due to insufficient insulin production	Caused by the body not responding to insulin
Abrupt onset	Slow onset and progression
Must take insulin	Controlled with oral hypoglycemic and diet

Hyperglycemia vs. Hypoglycemia

Hyperglycemia	Hypoglycemia
Polyuria	Diaphoresis/syncope
Polydipsia	Tachycardia/palpitations
Polyphagia	Hunger
Weight loss	Anxiety/irritability
Fatigue	Tremors/seizures/mental confusion
Blurred vision	Weakness

ACUTE KIDNEY INJURY (AKI)

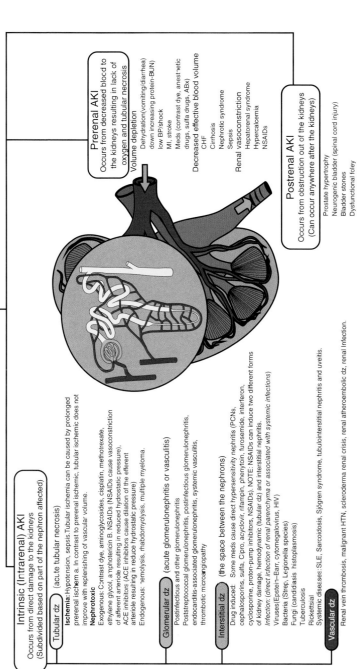

Intrinsic (Intrarenal) AKI
Occurs from direct damage to the kidneys
(Subdivided based on part of the nephron affected)

Tubular dz (acute tubular necrosis)

Ischemia: Hypotension, sepsis. Tubular ischemia can be caused by prolonged prerenal ischem a. In contrast to prerenal ischemic, tubular ischemic does not improve with replenishing of vascular volume.

Nephrotoxic
Exogenous: Contrast dye, aminoglycosides, cisplatin, methotrexate, ethylene glycol, a mphotericin B. NSAIDs (NSAIDs cause vasoconstriction of afferent arteriole resulting in reduced hydrostatic pressure), ACE inhibitors (ACE inhibitors cause dilation of the efferent arteriole resulting in reduce hydrostatic pressure)
Endogenous: 'nemolysis, rhabdomyolysis, multiple myeloma.

Glomerular dz (acute glomerulonephritis or vasculitis)

Postinfectious and other glomerulonephritis
Poststreptococcal glomerulonephritis, postinfectious glomerulonephritis, endocarditis-associated glomerulonephritis, systemic vasculitis, thrombotic microangiopathy

Interstitial dz (the space between the nephrons)

Drug induced: Some meds cause direct hypersensitivity nephritis (PCNs, cephalosporins, sulfa, Cipro, acyclovir, rifampin, phenytoin, furosemide, interferon, cyclosporine, proton-pump inhibitors, NSAIDs), NOTE: NSAIDs can induce two different forms of kidney damage, hemodynamic (tubular dz) and interstitial nephritis.
Infection: (direct infection of renal parenchyma or associated with systemic infections)
Viruses(Epstein–Earr, cytomegalovirus, HIV)
Bacteria (Strep, Legionella species)
Fungi (candidiasis histoplasmosis)
Tuberculosis
Rickettsial
Systemic diseases: SLE, Sarcoidosis, Sjögren syndrome, tubulointerstitial nephritis and uveitis.

Vascular dz

Renal vein thrombosis, malignant HTN, scleroderma renal crisis, renal atheroembolic dz, renal Infection.

Prerenal AKI
Occurs from decreased blood to the kidneys resulting in lack of oxygen and tubular necrosis

Volume depletion
Dehydration(vomiting/diarrhea)
down increasing protein-BUN)
low BP/shock
MI, stroke
Meds (contrast dye, anesthetic drugs, sulfa drugs, ABx)
Decreased effective blood volume
CHF
Cirrhosis
Nephrotic syndrome
Sepsis
Renal vasoconstriction
Hepatorenal syndrome
Hypercalcemia
NSAIDs

Postrenal AKI
Occurs from obstruction out of the kidneys
(Can occur anywhere after the kidneys)

Prostate hypertrophy
Neurogenic bladder (spinal cord injury)
Bladder stones
Dysfunctional foley

AV Fistula

An arteriovenous (AV) fistula is an abnormal connection between an artery and a vein. They can occur in the body as a result of trauma, iatrogenically, or from degenerative aneurysmal changes.

AV fistulas are artificially created in diabetics who are going on dialysis. The usual location is in the arm for easy access. An artery is anastomosed with a vein, resulting in the vein becoming larger over time. Under certain circumstances, an AV fistula is created with a synthetic graft consisting of a piece of tubing. This is done in cases where the patient does not have healthy or well-sized vessels.

The purpose of this enlarged area is to accommodate the needle, usually 14 to 17 gauge. This enlarged vein provides easier access for the rather large needles and better flow rate required for dialysis treatment. It usually takes about 6 weeks for the vein to mature to a point where dialysis can be started. During dialysis, two needles are inserted into the fistula, one drawing the blood out, and one putting it back.

Rule of 6's (tells you if you have a mature ready-to-use AV fistula)
  1. At least 0.6 cm in width
  2. 0.6 cm or less from surface
  3. Flow of at least 600 mL/min by 6 weeks postfistula creation
  4. Linear segment of at least 6 cm (ideally 10 cm)

LAB EVALUATION OF ACUTE KIDNEY INJURY

AKI	BUN:Cr	Urine Na (mEq/L)	Fractional Excretion of Sodium (FE Na)	Urine Sediment
Prerenal	>20:1	<20	<1%	Normal
Postrenal	>20:1	>20	Variable	Normal or RBCs
Intrinsic-Tubular	<10:1	>40	>2%	Muddy brown casts; tubular epithelial cells
Intrinsic-Interstitial	<20:1	>20	>1%	WBCs, WBC casts
Intrinsic-Glomerular	Variable	<40	<1%	RBCs, eosinophils
Intrinsic-Vascular	Variable	>20	Variable	Normal or RBCs

CHRONIC KIDNEY DISEASE (CKD)

Leading causes: type 2 diabetes (42%), HTN (28%), glomerular nephritis (7%), type 1 diabetes (4%), tumors, cystic and tubu-lointerstitial nephropathies

Drugs to Avoid in Kidney Disease

Tetracyclines (except doxycycline), sulfonamides, cephalosporins, vancomycin, metronidazole, aminoglycosides (gentamycin), penicillins, NSAIDs, clindamy-cin, amphotericin B, lithium, digoxin, immunosuppressants (cyclosporine), anticancer drugs (cisplatin), macrolides (Erythro-mycin), rifampin

Diagnosing Diabetes

FPG (fasting plasma glucose)
    Less than 100 mg per dL is
        normal.
    100 to 125.99 mg per dL is
        prediabetic.
    Greater than 126 mg per dL is
        positive for diabetes.
OGTT (oral glucose tolerance test)
    Less than 140 mg per dL is
        normal.
    140 to 199.9 mg per dL is
        prediabetic.
    200 mg per dL and up means
        diabetes.
A1C
    Less than 5.7% is normal.
    Between 5.7% and 5.99% is
        prediabetic.
    6.5% and up is diabetic.

Factors That Put Diabetics at Risk for Foot Ulcers

Immunocompromised

Defective PMN function resulting in an increased risk of infection

Angiopathy

Blood vessels in the diabetic are subject to accelerated atherosclerosis, increased clotting, and thrombosis formation.

Neuropathy

Diabetic peripheral neuropathy is caused by direct metabolic damage to nerves. Diabetic peripheral neuropathy affects all nerves: sensory, motor, and autonomic.

Sensory Neuropathy

Sensory impairment typically precedes motor dysfunction. Classically, it begins in the lon-gest nerves of the body and so affects the feet and later the hands. This is sometimes called the "stocking-glove" pattern. Protective threshold and proprioception (loss of balance) are lost.

Motor Neuropathy

Motor deficit affects the intrinsic muscles of the foot, leading to digital deformities.

Autonomic Neuropathy

Autonomic nerves to the sweat glands are damaged, causing anhidrosis (inability to sweat normally). This results in dry scaly feet, which are prone to fissuring. Other autonomic neuropathic symptoms include a hot, hyperemic foot; increased arteriovenous shunting; reduced capillary flow; and bounding pulses.

Dialysis

When is the best time for surgery? Soon after when blood is clean.

What are AV fistulas, and why are they surgically created in the arm of diabetics?

They are a connection between an artery and a vein. They cause the vein to grow larger and stronger, making it easier to access the blood.

WOUND CLASSIFICATIONS

Wagner Diabetic Ulcer Classification

Wagner Classification

GRADE	DESCRIPTION
0	Intact skin
1	Superficial ulcer (not extending to tendon, capsule, or bone)
2	Deep ulcer (extending to tendon, capsule, or bone)
3	Ulcer with bone involvement
4	Forefoot gangrene
5	Full-foot gangrene

Knighton Classification

KNIGHTON CLASSIFICATION

Level	Description
I	Partial-thickness (not extending into subQ)
II	Extending into subQ
III	Extending into tendon, ligament, joint, or bone
IV	Level III + abscess or osteomyelitis
V	Level III + necrotic tissue in wound
VI	Level III + gangrene

University of Texas Wound Classification System (Wound Grade and Stage Classification)

University of Texas Wound Classification System

STAGE		GRADE			
		0	**1**	**2**	**3**
	A	Pre- or post-ulcerative lesion. Completely epithelialized.	Superficial wound not involving tendon, capsule, or bone.	Wound penetrating to tendon or capsule.	Wound penetrating to bone or joint.
	B	Pre- or post-ulcerative lesion. Completely epithelialized with infection.	Superficial wound not involving tendon, capsule, or bone with infection.	Wound penetrating to tendon or capsule with infection.	Wound penetrating to bone or joint with infection.
	C	Pre- or post-ulcerative lesion. Completely epithelialized with ischemia.	Superficial wound not involving tendon, capsule, or bone with ischemia.	Wound penetrating to tendon or capsule with ischemia.	Wound penetrating to bone or joint with ischemia.
	D	Pre- or post-ulcerative lesion. Completely epithelialized with infection and ischemia.	Superficial wound not involving tendon, capsule, bone with infection and ischemia.	Wound penetrating to tendon or capsule with infection and ischemia.	Wound penetrating to bone or joint with infection and ischemia.

National Pressure Ulcer Advisory Panel (NPUAP)

NPUAP Pressure Ulcer Staging System

STAGE	DESCRIPTION
I	Nonblanchable erythema of intact skin
II	Partial-thickness skin loss involving epidermis and/or dermis
III	Full-thickness skin loss involving damage or necrosis of subcutaneous tissue that may extend to, but not through, underlying fascia
IV	Full-thickness skin loss with extensive destruction, tissue necrosis, or damage to muscle, bone, or supportive structures

PEDIS: Diabetic Foot Ulcer Classification

	P	E	D	I	S	
Grade	Perfusion	Extent	Depth	Infection	Sensation	Score
1	No PAD	Skin intact	Skin intact	None	No loss	0
2	PAD, no CLI	<1 cm²	Superficial	Surface	Loss	1
3	CLI	<1–3 cm²	Fascia, muscle, tendon	Abscess, fasciitis, septic arthritis		2
4		>3 cm²	Bone or joint	SIRS		3

PAD, peripheral arterial dz; CLI, critical limb ischemia; SIRS, systemic inflammatory response syndrome.

Record a score for each column. Add up the score and this is the PEDIS score. The higher the score, the worse the prognosis for healing the ulcer.

SVS WIFI WOUND CLASSIFICATION

The Society for Vascular Surgery (SVS) developed a wound classification system that took into account not just the wound size but also ischemia and infection—WIfI (Wound, Ischemia, and foot Infection). This classification system is widely used by vascular surgeons.

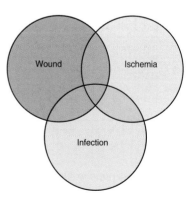

Wound Grade		Ischemia Grade		Infection Grade	
0	No wound	0	TP >60 mm Hg ABI >0.8 ASP >100 mm Hg	0	No symptoms or signs of infection
1	Small, shallow ulcer No exposed bone, unless limited to distal phalanx No gangrene	1	TP >40–59 mm Hg ABI 0.6–0.79 ASP 70–100 mm Hg	1	Local infection involving only skin and the subcutaneous tissue
2	Deeper ulcer with exposed bone, joint, or tendon, not involving tissue heel Shallow heel ulcer without calcaneal involvement Gangrene limited to digits	2	TP 30–39 mm Hg ABI 0.4–0.59 ASP 50–70 mm Hg	2	Local infection with erythema > 2 cm or involving structure deeper than skin and subcutaneous tissues- (e.g., abscess osteomyelitis)
3	Extensive, deep ulcer involving forefoot/midfoot Deep, full-thickness heel ulcer and/or calcaneal involvement Extensive gangrene involving forefoot/midfoot Full-thickness heel necrosis and, calcaneal involvement.	3	TP <30 mm Hg ABi <0.39 ASP <50 mm Hg	3	Local infection with signs of SIRS

ABI, ankle–brachial index; ASP, ankle systolic pressure; SIRS , systematic inflammatory response syndrome; Tp, toe pressure.
If ABI and TP result in different grades, TP is recommended to determine grade.

Estimate risk of amputation at 1 year for each combination

	Ischemia—0				Ischemia—1				Ischemia—2				Ischemia—3			
W-0	VL	VL	L	M	VL	L	M	H	L	L	M	H	L	M	M	H
W-1	VL	VL	L	M	VL	L	M	H	L	M	H	H	M	M	H	H
W-2	L	L	M	H	M	M	H	H	M	H	H	H	H	H	H	H
W-3	M	M	H	H	H	H	H	H	H	H	H	H	H	H	H	H
	fl-0	fl-1	fl-2	fl-3	fl-0	fl-1	fl-2	fl-3	fl-0	fl-1	fl-2	fl-3	fl-0	fl-1	fl-2	fl-3

fl = foot infection; H = high-risk; L = low-risk; M = moderate-risk; VL = very low-risk; W = wound

Estimate likelihood of benefit of/requirement for revascularization

	Ischemia—0				Ischemia—1				Ischemia—2				Ischemia—3			
W-0	VL	VL	VL	VL	VL	L	L	M	L	L	M	M	M	H	H	H
W-1	VL	VL	VL	VL	L	M	M	M	M	H	H	H	H	H	H	H
W-2	VL	VL	VL	VL	M	M	H	H	H	H	H	H	H	H	H	H
W-3	VL	VL	VL	VL	M	M	M	H	H	H	H	H	H	H	H	H
	fl-0	fl-1	fl-2	fl-3	fl-0	fl-1	fl-2	fl-3	fl-0	fl-1	fl-2	fl-3	fl-0	fl-1	fl-2	fl-3

fl = foot infection; H = high-risk; L = low-risk; M = moderate-risk; VL = very low-risk; W = wound

Other less popular ulcer classifications include:
DUSS (Diabetic Ulcer Severity Score)
SINBAD (Site, Ischemia, Neuropathy, BActerial infection, Dept)

Amit Jain's Classification
Slough—moist, yellow or tan, thin, stringy or mucinous consistency shedding of cells
Exudate—fluid leakage from tissue

ULCER EXAMINATION

TIME

TIME is an acronym for a wound care clinical decision support tool to help guide wound bed preparation, dressing selection, and wound management.

T is for Tissue

Both in and around the wound. Epithelial, granulating, slough, necrosis, black, beefy red

I is for Infection/Inflammation

Any open area always has the potential for infection.

M is for Moisture (Exudate)

This determines the type of dressing needed to maintain balance.

E is for Edges

Are they contracted, rolling, undermining?

Ulcer Description Terminology

Boggy—abnormal texture of tissues from high fluid content presenting as spongy and mushy.

Slough—moist, yellow or tan, thin, stringy or mucinous consistency shedding of cells. Liquified or wet dead tissue. Yellow or white tissue that adheres to the ulcer bed in strings or thick clumps, or in mucinous.

Exudate—fluid leakage from tissue

Types: Serous—clear, amber, thin, and watery

Fibrinous—cloudy and thin, with strands of fibrin

Serosanguineous—clear, pink, thin, and watery

Sanguineous—reddish, thin, and watery

Seropurulent—yellow or tan, cloudy, and thick

Purulent—opaque, milky, sometimes green

Hemopurulent—reddish, milky, and viscous

Hemorrhagic—red, thick

Granulation—new red connective tissue

Erythema—redness of skin

Eschar—A black necrotic tissue that may be either soft or hard. Dead tissue that sheds of falls off. Usually brown or black. Black, brown, or tan tissue that adheres firmly to the wound bed or ulcer edges, may be softer or harder that surrounding skin.

Blanching—Skin turns white when palpated firmly

Tunneling—A narrow opening or passageway extending through soft tissue, resulting in a dead space that can develop into an abscess. Also called a *sinus tract*.

Undermining—The destruction of underlying tissue surrounding the wound margins

Dehiscence—Separation or splitting open of layers of a surgical wound

Kennedy terminal ulcer (Kennedy ulcer)—A skin wound that appears in some patients during their final weeks of life. The exact cause is unknown, but organ failure may be a factor. They differ from pressure ulcers in that they develop over hours vs. days with a pressure ulcer.

Wounds should be at least 30% smaller by week 4 to consider on a healing trajectory.

Proper Wound Measuring Technique

Measure the longest length and then the greatest width perpendicular to the longest length. If there is undermining, imagine a clock face over the wound with 12 o'clock being toward the head and 6 o'clock toward the toes. Describe the location of the undermining by the numbers on the clock. In this example, the undermining would be documented as extending to 7 o'clock.

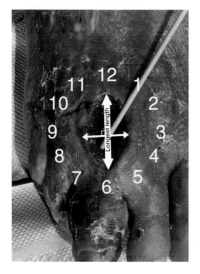

Systemic Signs

Rule out sepsis. Assess for fever, chills, sweats, lethargic, general malaise, and elevated pulses. Sepsis is a medical emergency, and patient should be admitted.

Vascular

Establish adequate perfusion. A toe systolic pressure of at least 30 mm Hg is required to heal a foot ulcer.

Neurologic

Establish adequate protective threshold. Semmes–Weinstein monofilament assesses sensory integrity. Gently press the monofilament perpendicular to the skin with enough pressure to cause the filament to bend.

Musculoskeletal

Assess bony prominences that may be the cause of ulcers.

Dermatologic

Assessing Ulcer

Depth (probe with Q-tip)
Diameter (measure)
Base (necrotic, granular, beefy red, macerated, fibrotic)
Margins (keratolytic, usually neuropathic in origin)
Drainage (purulent, clear, red, brown)
Odor (fecal smell—anaerobes; fruity [sickly sweet] smell— pseudomonas; ammonia-like smell—Proteus)

Assessing Surrounding Tissue

Temperature (warm to touch)
Erythema, note distribution and rate of progression (draw margins of erythema directly on skin). Rule out cellulitis and necrotizing fasciitis.
Edema, note pitting vs. nonpitting and extent
Lymphangitis/lymphadenopathy
Red streaks up leg
Tender palpable regional lymph nodes

Venous vs. Arterial Ulcers

	Arterial Ulcer	Venous Ulcer
Etiology	Arterial insufficiency	Venous insufficiency
Location	Distal toes, heels Lateral malleolus Areas of trauma	Medial malleolus Medial lower leg Areas of trauma
Pain	Severe, increases with elevation, decreases with dependence, intermittent claudication	Mild to moderate, relieved by elevation and compression
Drainage	Little to none	Moderate to heavy Venous weeping
Wound presentation	"Punched-out" deep round smooth ulcers Pale granulation tissue if present Gangrene	Shallow Irregular shape
Associated findings	Thin, shiny skin Loss of hair Thick yellow nails	Stasis dermatitis Hemosiderin deposits Cellulitis
Edema	No	Yes
Ulcer	Black eschar	Fibrous yellow or glossy coating over wound bed Ruddy granular tissue
Pulses	Decreased or absent	Normal or decreased due to edema

Diabetic Foot Infections

Most diabetic foot ulcers are polymicrobial (usually two to five mixed aerobic and anaerobic bacteria).

Bacterial count of $>10^5$ per g of tissue in a healthy adult can cause infection.

The most common organisms infecting superficial diabetic wounds are as follows:

Staphylococcus aureus
Staphylococcus epidermidis
Group A and B streptococci
Proteus spp.
Escherichia coli
Enterococcus
Klebsiella/Enterobacter spp.
Pseudomonas spp.
Bacteroides and other anaerobes

LABS

BACTERIAL BURDEN

Contamination: All chronic wounds are contaminated, which means they have nonreplicating microorganisms on the wound surface. These wounds heal in spite of the presence of bacteria.

Colonization: Colonization is the presence of replicating microorganisms within a wound, but their numbers are not sufficient to elicit a host response. Wounds can go on to heal, while they are actively colonized.

Critical colonization: A point where the bacterial burden has reached a point where the host is not able to maintain a healthy wound. The bacterial count at critical colonization is 10^5 colony-forming units per gram of tissue (100,000 viable organisms per gram of tissue). This is the "critical" point between colonization and infection. At this point, there are subtle, covert, signs of infection, such as absent or abnormal granulation, increased drainage, and increased pain.

Infection: With bacterial numbers $>10^5$, the wound is considered infected.

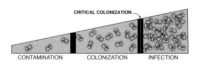

CONTAMINATION   COLONIZATION   INFECTION

Cultures

Levine swab technique: Cleanse/irrigate with saline, firmly press swab tip in cleanest portion of wound base, rotate 360°, transport media.

Culture and Sensitivity (C&S)

C&S consists of two parts:

Culture: Determines definitive identification of the organism, genus, and species. This is based on Gram stain, morphology, and biochemical profile. The Gram stain usually comes back first, which can help guide initial ABX therapy.

Sensitivity: Gives information on the best antibiotic to use. The sensitivity test consists of a minimal inhibitory concentration (MIC) of common antibiotics. The MIC is the lowest concentration (in µg/mL) of an antibiotic that inhibits the growth of a given strain of bacteria. Somewhat counterintuitive, but the lower the MIC, the more effective the antibiotic. Results show as either S (sensitive), I (intermediate), or R (resistant) followed by the MIC in µg/ml. "Intermediate" drugs may still be used but will require higher concentrations. They should only be used as a second choice if there are allergies to "sensitive" antibiotics. Resistant antibiotics are of no use.

Blood cultures (when sepsis is suspected)

Blood cultures require three samples, each from a different location or from the same spot 10 minutes apart. Best to obtain blood when the patient is spiking a fever.

Blood Tests

CBC With Diff

WBC $>10,000$ indicates an infection.

An acute infection will show an increase in immature leukocytes called a *left shift*.

Check for anemia, which is often associated with diabetic infection.

ESR and C-Reactive Protein
Used to follow progression and regression of infection

Hemoglobin A1C
Determines long-term control of diabetes

Glucose
Hyperglycemia, despite using the normal dose of insulin, may indicate an infection.
Values >250 mg per dL have a negative effect on wound healing.

Types of Debridement
Surgical (Sharp) Debridement
Sharp or surgical procedure that is mostly selective, causing little or no damage to healthy tissue. Performed with a scalpel or curette. Debridement turns a chronic wound into an acute wound. SELECTIVE

Mechanical Debridement
Nonselective procedure performed by changing wet-to-dry gauze dressings or hydrotherapy. As the gauze is removed, necrotic tissue comes along with it; drainage and debris are stuck to the dressing. NONSELECTIVE

Enzymatic or Chemical Debridement
A process requiring topical exogenous enzymes capable of degrading eschar, protein, and other nucleic agents (collagenase [Santyl]). MOST SELECTIVE

Autolytic Debridement
The body's own phagocytic debridement, which is encouraged by a moist occlusive dressing such as hydrogel. SELECTIVE

THREE PHASES OF WOUND HEALING
Inflammatory Phase (Injury to 2 to 5 days)
Also known as substrate phase, lag phase
Influx of platelets and leukocytes
Release of cytokines and mediators
Coagulation

Proliferative Phase (2 days to 3 weeks)
Also known as fibroblastic phase, repair phase
Collagen fibers are produced (fibroplasia), causing wound contraction and strength.
Reepithelialization (some describe epithelialization as a separate phase between proliferation and remodeling)
Epithelialization, angiogenesis, granulation

Remodeling Phase
Also known as maturation phase
3 weeks to 2 years
Deposition of matrix materials
Collagen deposition and remodeling
Return to preinjury state
As long as the scar or past ulcer site is erythematous, remodeling is occurring.

COLLAGEN
Collagen is a fibrous protein produced by fibroblasts that make

up connective tissue. It is the most abundant protein in the body. It provides structural support to cells and tissues. There are over 20 types.

Type I: Type I collagen is the strongest and the most abundant type of collagen found in the body. Approximately 90% of the body's collagen is type I. Type I collagen is the major component of extracellular matrix in skin and the primary collagen in a healing wound. Bones are also made of type I collagen and everything that attaches to the bone: ligaments, tendons, and menisci. A genetic defect in type I collagen is the cause of osteogenesis imperfecta and a form of Ehlers–Danlos syndrome.

Type II: Type II collagen is found in hyaline cartilage. Approximately 95% of hyaline cartilage is type II. A genetic defect in type II collagen will result in spondyloepiphyseal dysplasia (SED).

If hyaline cartilage is damaged, it cannot regenerate; however, it can be replaced by fibrocartilage. Fibrocartilage development is encouraged by subchondral drilling. This subchondral drilling causes the underlying bone to develop fibrocartilage using its type I collagen. Therefore, fibrocartilage is composed of mostly of type II collagen.

Type III: (10% to 20%) Found in the blood vessels and the skin. Seen in early phases of wound healing. Normally present in skin, becomes more prominent and important during wound healing. A type III collagen defect is responsible for a form of Ehlers–Danlos syndrome. Plantar fibromatosis and Dupuytren contracture are conditions where type I collagen is replaced by type III collagen.

Type IV: Found in the lungs and tissue around heart and intestines. Main component of basement membrane together with the lamina.

NOTE: Ehlers–Danlos syndrome is a group of inherited connective tissue disorders that results from a defect in synthesis of either type I, III, or V collagen.

OSTEOMYELITIS

Osteomyelitis is a bone infection. Definitive diagnosis requires a bone biopsy. Some clinicians consider any exposed bone to be clinical osteomyelitis.

Infectious Organisms in Bone	
Osteomyelitis in...	Most Common Organism
Healthy adults and children	*S. aureus*
Drug addicts	*Pseudomonas*
Sickle cell disease	*Salmonella*
Cat or dog bites	*Pasteurella*

Bone Becomes Infected by One of Three Ways

Hematogenous—enters bone via the bloodstream (most common)

Contiguous—spread from adjacent soft tissue

Direct inoculation—trauma or surgical

Acute Osteomyelitis

Occurs from the time the bone becomes infected until the portions of the bone become necrotic. The earliest radiographic signs of osteomyelitis are usually osteolysis, cortical erosions, and periosteal reaction.

Chronic Osteomyelitis

Involves necrotic bone. Once a chronic osteomyelitis develops, antibiotics alone are rarely effective and must be combined with surgical debridement of necrotic bone.

X-Rays

Take on initial presentation to use as a baseline for osteomyelitis. Bony changes take about 2 weeks to show up on x-ray after there has been a 50% loss of bone. Osteomyelitis usually initially presents as osteolysis along with periosteal reaction and cortical erosions. Soft-tissue swelling should be evaluated along with gas in the tissues.

As osteomyelitis progresses, areas of both osteolucency and sclerosis may develop along with gross remodeling of bone.

A *sequestrum* is a complication of osteomyelitis, where a portion of dead bone becomes separated from the surrounding bone and is found "floating" within an area of necrosis and resorbed bone. Over time, the sequestrum may become encased in a cloak of living bone formed from periosteal reaction called an *involucrum*. An opening may develop in the involucrum, allowing the necrotic purulent material out of the bone. This opening is called a *cloaca*. If the cloaca extends to skin, it is called a *sinus tract*.

Diagram:

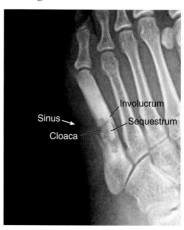

Involucrum—thickened periosteum
Sequestrum—dead bone
Cloaca—pus-filled space where the sequestrum resides
Sinus tract—opening to the outside

Brodie Abscess

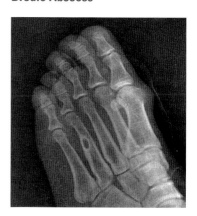

A form of *subacute osteomyelitis* without involucrum and usually with no sequestrum. A Brodie abscess is usually found in the metaphysis of long bones. A Brodie abscess is essentially a mild form of osteomyelitis due to decreased organism virulence. The infection becomes walled off by reactive bone and may remain dormant for years or indefinitely. Radiographically, it takes the form of a radiolucent cavity surrounded by dense sclerotic bone and fibrous tissue. Often misdiagnosed as an osteoid osteoma. Most commonly occurs in the tibia. This condition may be subclinical on examination, and patients may be asymptomatic or have only mild local pain.

Bone Scans

Tc-99 bone scan is positive in all phases, especially the third phase, which is highly sensitive for osteomyelitis. In most cases, bone scans are positive within 48 to 72 hours of infection.

MRI

Most specific and most sensitive modality for diagnosing osteomyelitis. Can detect osteomyelitis as early as 3 to 5 days after the onset of infection.

Treatment

Patients presenting with gas in the tissue, necrotizing fasciitis, or overt clinical signs of infection such as fever, chills, and streaking up the leg should be considered a medical emergency. These situations require the patient to be admitted to the hospital and prompt surgical intervention and/or antibiotic therapy. Antibiotic treatment for osteomyelitis should continue for at least 6 weeks. Antibiotics alone, for osteomyelitis, may be effective if started in the acute phase. Chronic osteomyelitis involving necrosis of bone requires surgical excision. Dead bone has no blood flow, and the antibiotics cannot reach it.

Surgery involves I&D, with excision of infected bone. In the foot, this may require partial amputation. All necrotic materials should be cut out along with drainage of any abscess. Following I&D, the surgical site is packed and left open to drain. If the entire infected site has been removed, as with an amputation, the site may be primarily closed. In instances where the entire infected site has been removed via amputation, postoperative antibiotics may not be required. Deep cultures should be taken intraoperatively. Vascular status should be assessed to assure adequate healing. Vascular status may dictate the level of amputation.

Antibiotic Beads

Following surgical I&D for osteomyelitis, antibiotic impregnated beads can be used in conjunction with other therapy. Antibiotic-impregnated beads are made from bone cement, which is composed of polymethylmethacrylate (PMMA). The bone cement is mixed intraoperatively from a kit containing powdered polymer and a liquid monomer to form a solid structure. As the mixture hardens, the beads are made by hand or with a mold.

During the process of making PMMA beads, antibiotics can be mixed with the beads. PMMA heats up as it hardens, so the antibiotics must be heat stable. Heat-stable antibiotics include;

Aminoglycosides (tobramycin, gentamicin)

β-Lactam antibiotics (cephalosporins, meropenem)

Vancomycin

Ticarcillin

Antibiotics are mixed into the PMMA, and the cement is rolled into pea-sized balls and packed in the surgical site. The beads are usually strung together on a piece of nylon suture in a "string of pearls" manner before insertion. This makes them easier to remove at a later date. The number of beads inserted should be counted and put in the operative report; so when they are removed, the surgeon knows how many to look for.

The amount of antibiotics used varies widely but generally 2 to 4 g of antibiotics per 40 g of cement. There are also commercially available antibiotic beads that come with the antibiotics already in the set, and there are also biodegradable (calcium sulfate) antibiotic beads available.

Antibiotic beads can achieve 200 times the antibiotic concentration achieved with IV administration. Beads are closed in the wound primarily and removed 2 to 4 weeks later. Antibiotic beads can be left in much longer, but in theory after all the antibiotics have leached out of the cement, the beads themselves become a place for bacteria to hide and multiply.

CHARCOT FOOT

General

A destructive arthropathy resulting from *impaired pain perception* and *increased bone blood flow* from reflex vasodilation. With increased bone blood flow, the bone becomes washed out and weak, and with impaired deep pain sensation on proprioception, small periarticular fractures go unnoticed until the entire joint is destroyed. Diabetes is the leading cause of Charcot foot. The majority of Charcot joints are the result of trauma and impaired sensation caused by neuropathy. Male-to-female ratio is equal, and it is bilateral in 30% of cases. Painless swelling is the hallmark sign of Charcot foot; however, about half of the patients present with a chief complaint of pain. Most feet with Charcot joint involve the midfoot.

Cause

Diabetes, alcoholism, syphilis, Hansen dz, syringomyelia, cerebral palsy, hereditary insensitivity to pain, myelodysplasia, poliomyelitis, spina bifida, meningomyelocele, spinal or peripheral nerve injury

Stages

Stage I (fragmentation)
  Acute inflammatory process
  Foot is hyperemic, swollen, red, and hot.
  Dissolution, fragmentation, and dislocation
Stage II (coalescence)
  Beginning of the reparative process
  Decreased edema, warmth and redness
  Radiographically, there are signs of new bone formation.
Stage III (remodeling)
  Marked by bony consolidation and healing
  Residual bony deformity is common, most notably collapse of the longitudinal arch resulting in the classic "rocker-bottom" foot.

Bony protuberances are clinically important because they may develop sites for future neuropathic pressure ulcers.

Treatment

Patients should be instructed to remain totally non–weight bearing immediately upon diagnosis to prevent further bone destruction. Treatment for Charcot foot also includes rest, elevation, and cast immobilization. Once bony consolidation has begun and the foot has stabilized, a custom-molded accommodative insert is indicated or a pair of custom-molded shoes depending on the extent of the deformity. Surgery on the Charcot foot is aimed at removing either bony prominences or arthrodesis to realign and stabilize the architecture of the foot.

TYPES OF WOUND CLOSURE

Primary closure	Wound is immediately sutured; must be a clean wound. Results in a pleasing linear scar.
Secondary closure/intension	Infected or dirty wounds are left open and allowed to granulate in from the bottom up; results in a less pleasing scar.
Delayed primary closure	Infected or dirty wound is left open until immediate threat of infection has passed (days to weeks) and then later the wound is closed primarily with sutures.

WOUND DRESSING

Primary Dressing

Comes in direct contact with wound

Secondary Dressing

Placed over primary dressing to improve protection

Nonadherent Dressings

These are mesh gauze dressings that are impregnated with petroleum to prevent them from sticking to the ulcer site during dressing change.

Adaptic—gauze with petroleum impregnated

Xeroform—gauze with petroleum impregnated and 3% bismuth tribromophenate. The bismuth adds a bacteriostatic component to the dressing.

Dressings From Least Absorptive to Most Absorptive

Wound dressings in order of their ability to absorption drainage

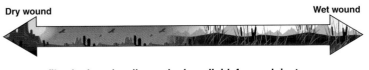

Dry wound   **Wet wound**

film, hydrogel, collagen, hydrocolloid, foam, alginate
Less absorptive   *More absorptive*

Film

Composed of a thin transparent adhesive polyurethane membrane. Provides a moist wound healing environment by trapping moisture. Should not be used on exudative wounds because it holds no properties to absorb wound drainage. Commonly used to cover IV catheters and as a post-op dressing. Also useful for minor burns, simple injuries, and treatment of superficial pressure area. Examples include OpSite and Tegaderm.

Hydrogel

Hydrogels are indicated for dry wounds where rehydration of eschar is desired. Also useful in deeper wounds where structures such as tendons need to be kept moist.

Hydrocolloid

Hydrocolloid dressings are designed to maintain a moist wound environment while absorbing excess drainage and exudate. They come as a flexible, waterproof, self-adhesive wafer that, when combined with water (exudate), forms a soft gel mass. Hydrocolloid dressings are made from materials such as gelatin or pectin that contain hydrocolloid granules or powder. Available as free granules or attached to polyurethane foam or film backing. Examples include DuoDerm.

Foam

Foam dressings have a very high absorbency and can be used on infected wounds. They maintain a moist wound environment, but if a wound has too little exudate, the wound can dry out. Foam dressings also raise the core temperature of the wound.

Alginate

Alginates are a highly absorbent dressing made from seaweed that osmotically dries out wounds. They also have a hemostatic effect and are used at donor sites postsurgically and other bleeding areas.

Enzymatic Debriders

Enzymatically debrides necrotic tissue from the wound

Panafil, Collagenase, Santyl, Accuzyme

Growth Factors

Growth factors incorporated into gel

Procuren, Regranex

Bioengineered Dressings

Apligraf, Dermagraft, SIS graft, Mediskin

Silver Dressings

Silver has been used for years in various forms of wound treatment. It has broad antimicrobial activity, including MRSA and VRE.

Acticoat, Sulfadiazine cream, Polymem Silver, Actisorb Plus

Negative-Pressure Wound Therapy (NPWT)

A type of closed active drain system. It has been shown to improve wound profusion. NPWT decreases interstitial edema, stimulates fibroplasia, and enhances angiogenesis. A pressure of −125 mm Hg increases micro-vascular blood flow and is the optimal pressure. Pressures > −400 mm Hg inhibits blood flow and should not be used. The recommended pressure for use over a skin graft is lower, −65 to −75 mm Hg.

PRESSURE ULCERS

Pressure ulcers are also called *bed-sores or decubitus ulcers.* They are an area of unrelieved pressure over a defined area. Pressure to the tissue causes ischemia and necrosis. Ischemia occurs after 2 to 6 hours of unrelieved pressure, and necrosis occurs after 6 hours of continuous pressure. Patients at risk for pressure ulcers should be turned or re-positioned every 2 hours. (NOTE: This is the same length of time tour-niquets can be inflated.)

The most common sites for pressure ulcers are the occiput, scapula, elbows, sacrum, trochan-ter, ischium, and heels. The ischium is the most common pressure sore found in wheelchair-bound pa-tients. The sacrum is the most com-mon site for bedridden patients in the prone position and the trochan-ter for the lateral position.

Stages of Pressure Ulcers

Stage I	Nonblanchable erythema, epidermis intact
Stage II	Partial-thickness loss of skin involving the epidermis and possibly into the dermis
Stage III	Full-thickness destruction into subcutaneous tissue
Stage IV	Deep tissue destruction extending to fascia, muscle, bone

FORMAL ASSESSMENT TOOLS
Norton Scale

A risk assessment evaluation form is used to estimate a patient's risk for developing pressure ulcers. The patient is rated from 1 to 4 on five different factors (physical condi-tion, mental condition, activity, mo-bility, and incontinent). A score of ≤14 indicates high risk.

Low/no risk	≥18
Medium risk	14–18
High risk	10–14
Very high risk	≤10

Braden Scale

A risk assessment evaluation form is used to estimate a patient's risk for developing pressure ulcers. The patient is rated from 1 to 3 or 4 on six different categories (sensory perception, moisture, activity, mo-bility, nutrition, and friction/shear). Score can range from 6 to 23. A score of ≤12 indicates high risk.

Low/no risk	≥19
At risk	15–18
Moderate risk	13–14
High risk	10–12
Very high risk	≤9

AMPUTATIONS
Metatarsophalangeal Amputation

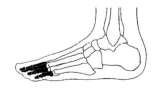

Transmetatarsal Amputation

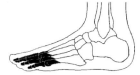

Lisfranc Amputation

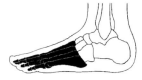

Chopart Amputation

In addition to Achilles tenotomy, the tibialis anterior tendon is reattached through a drill hole in the neck of the talus to prevent equinovarus deformity.

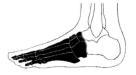

Syme Amputation

Flaps should be planned such that the WB surface is sensate skin.
Use a drain.
Two-stage Syme amputation
Performed when there is an infection
Same as one-step Syme amputation but split into two steps
    Stage I: After the talus and calcancus are removed, the void is temporarily packed and partially sutured with retention sutures.
    Stage II: Performed 3 to 5 days later when the immediate threat of infection has decreased. The malleoli and distal tibia are resected, and the procedure is completed.

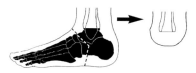

Variations of the Syme Procedure

Both use a piece of the calcaneus to maintain limb length.

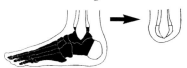

Pirogoff Amputation

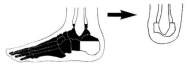

Boyd Amputation

COMPRESSION THERAPY

Compression therapy is contraindicated in patients with an ABI of <0.8.

Stockings (Jobst, TED, Sigvaris)

Type of Stocking	Pressure (mm Hg)	Uses
Antiembolism stockings	16–18	DVT prophylaxis
Low compression stockings	18–24	Nonambulatory patients
Low-to-moderate compression stockings	25–35	Edema secondary to venous insufficiency
Moderate compression stocking	30–40	Edema with or without ulcer
High compression stocking	40–50	Severe venous insufficiency, lymphedema

Four-Layer Bandage (Profore)

Provides a graduated sustained compression using four layers of bandage. If applied correctly, the bandages start with 40 mm Hg at the ankle and decrease to 17 mm Hg at the calf.

Unna Boot

An Unna Boot is a soft compression dressing often applied to the foot and ankle. The active ingredients in an Unna boot is zinc oxide that helps ease skin irritation and keeps lesions moist. Zinc oxide is also the active ingredient in calamine lotion and some Unna boots are pink from the calamine lotion. They are commonly used for diabetic ulcers, burns, and swelling.

Compression Pump

A programmable leg sleeve is periodically inflated and "milks" edema from the leg.

OFFLOADING

Total Contact Cast

TCC has long been considered the gold standard for offloading diabetic foot ulcers. TCCs consist of a well-molded cast that maintains contact with the entire plantar aspect of the foot and lower leg. Body weight is redistributed over a larger surface area, resulting in alleviating pressure from the ulcer site. Although they are excellent for offloading, they are difficult and time-consuming to apply and have very low reimbursement.

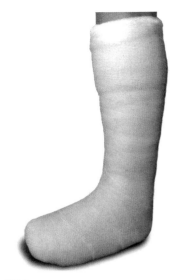

iTCC

Instant total contact cast. An instant total contact cast basically consists of a CAM walking boot with cast material wrapped around it to prevent removal and force compliance.

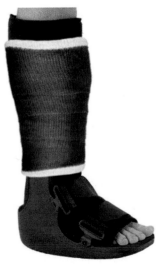

Football Dressing

A football dressing is a bulky dressing used in lieu of a total contact cast (TCC) as an offloading modality for neuropathic plantar foot ulcers. It consists of about three rolls of 4-inch cast padding, one roll of 4-inch gauze, and one roll of 4-inch Coban.

Felted Foam Dressing

Foam and felt are applied directly to the entire bottom of the foot with a cut out for the ulcer. A secondary dressing is applied, and the patient is put in a post-op shoe.

Prefabricated Walker

Also known as a CAM (controlled ankle motion) walking boot. They were originally designed to treat fractures and sprains but are often used, along with padding, as offloading treatment for diabetic ulcers.

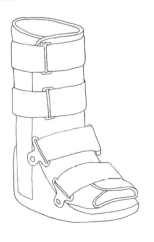

Ossur Active Offloading Walker

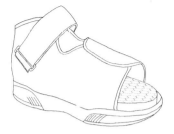

Very similar to the prefabricated walker, except that the floor of the device has small removable octagonal ulcer cushion pieces to accommodate ulcerations

Bledsoe Boot

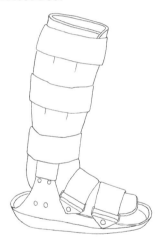

There are several different types, but they are all designed to replace TCCs for the treatment of ulcerative or preulcerative conditions of the bottom of the foot. Appears very similar to a prefabricated walker, but the foot plate of the boot is designed to function more like a TCC. The special insoles are designed to evenly distribute body weight across the entire bottom and sides of the foot to mimic a TCC.

IPOS Shoe

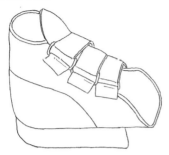

IPOS (Integrated Prosthetic and Orthotic System) shoes are a wedge shoe designed for forefoot ulcerations. They are a half-shoe, with 10° dorsiflexion and a 4-cm lift. Nothing touches the forefoot. A walker is recommended to assist in the stability for this shoe.

Orthowedge Shoe

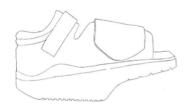

Orthowedge shoes are wedge shoes designed for forefoot ulcerations. Similar to the IPOS shoe, but the sole extends to the toes. Wedge in sole to relieve forefoot pressure. A walker is recommended to assist in the stability for this shoe.

Reverse IPOS

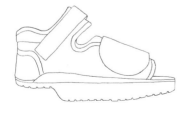

Reverse IPOS shoes are designed for heel ulcerations. The shoe design is open at the back and angled in 10° plantar flexion. A walker is recommended to assist in stability for this shoe.

Charcot Restraint Orthotic Walker (CROW) Boot

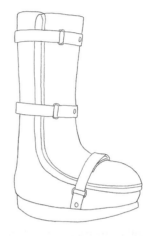

A total contact custom orthotic with a rocker-bottom sole. Also called a *Clamshell* or *bivalved AFO* (BAFO). It is essentially a removable TCC. Excellent for diabetic foot ulcers and designed to accommodate and support a Charcot foot. May be used during the second and third stages of Charcot.

MABAL Shoes

A fiberglass cast of the foot with padding inside that can be taken off and on like a shoe. Main advantage is that it allows ankle motion.

Healing Sandal

The Healing Sandal, also called the *Carville Sandal*, is a custom-molded accommodative orthotic made from

Plastazote, which is then made into a sandal or placed in a surgical shoe.

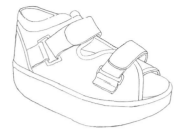

Ankle Contracture Boot

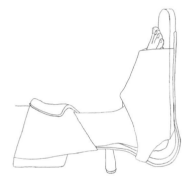

Also called *L'Nard Splints* or *Multi Podus Boots.* They are used to treat equinus deformities that develop in bedridden patients. They are also designed to alleviate pressure from the heel by suspending the foot. It is intended for patients who are mostly bedridden. There is a swing-out antirotational bar and height-adjustable footplate that prevents pressure from bedding on the toes.

Football Dressing

A football dressing relies on volume of padding to protect the foot. Several bulky layers of cast padding are applied dorsally on the foot and wrapped over the distal aspect of the toes onto the plantar foot. This is held in place with a second bulky circumferential wrapping of cast padding around the foot and then anchored around the ankle. This is then held in place with Coban or an Ace wrap.

DIABETIC EDUCATION

Wear soft moldable uppers (always with socks).
Break new shoes in slowly by wearing only 2 hours at a time initially.
Buy shoes at the end of the day when feet are most swollen.
Avoid socks with mends and seams.
Feel inside shoes for seams or folds.
Avoid pads or devices not custom made.
Avoid constrictive bandages.
Never place bandaged foot in closed shoe.
Proper nail care.
Nightly inspection of feet including between toes.
Inspect inside of shoe for sharps.
Never go barefoot.
Avoid open-toed or open-backed shoes.
Never trim callus.
Beware of tapes, adhesives on risk areas.
Check bath temperature with elbow.
Protect feet from sunburn.
Beware of hard floors.
Beware of corn remedies.
Never use OTC corn remedies.
Dry feet completely, especially between toes.
Buy shoes with a good fit (excessive width or length can lead to friction, causing blistering and ulceration).

High toe box and a rounded toe (to accommodate HT, orthotics, and HM).

Rigid counter to support heel.

Wide toe box with extra depth.

Rigid shank to support arch.

Soft insert to accommodate any plantar lesions.

No cracks or breaks in the inserts or seams.

Apply a light water-based lotion daily without moistening between the toes.

Refrain from applying adhesive tape or chemical agents for removing corns/callus.

Patients with impaired vision should have a family member inspect their feet daily.

Professional nail care with regular follow-ups.

HYPERBARICS

Hyperbaric oxygen treatment (HBO) has been shown to be an effective treatment in hypoxic ulcers (i.e., ulcers due to diabetes or arterial insufficiency). Repeated dives in the chamber over a period of time increase the oxygen concentration in the blood. As a result, angiogenesis and fibroblast production occurs, which help collagen synthesis and epithelial closure. During the HBO treatment and for 3 to 4 hours after treatment, the O_2 is dissolved in the plasma to help oxygenate the hypoxic area. This elevates the O_2 levels surrounding the ulcer site to speed the healing time.

Patients who will benefit from hyperbarics must have a serious problem with their oxygen gradient in the tissue around the ulcer. This oxygen gradient is quantified in a measurement called *transcutaneous oxygen monitor* (TCOM). TCOM uses a series of electrodes adjacent to the patient's wound to measure the oxygen tension in periwound tissue. A normal value is 50 mm Hg. If the TCOM reading is $<$30 to 40, the patient has a problem involving oxygen transport that is serious enough to consider hyperbaric oxygen therapy.

If TCOMs are low, a trial hyperbaric oxygen treatment is performed at 2.4 atm of 100% oxygen. TCOMs are measured again in the hyperbaric oxygen environment. If hyperbaric therapy is going to help the patient, the TCOMs should rise from 30 to 40 to over 200.

Patients are typically placed in the hyperbaric chambers between 2 and 2.4 atm of 100% oxygen for 90 minutes. Treatment does not generally exceed 90 minutes because 100% oxygen can cause convulsions and oxygen toxicity. The peak effects of hyperbarics are between 18 and 23 dives, at which time TCOMs should improve as a result of angiogenesis.

Other indications for hyperbaric oxygen treatment include chronic refractory osteomyelitis, necrotizing infections, burns, crush injuries, compromised or failed flaps, and soft-tissue radionecrosis.

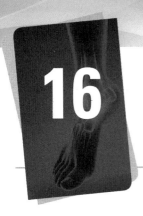

16 NAILS

NAIL ANATOMY

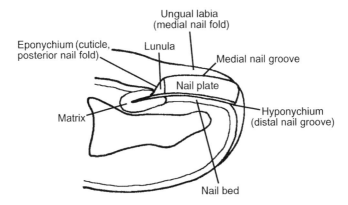

NAIL PATHOLOGY

Anonychia: Absence of nail. Describes a nail that has failed to develop.

Beau lines: Horizontal depression across a nail plate caused by transient arrest of nail growth.

Causes could include any stressful event such as MI, PE, or high fever.

Blue nails: Causes include antimalarial drugs, minocycline (a tetracycline), hemochromatosis (an iron metabolism disorder), Wilson dz, ochronosis (a metabolic disorder), and exposure to silver nitrate

Brown nail: Occurs in Addison dz, hemochromatosis, gold therapy, arsenic intoxication, malignant melanoma, and Nelson syndrome

Dystrophic nail: A nail disorder due to faulty nutrition

Gray nail or gray lunula: Occurs in argyria (prolonged ingestion, injection, or mucosal absorption of silver nitrate)

Green nail: *Pseudomonas* infection

Hapalonychia: A rubbery and pliable nail plate usually caused by hyperhidrosis or endocrine disorders

Herpetic whitlow: Usually severely painful herpetic (viral) infection of the distal phalanx. Erythematous streaking of the extremity and enlarged lymph nodes may be noted.

Hippocratic nails (clubbing): Positive clubbing is noted when the Lovibond angle is >180°. Lovibond angle is the angle between the nail plate and the proximal nail fold. Occurs in cardiac disease (cyanotic heart disease, bacterial endocarditis), pulmonary disease (primary and metastatic cancer, bronchiectasis, lung abscess, mesothelioma), or GI disease (enteritis, ulcerative colitis, and hepatic cirrhosis).

Intraungual hematoma: Hematoma within the body of the nail, due to trauma to the proximal nail fold. May take several weeks to develop because the nail must grow out.

Koilonychia (spoon nail): Seen in long-standing iron deficiency anemia or Plummer–Vinson syndrome (a combination of koilonychia, dysphagia, and glossitis primarily seen in middle-aged women). Also known as Plummer nails.

Leukonychia: Nails exhibiting white spots (punctata) and/or striata

Lindsay nail (half and half nails): The distal half is pink or brown and is sharply demarcated from the proximal half, which is dull and white and obliterates the lunula. Seen in liver disease and azotemia (uremia).

Macronychia: Abnormally large nail

Mees lines: Single transverse white band associated with arsenic poisoning. A variation of Beau lines can also be seen following stressful events.

Melanonychia: Pigmented longitudinal bands in the nails. Normal variant usually seen in darker skinned individuals.

Micronychia: Abnormally small nail

Muehrcke nails: Paired narrow horizontal white bands, separated by normal color, that remain immobile as the nail grows. Seen in hypoalbuminemia associated with nephrotic syndrome.

Onychatrophia: Atrophy of the nail

Onychauxis: Hypertrophy of the nail (thick nail)

Onychia: Inflammation of the matrix of the nail

Onychoclasis: Breaking of a nail

Onychocryptosis: Ingrown nail

Onychogenic: Producing nail substance

Onychogryphosis: A type of onychauxis (rams horn nail)

Onychoheterotopia: Abnormally placed nail on the digit as a result of displaced matrix material

Onycholysis: Separation of the nail plate from the nail bed. Begins distally and progresses proximally. Associated with many systemic diseases.

Onychomadesis: Separation of the nail from the nail bed, beginning proximally and progressing distally. Typically results in shedding of the nail. Seen in pemphigus vulgaris and hand, foot, and mouth disease.

Onychomalacia: Softening of the nail

Onychomycosis: Fungal nail

Onychophagia: Nail biting

Onychophosis: A callus in the nail groove

Onychopuntata: Pitting of the nails. Seen in psoriasis, alopecia areata, lichen planus

Onychorrhexis: Abnormal brittle nails with <16% water in nail. Normal nail hydration is between 16% and 30%.

Onychoschizia: Splitting or lamination of the nail plate into layers that flake off

Onychotillomania: Neurotic picking or tearing at the nail

Paronychia: Inflammation involving the folds of tissue around the nail

Pterygium: The overgrowth of cuticle. May be normal variant or caused by lichen planus, dermatomyositis, or scleroderma.

Racquet nail: A short fat nail

Red lunula: Right-sided CHF

Splinter hemorrhages: Seen in subacute bacterial endocarditis and trichinosis, which is a disease from eating inadequately cooked meet infected with *Trichinella spiralis*. Patients will also have diarrhea, nausea/vomiting, and fever.

Subungual hematoma: Associated with acute trauma (dropping something on the toe). Hematoma develops instantly beneath the nail plate. Often, there is severe pain from the pressure of the blood beneath the nail plate, which can lead to increased necrosis of tissue. Drilling a hole in the nail or avulsing the nail may be necessary to relieve pressure.

Telangiectatic posterior nail folds: Proximal nail fold becomes tortuous and dilated. Indicative of connective tissue disease (lupus and dermatomyositis).

Terry nails: Proximal 2/3 of the nail plate is white, whereas the distal 1/3 shows the red color of the nail bed. Seen in hypoalbuminemia associated with hepatic cirrhosis.

Yellow nail syndrome: Nails grow slow, thick, and with increased longitudinal curvature with some onycholysis. Usually associated with pulmonary disease and lymphedema.

CHEMICAL MATRIXECTOMY

Also called *phenol and alcohol matrixectomy* (P&A)

Standard foot prep and digital block are performed.

Tourniquet is applied (phenol must be applied to a bloodless field).

A 2- to 3-mm strip of nail is removed from the offending border.

Next, scrape the matrix epithelium with a small curette to further destroy matrix cells.

Three thirty-second applications of 89% phenol are applied to the nail matrix with an applicator.

Next, lavage the entire field with 70% isopropyl alcohol to flush the remaining phenol from the tissue.

10% sodium hydroxide can be used instead of phenol and lavage with acetic acid—success rate parallels phenol.

SURGICAL MATRIXECTOMIES

Partial Matrixectomies

Frost

An inverted "L" incision is made through the long axis of the nail and carried about 1/16 of an inch beyond the proximal and distal ends of the nail, being vertical in nature, and carried down to the periosteum. The base of the "L" is an incision just through the dermis down to, but not into, the nail root.

The base of the "L" becomes a skin flap, which is dissected free of the nail matrix and reflected.

The next incision is parallel to the first incision beneath the skin flap and becomes semielliptical distally to join the first incision.

The tissue sliver is dissected free of the periosteum and dissected proximally back onto the base of the phalanx until this portion of the nail root is freed.

The flap at the base is now reapproximated.

When the Frost technique was first described, no sutures were advised because it was thought to compromise blood flow.

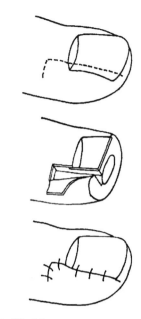

Modified Frost

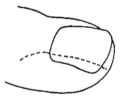

The procedure is basically the same as a Frost, except it involves altering the "L" flap to a curved incision.

Plastic Lip

Involves excision of a pie-shaped wedge of tissue taken from the side of the toe. Useful only in cases of hypertrophy of the ungualabia.

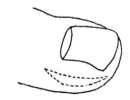

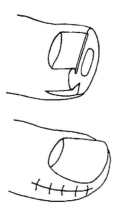

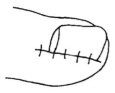

Total Matrixectomies

Kaplin

This is a modification of the Zadik.
Nail plate is avulsed.
Two incisions are made from the corners of the eponychium extending each nail groove proximally, forming a tissue flap (as in the Zadik).
The leading edge of the eponychium is trimmed.
The entire matrix is excised, along with the entire nail bed, down to the periosteum of the phalanx.
The incisions into the eponychium are sutured, but the exposed phalanx is left open and allowed to granulate in by secondary intention.

Winograd

A longitudinal incision is made through the nail and nail bed ~4 mm from the affected margin, then through the skin over the nail matrix and the matrix itself, extending 1 cm proximal to the eponychium.
A second incision is made in the skin at the nail fold, completing an ellipse with the first incision.
A wedge of tissue is then removed down to the periosteum, and the wound is curetted.
The edges are reapproximated and sutured.

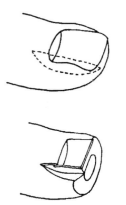

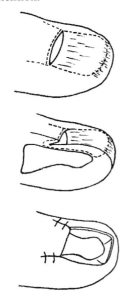

Suppan (Technique #2)

Nail is avulsed.

Using a blade, the entire matrix is excised down to periosteum in toto from under the eponychium without any skin incisions.

The posterior nail fold is then sutured to the proximal nail bed.

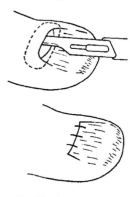

Syme (Lapidus)

An elliptical incision is made around the entire nail and nail bed (the proximal curve of the incision should be distal to the IPJ and the distal curve in a fish-mouth incision carried around the sides and across the tip of the toe).

The distal half of the distal phalanx is then cut so that the nail, nail bed, and the terminal half of the proximal phalanx are removed as a single unit.

The plantar flap is then pulled up over the remaining phalanx and sutured to the dorsal skin.

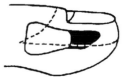

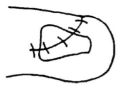

Whitney

Nail is avulsed.

Frost type incisions are made in the eponychium.

The flaps are undercut and retracted.

Leading edge of the eponychium is trimmed.

The central eponychium skin flap should now be freed and retracted proximally to expose the entire matrix.

A circumferential, transverse incision carried down to bone encompassing the lunula and entire matrix is made at this time.

This tissue is then freed of its attachments and removed.

The three skin flaps are then reapproximated and sutured; the eponychial flap is sutured to the proximal edge of the nail bed.

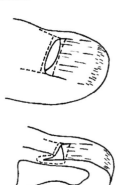

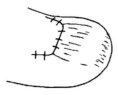

Zadik

Nail plate is avulsed.

Two incisions are made from the corners of the eponychium extending each nail groove proximally, forming a tissue flap.

The leading edge of the eponychium is trimmed.

A strip of tissue is excised from just distal to the lunula laterally into the nail folds and proximal ~3 to 5 mm under the proximal nail fold. The tissue to be excised should extend down to periosteum, and care should be taken to include the under surface of the proximal nail fold.

The proximal nail fold is then advanced distally where it meets the proximal end of the nail bed and is sutured.

If the lateral nail furrows are deep, Zadik advises excising the lateral nail folds and suturing them to the nail bed.

SUBUNGUAL EXOSTOSIS

A benign bony lesion, which protrudes from the dorsal surface of the distal phalanx. Most commonly seen in the hallux. This condition is usually painful and causes the nail to become deformed. Radiographs are often unhelpful as the protuberance may have a cartilaginous cap, which will not show on x-ray. Treatment of choice is excision of the lesion.

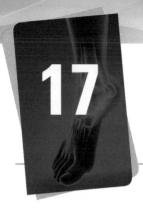

17

HEEL CONDITIONS

PLANTAR FASCIITIS (HEEL SPUR SYNDROME)

Description

Plantar fasciitis is a condition resulting in pain and inflammation of the plantar fascia. The plantar fascia, also called the *plantar aponeurosis*, is a thick band of connective tissue originating on the calcaneus and inserting into the ball of the foot. The plantar fascia is composed of three distinct structural components: the medial, central, and lateral bands. The medial band is a small slip of fascia that originates off the central band and overlies the abductor hallucis muscle. The central band comprises the majority of the plantar fascia and overlies the flexor digitorum brevis muscle.

The lateral band is a separate and distinct band that originates off the lateral process of the calcaneal tuberosity and overlies the abductor digiti minimi muscle.

Although pain may occur along the entire course of the plantar fascia, it is usually limited to the inferior medial aspect of the calcaneus, at the medial process of the calcaneal tubercle. Plantar fasciitis often presents as "first-step pain," which is pain when the patient first gets out of bed in the morning or gets up after periods of rest.

A heel spur may or may not be present but is rarely the source of the pain. The spur is actually located at the origin of the flexor digitorum brevis muscle, which is deep to the plantar fascia.

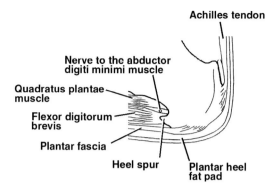

Achilles tendon

Nerve to the abductor digiti minimi muscle

Quadratus plantae muscle

Flexor digitorum brevis

Plantar fascia

Heel spur

Plantar heel fat pad

Causes

Causes include poor foot mechanics due to pes planus or pes cavus, obesity, inappropriate footwear, tight triceps surae, fat pad atrophy, and repetitive microtrauma.

Signs/Symptoms

Women more commonly affected than men (3:1)

Bilateral in 10% of cases

Described as a deep aching pain; feels like a stone bruise

Direct palpation of the medial calcaneal tuberosity often elicits pain.

Pain may be elicited by evoking the "windlass mechanism" with passive dorsiflexion of the MPJs.

Treatment

Conservative (90% of cases improve with nonsurgical treatment)

NSAIDs
  Low-dye strap
  Orthotics
  Avoid barefoot walking
  Decrease activity level
  Daily tendoachilles and plantar fascial stretching

Ice
Night splints
Corticosteroid injection
Therapeutic ultrasound
Short leg walking cast for 4 to 6 weeks
Surgical
  Plantar fasciotomy
  Orthotripsy

INFRACALCANEAL HEEL SPUR

Infracalcaneal heel spurs develop at the origin of the flexor digitorum brevis muscle, not at the origin of the plantar fascia. They are thought to be caused from poor foot mechanics, resulting in greater intrinsic muscle activity. This leads to excessive traction on the calcaneal tubercle. Over time, this enthesopathy leads to periostitis, and ultimately, a spur develops.

Conditions Producing Sharp Well-Defined Heel Spur

RA, may also be associated with a spur at the Achilles insertion with posterosuperior calcaneal erosions

Normal variants

DJD

Acromegaly

DISH, large well-defined spur irregular in outline. Spurs may also occur at the Achilles insertion.

Reiter syndrome

Conditions Producing Fluffy III-Defined Heel Spur

An ill-defined heel spur occurs with seronegative arthropathies as a result of enthesopathy.

Psoriasis

Reiter syndrome (reactive arthritis)

Ankylosing spondylitis

RA

Hyperparathyroidism

BAXTER NEURITIS

Often misdiagnosed as plantar fasciitis. The Baxter neuritis is an entrapment neuropathy of the first branch of the lateral plantar nerve. Also called the *nerve to the abductor digiti quinti muscle*. As compared with plantar fasciitis, there is usually pain after activity vs. first-step pain. Also, pain may be present on palpation of the medial aspect of the heel along the course of the nerve.

The nerve travels between the abductor hilluces and quadratus plantae muscles medially and between the flexor digitorum brevis and quadratus plantae muscles plantarly. Baxter neuritis develops when the nerve becomes compressed between the fascia of the abductor hallucis muscle and the

medial side of the quadratus plantae muscle. Conservative treatment is much the same as with plantar fasciitis, but if surgery is considered, the procedure of choice is neurolysis. Through a medial incision, bluntly dissect down to the superficial and deep fascia of the abductor hallucis muscle, perform a vertical incision through the abductor hallucis fascia, and remove a segment of tissue. Follow the nerve plantarly, and resect a portion of the plantar fascia. If a spur is present, resect it. The nerve is just superior to the spur.

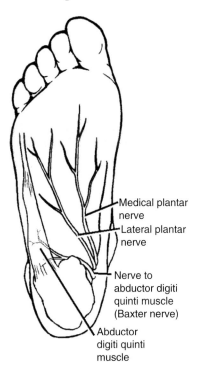

Medical plantar nerve

Lateral plantar nerve

Nerve to abductor digiti quinti muscle (Baxter nerve)

Abductor digiti quinti muscle

Baxter neuritis

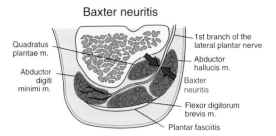

Quadratus plantae m.

Abductor digiti minimi m.

1st branch of the lateral plantar nerve

Abductor hallucis m.

Baxter neuritis

Flexor digitorum brevis m.

Plantar fasciitis

RETROCALCANEAL BONE SPUR

Also called *retrocalcaneal exostosis*. Usually occurs in middle-aged to elderly patients. Retrocalcaneal bone spurs occur at the insertion of the Achilles tendon and are often associated with intratendinous calcifications. Conservative treatment includes strengthening exercises, ROM exercises, and eccentric exercises. Surgical treatment involves excision of the spur, which requires at least partial detachment of the Achilles tendon.

CALCANEAL BURSITIS

Types

Subcutaneous Calcaneal Bursitis

Subcutaneous calcaneal bursa is an adventitious bursa. An adventitious bursa is a non-native bursa that develops over areas of repeated insult. In the heel, they develop posteriorly in the subcutaneous layer between the Achilles tendon and the skin. This bursa can often be palpated as a fluctuant mass just below the skin over the Achilles tendon. It is often associated with localized erythema and warmth.

Subtendinous Calcaneal Bursitis (Achillodynia, Albert Disease, Retrocalcaneal Bursitis, Anterior Achilles Bursitis)

Located between the Achilles tendon and the calcaneus. A diagnostic maneuver is to squeeze the back of the heel with the thumb and index finger just superior to the insertion of the Achilles tendon. With subtendinous calcaneal bursitis, this maneuver will elicit pain, and one can often feel fluid within the subtendinous bursa. This condition is often present as part of the sequela of Haglund deformity.

Bursitis develops in response to an area of repeated irritation or insult such as trauma, poorly fitting shoes, arthritis, or certain sports activities.

Treatment includes RICE, NSAIDs, padding, corticosteroid injections, and heel lifts.

HAGLUND DEFORMITY (PUMP BUMP)

A painful bony prominence at the posterior superior or posterior superior lateral aspect of the calcaneus above the insertion of the Achilles tendon. Also called a "pump bump." It is more common in females. The pain stems from an impingement of the Achilles tendon over the posterior superior aspect of the calcaneus. This impingement can occur due to an enlarged bony prominence at the posterior superior aspect of the calcaneus or from a high calcaneal inclination angle. Haglund deformity usually involves the retrocalcaneal bursa that is located just superior and anterior to the insertion of the Achilles, between the posterior superior calcaneus and the Achilles tendon. An adventitious bursa between the Achilles tendon and the skin may also develop. The most common cause is a high calcaneal inclination angle; thus, the condition is commonly seen with a cavovarus foot type.

Signs and Symptoms

Bony prominence at the posterior superior lateral aspect of the calcaneus
Pain (worse in shoes) and tenderness that worsen with activity
Radiographically, the Fowler–Philip angle, parallel pitch lines, calcaneal inclination angle, and the total angle of Ruch are all useful tools for diagnosing Haglund deformity.

Treatment

Conservative
    Heel lifts, to elevate the prominence above shoe counter
    RICE
    NSAIDs

Steroid injections, use caution around the Achilles tendon
Orthotics, to control rearfoot motion to prevent friction against shoes
Bursal aspiration
Surgical
Surgical correction involves excision of the bony prominence and removal of the inflamed bursa.
An alternative surgical technique is the Keck and Kelly osteotomy. This procedure effectively decompresses the posterior/superior aspect of the calcaneus without the need for dissection around the Achilles insertion.

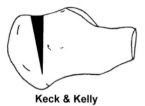

Keck & Kelly

CALCANEAL APOPHYSITIS

Calcaneal apophysitis is an inflammatory condition of the secondary calcaneal growth plate located at the posterior heel. The calcaneal apophysis serves as the attachment site for the Achilles tendon. As the gastrocnemius contracts, traction on the apophysis causes micromotion between the apophysis and the body of the calcaneus, resulting in inflammation and arthritic-type pain. Pain is located at the posterior aspect of the heel and is worse after activity. Calcaneal apophysitis is an overuse injury common in young athletes between the ages of 8 and 14 years. Causes usually involve overuse and stress most commonly from sports. The condition is usually self-limiting and goes away with rest or when the ossification center fuses. In extreme cases, the apophysis becomes necrotic and turns into Sever disease.

Treatment

RICE
NSAIDs
Physical therapy
Heel lefts

18 SOFT-TISSUE MASSES

FIBROUS TISSUE ORIGIN

Fibroma

Fibroma is a general term for a be-nign tumor composed of connec-tive tissue. They can grow almost anywhere in any organ, arising from mesenchyme tissue. When found in the soft tissue, they are generally self-limiting and present as painless, slow-growing, fairly well-demar-cated, firm, encapsulated tumors. There are many types of fibroma based on what other elements are involved (e.g., fibrolipoma, fibroker-atoma, angiofibroma, fibromyxoma, xanthofibroma, neurofibroma).

Surfer knob is a type of fibromas found on the dorsum of the feet or at the tibial tuberosity as a result of repeated physical trauma from a surfboard.

Fibrosarcoma

Extremely rare sarcoma that arises from fascial or aponeurotic struc-tures of the deep soft tissue. This should be ruled out when evaluat-ing plantar fibromatosis.

Dermatofibrosarcoma Protuberans (Darier Tumor)

A slow-growing cutaneous tumor of intermediate malignancy (can become metastatic)

Usually presents as a somewhat elevated, slightly protruding structure that is fixed to the skin and may have hyperpigmented and somewhat violaceous over-lying skin. Most commonly seen in patients aged 30 to 50 years. Males are affected more than females. Treatment involves excision with surrounding tissue; frozen sections may be necessary.

Periungual Fibroma

Periungual fibromas are benign fibrous tumors seen in and around the nail bed and nail folds. They are slow-growing flesh-colored, usually painless, nodular tumors that usually do not develop until puberty. These lesions are common in patients with *tuberous sclerosis* where they are called *Koenen* tumors.

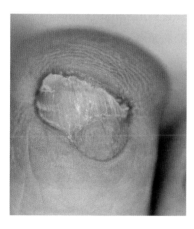

Fibrosarcoma

A fully malignant, infiltrative, metastatic tumor of fibroblastic origin. Presents as a slow-growing, lobulated, rubbery, firm mass with or without ulceration. Pain may or may not be present. They tend to metastasize to regional lymph nodes and have a high reoccurrence rate. Most often seen between the ages of 40 and 60 years in the thigh, knee, trunk, and forearm.

Treatment includes wide excision with surrounding normal tissue, chemotherapy, and irradiation.

Amputation may be required. Survival depends on the histologic grade of the neoplasm.

Fibromatosis (Desmoid Tumor)

Benign, deep-seated, well-circumscribed mass arising from muscular aponeurosis. Most patients are <40 years and present with a deep painful mass. Fibromatosis usually affects the larger muscles close to the trunk, shoulder girdle, upper arms, thigh, and buttock. It rarely affects the feet.

Plantar Fibromatosis (Ledderhose Disease)

Plantar fibromatosis is a benign reactive lesion of fibrous tissue. Usually presents as firm, single or multiple, lobular nodules, involving the medial aspect of the central bands of the plantar fascia of the foot. Plantar fibromatosis is more common in males and can be associated with other forms of fibromatosis such as its palmer equivalent Dupuytren disease and Peyronie disease, which is penile fibromatosis. While there are no clear pathophysiologic predictors for the condition, plantar fibromatosis may be associated with areas of repeated trauma, epilepsy, alcoholism, hypothyroidism, hypothyroidism, diabetes mellitus, and especially hereditary factors. Treatment is necessary only if the lesion is painful from pressure on surrounding structures. Conservative treatment includes padding and cortisone injections. Surgery involves radical resection with large margins of normal-appearing plantar fascia; reoccurrence rate is high.

Plantar fibromatosis

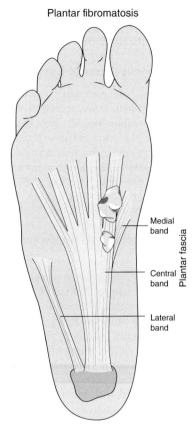

Medial band

Central band

Lateral band

Plantar fascia

Nodular Fasciitis (Pseudosarcomatous Fasciitis)

Nodular fasciitis is a benign, self-limiting, fibroblastic proliferation most commonly seen in the forearm; lower extremity involvement is relatively uncommon. Lesions present as rapidly growing, firm, soft-tissue nodules in the subcutaneous tissue. Symptoms are nonspecific and may be difficult to differentiate from fibrosarcoma. Occurs predominantly in patients aged 20 to 40 years. Pain may be present depending on involvement. Wide surgical excision to prevent reoccurrence is advised.

SMOOTH MUSCLE ORIGIN

Leiomyoma

Leiomyomas are benign smooth muscle tumors found almost exclusively in adults. They are far more frequent in organ systems such as the gastrointestinal tract and the female genital system. When found in the soft tissue, leiomyomas are confined to the superficial subcutaneous tissue and skin. Treatment usually involves excision with surrounding normal tissue.

SKELETAL MUSCLE ORIGIN

Rhabdomyoma

Rhabdomyomas are extremely rare benign tumors occurring in striated muscle. Striated muscle means either skeletal or cardiac, smooth muscle is not striated. Cardiac rhabdomyomas are the most common tumors found in the heart, and extracardiac rhabdomyomas usually occur in the neck region (tongue, neck muscles, larynx uvula, nasal cavity, axilla) or the vulva.

Rhabdomyosarcomas

The malignant form of rhabdomyoma. Rhabdomyosarcomas are the most common soft-tissue sarcoma in children. Relatively uncommon in adults and uncommon in the foot. High potential for metastasis.

Myositis Ossificans (Munchmeyer Disease)

A self-limiting, benign ossifying lesion that can occur in many different types of tissue but most commonly occurs in muscle. It is a reactive lesion resulting from trauma. Older lesions once ossified will show on radiograph.

ADIPOSE TISSUE ORIGIN

Lipoma

Lipomas are benign, slow-growing tumors composed of fat cells, usually painless unless they begin to push on nearby structures. They present as soft (doughy), freely moveable, lobulated masses that usually arise superficially in the subcutaneous tissue. They are the most common benign soft-tissue tumor in adults and usually occur between the ages of 50 and 60 years. Lipomas can occur anywhere, although neck, shoulder, arms, and trunk are most common, rarely found in the foot. Diagnosis is easily made with MRI.

Lipoma

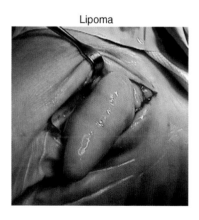

Very rarely can transform into liposarcomas. If painful, they can be surgically excised or removed by liposuction. A hibernoma is a rare type of lipoma composed of vestigial fetal brown fat. It usually occurs between the ages of 20 and 40 years and is benign and presents much the same as lipoma.

Liposarcoma

Liposarcomas are a slow-growing malignant tumor of adipose tissue seen most commonly between the ages of 40 and 60 years. Usually arising from deep in the subcutaneous tissue or between the fascial planes of major muscle groups. Pain may be present depending on involvement. Liposarcomas may occur almost anywhere but are most commonly seen in the upper thigh, buttocks, or back. With few exceptions, they are not derived from preexisting lipomas. Compared with lipomas, liposarcomas tend to be somewhat more firm, less compressible, and less freely moveable and are found deeper in the tissue than benign lipomas. Treatment may include amputation, chemotherapy, and irradiation; check for metastasis. One of the most common soft-tissue sarcomas in adults; however, it is still about 100 times less common than a benign lipoma.

Angiolipoma

Angiolipomas are essentially the same as lipomas but have a vascular component and are painful. They are composed of mature fat with multiple vascular channels. Besides the vascular channels, they differ from lipomas in that they rarely grow >2 cm and they are painful.

Piezogenic Pedal Papule

Benign herniation of subcutaneous fat into the dermal connective tissue found frequently on the lateral and medial aspect of the weight-bearing heel. Piezogenic pedal papules usually measure

<10 mm in diameter and tend to be more common in obese patients due to pressure. Depending on where they are located, they may become painful or necrotic. When multiple lesions are present, they may give "cobblestone" appearance. When symptomatic, treatment involves heel-cupping orthoses and weight loss programs.

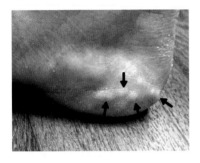

NERVE TISSUE ORIGIN

Neurilemmoma

Also known as a *schwannoma*, a neurilemmoma is a benign slow-growing neoplasm arising from Schwann cells. They appear around ages 20 to 50 years. Neurilemmomas present as a solitary, painless, fusiform, round, or oval mass that is sharply circumscribed and encapsulated. Tumors develop along the course of digital nerves and tend to favor the flexor surfaces of the extremity. Malignant transformation is extremely rare. Due to their encapsulated *eccentric location*, the nerve is rarely damaged during excision.

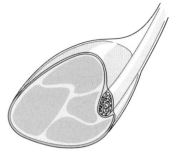

Eccentric lesion
(Neurilemmoma)

Neurilemmomas (schwannomas) are associated with neurofibromatosis type 2.

Neurofibroma

An autosomal dominant disorder occurring around ages 20 to 30 years. Solitary neurofibromas are usually small, superficial nodules that are asymptomatic. They have a *central location* in the nerve. This means if the neurofibroma is excised, the entire segment of nerve must be sacrificed. They have a very low risk of becoming malignant. Unlike neurilemmomas, neurofibromas contain cells other than Schwann cells, such as fibroblasts.

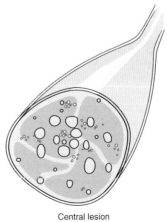

Central lesion
(Neurofibroma)

Multiple neurofibromas are associated with neurofibromatosis. Neurofibromatosis is an autosomal dominant disorder. The biggest risk factor associated with developing neurofibromatosis is a positive family history. There are two types of neurofibromatosis type 1 and type 2.

Neurofibromatosis

Type 1 (von Recklinghausen dz)	Type 2
Diagnosed at birth or early childhood	Develop during late teen and early childhood
Multiple neurofibromas	Schwannomas in the inner ear*
Associated with Café-au-lait spots and scoliosis	Less common than type 1

*Vestibular schwannomas: benign, slow-growing tumors in the ear causing hearing loss.

von Recklinghausen Dz

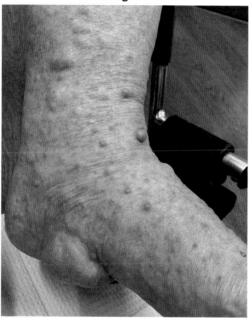

Schwannomatosis

Schwannomatosis is a rare disorder with many shared features with neurofibromatosis but is a distinct genetic disorder. It is sometimes referred to as neurofibromatosis type 3. Affects people after age 20, usually between 25 and 30. Characterized by benign schwannomas and chronic pain.

SYNOVIAL TISSUE ORIGIN

Ganglion Cyst (Tenosynovial Cyst, Synovial Cyst)

Common benign soft-tissue lesion produced from an outpouching or herniation of a joint capsule or synovial tendon sheath. Common in the feet and hands. The cyst is filled with synovial fluid, forming a fluctuant mass that readily transmits light. A pen light placed on the side of the ganglion will cause the whole cyst to glow (transilluminate). Pain may be present due to pressure from shoes or local tissues. Although the skin is freely moveable over the ganglion, the ganglion itself is usually firmly tied to its structure of origin so that it cannot be mobilized over the underlying bones and joints. The cyst contains a stalk or pedicle connecting it to the joint or tendon sheath.

Ganglion cyst

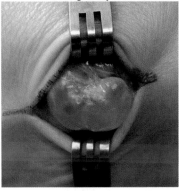

Baker cyst A Baker cyst is a common ganglion cyst that develops behind the knee in the popliteal fossa. Often presents as pain behind the knee. Differential diagnosis should include DVT.

Mucoid cyst A mucoid cyst is a small ganglion cyst that develops at the distal interphalangeal joint. These are often confused for bone spurs because they are harder and less fluctuant in this location. They may follow a course of increasing in size, bursting open and draining, crusting over, and then resolving for a period before this process repeats.

Treatment of synovial cysts includes aspiration with injection of corticosteroids; however, there is a high reoccurrence rate of about 70%. Local excision of the entire cyst with pedicle is curative.

Giant Cell Tumor of Tendon Sheath

Giant cell tumors of tendon sheaths are a relatively rare, benign, soft-tissue tumor. They are slow-growing, well-circumscribed, firm, solitary lesions attached to tendons. They may be, but not always, painful. Usually affect people between the ages of 30 and 50 years and affect females more than males (3:2). They are much more common in the hands than the feet. Erosion and invasion of local bones may be seen on radiograph. These lesions occasionally become malignant, and excision with surrounding normal tissue is treatment of choice. Even if benign, these lesions can be pseudometastatic; if cut, they can reseed locally. They are usually red brown in color due to the amount of hemosiderin found in the tissue. Histologically, these giant cell tumors of tendon sheath are identical to pigmented villonodular synovitis.

Mucoid cyst

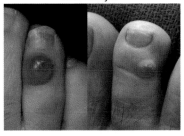

NOTE: In spite of their names, giant cell tumors of tendon sheath are in no way related to giant cell tumors of bone.

Pigmented Villonodular Synovitis

PVNS is a slow-growing, benign, reactive synovial proliferation characterized by proliferating of pigmented histiocytes and giant cells. PVNS is a benign inflammatory condition of unknown etiology. It is a condition that causes the synovium to thicken and overgrow. Most common in the knee (80%), followed by the hip. Also seen in the ankle and midfoot. The condition is benign but progressive, and slowly worsens and can lead to bony erosions and arthritis. Upon initial presentation, symptoms have often been present for years and include vague pain, joint swelling, and limited ROM. The symptoms arise from excessive fluid being produced in the joint. MRI is best diagnostic study.

Histologically, PVNS is identical to giant cell tumor of the tendon sheath. Treatment involves surgical excision of abnormal synovium. This often requires a complete synovectomy of the joint due to its high reoccurrence rate. As a result of the degree of tissue required to be removed in surgery, these joints often end up with an arthrodesis. Diagnosis can be made with an MRI and/or joint aspiration. The synovium will appear red brown in color due to the hemosiderin found in the tissue. Radiographic evidence of PVNS is subtle and shows mild subchondral well-defined osteolytic lesions on both sides of the joint. Reoccurrence rate is high.

CHANGING NOMENCLATURE

Tenosynovial giant cell tumor (TGCT) is a catchall term that includes both giant cell tumors of tendon sheath and pigmented villonodular synovitis. They are further broken down into localized (nodular) and diffuse forms.

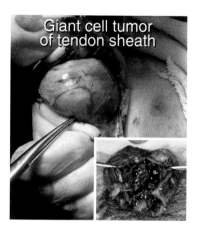

Giant cell tumor of tendon sheath

Synovial Sarcoma (Tenosynovial Sarcoma, Malignant Synovioma)

A rare, highly malignant soft-tissue sarcoma that occurs predominantly in young adults under 20 years of age. Despite its name, synovial sarcomas do not originate from synovial tissue. Early in the development, there may be no noticeable signs or symptoms and consequently the condition is often overlooked. As the tumor grows larger, a tender mass may develop. Tends to occur near, but not in, the large joints of the arms and legs, especially the knees. Due to its vague symptoms, it should be in the differential diagnosis for all deep pedal pain, especially in young adults. Treatment often necessitates amputation unless a large tumor-free area can be taken with the lesion. Treatment also includes radiation and chemotherapy. These patients should be evaluated for metastatic lesions.

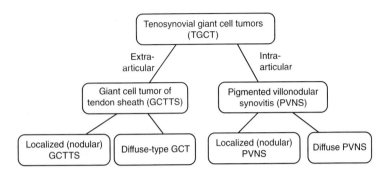

MISCELLANEOUS

Epidermal Inclusion Cyst (Epidermoid Cyst)

Common cyst that occurs in the skin secondary to traumatic implantation of the epidermis into the dermis; the implanted epidermal cells continue to grow and accumulate keratin within the dermis, forming a cyst. Epidermoid cyst presents as a slow-growing, round, firm, elevated subcutaneous lesion. A sinus tract may develop exuding a pasty, foul-smelling, cheese-like material. Most commonly found on the plantar surface of the foot. An infundibular cyst is an epidermal inclusion cyst originating from a hair follicle. Treatment of epidermal inclusion cysts usually consists of surgical excision.

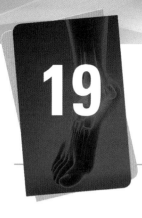

CHARTING

19

INPATIENT CHARTING

Admit Orders (ADCVANDILMAX)

ADMIT:	Admit to podiatry service.
DIAGNOSIS:	Fracture, osteomyelitis, ulcer
CONDITION:	Good, stable, fair, poor
VITALS:	How often, q8h, q-shift. May include criteria for notification of doctor
ACTIVITY:	Bed rest with bedside commode, bathroom privileges, NWB, bathroom privileges with use of crutches
NURSING:	Dressing changes, incentive spirometry, drain management
DIET:	Regular, diabetic, low sodium, NPO
I/O:	IV, Foley catheter
LABS:	C&S, Gram stain, anaerobic/aerobic cultures, blood cultures, med levels; ABG/O_2: If COPD
MEDICATIONS:	IV antibiotics, PRN meds for pain or nausea
ANCILLARY:	Consults (primary care for H&P, infectious disease, PT, social services)
X-RAY:	Baseline, R/O OM, gas gangrene, fractures

Admit Note/Inpatient Progress Note

Written upon admittance and twice a day thereafter (morning and evening rounds).
SOAP format.
DATE/TIME:

S   Patient visited at bedside, awake, alert, and oriented. Patient without
        complaints. Patient denies fever/chills, nausea/vomiting, calf/thigh pain,
        chest pain, and SOB. Good appetite, +void, +BM

O T_{max}: $T_{present}$:   BP: Pulse: Resp:
        Lungs: Clear B/L
        L foot: NVS intact wound edges appear healthy, viable, and well approximated
        with sutures. No drainage or erythema noted. Mild localized edema.
        Labs: C&S
        X-rays: OM

A   S/P bunionectomy with infection.
        Wound status improving. Low-grade fever (Vanco day #5), IDDM, blood glucose
        well controlled.

P   1. Dressing change performed.
        2. Continue daily wound care BID.
        3. Increase Vanco 750 mg q12h IV, check Vanco levels postinfusion, and report.
        4. Repeat CBC and wound cultures in AM.

Discharge Summary

Patient's Name:
Medical Record#:
Physician:
Admission Date:
Discharge Date:
Date of Surgery:

Admitting Diagnosis:	Infected 1st metatarsal left foot following bunion surgery.
Discharge Diagnosis:	S/P foot infection.
Procedures:	I&D 1st metatarsal head with bone biopsy.
History and Physical Examination:	Pertinent admission H&P and lab tests.
Course:	Summary of the treatment and progress during hospital stay.
Discharge Condition:	Good, stable, fair, guarded, critical, etc.
Medications:	Discharge meds with dosage, administration, refills.
D/C Instructions:	The patient was discharged home with the following instructions:

1. Keep the foot elevated during periods of rest.
2. Wear surgical shoe during all periods of ambulation, and avoid excessive ambulation.
3. Keep dressing dry and intact.
4. Contact Dr. _____ for all follow-up care and if any problems arise.

The patient was given written and oral instructions on wound care before discharge. Before discharge, the patient was noted to be afebrile, all vitals were stable, and they were ambulating well in post-op shoe. All the patient's questions were answered, and the patient was discharged in apparent satisfactory condition.

Follow-up: Follow-up appointment, emergency phone numbers, etc.

OUTPATIENT SURGERY CHARTING

Pre-op Check/Note

DATE/TIME:
SURGEON:
PRE-OP DIAGNOSIS:
PLANNED
PROCEDURE:
CONSENT: Signed and in chart.
ANESTHESIA: MAC (monitored anesthesia care).
PATIENT confirms NPO since midnight.
HISTORY AND PHYSICAL by _____, no contraindications to surgery:
PMH: Allergies
                  Medications
                  Illnesses
LABS:

$$\frac{Na^+ \mid Cl^- \mid BUN}{K^+ \mid CO^- \mid Creat} \diagdown Glu \qquad WBC \diagdown \frac{Hct}{Hgb} \diagdown Plat$$

Color turbidity	
Specific gravity	pH
Protein	WBC
Ketones	RBC
Glucose	Epi
Bilirubin	Bac

EKG: NSR (normal sinus rhythm).
CXR: Patient presented for _____ surgery. No contraindications to
                  surgery noted, no guarantees given or implied.

                                                          SIGNATURE

Operative Note (SAPPPPA HEMI)

DATE/TIME:	Operation start time
	Operation end time
SURGEON:	
ASSISTANTS:	
PREOPERATIVE DIAGNOSIS:	
POSTOPERATIVE DIAGNOSIS:	
PROCEDURE:	
PATHOLOGY:	Specimens taken, including type and analysis ordered. Pertinent intra-op findings (i.e., DJD)
ANESTHESIA:	MAC or IV sedation with local (amount)
HEMOSTASIS:	R/L pneumatic ankle/thigh cuff at 250/350 mm Hg (time inflated and deflated)
EBL:	Minimal
MATERIALS:	Anything left in the body
INJECTABLES:	Back table meds
PROCEDURE IN DETAIL:	*See examples at the end of the chapter.*
GENERAL STATEMENT:	The patient tolerated anesthesia and procedure well and left the OR for recovery with VSS (vital signs stable) and normal vascular status intact to the R/L foot as noted by immediate hyperemia to digits 1–5 R/L foot upon deflation of the ankle cuff.

SIGNATURE, DEGREE
RESIDENT, DEGREE
ATTENDING, DEGREE

Post-op Note (a.k.a. Post-op Check, Progress Note)

DATE/TIME:

S   Patient seen at bedside, resting comfortably, NAD
    If sleeping, were they easily aroused?
    Number of hours' s/p (name of procedure)
        If IV sedation with local is used, visit patient 1 to 2 hours post-op.
        If general anesthesia is used, visit patient 2 to 3 hours post-op.
    Questions to ask: (if yes, you must do an HPI for the problem)

1. Pain at surgical site	6. Groin pain on the side of surgery
2. Headache	7. Calf pain on the side of surgery
3. Chest pain	8. Appetite
4. Shortness of breath	9. Unable to void (urination)
5. Nausea or vomiting	10. Bowel movement

O   Vitals: Document the most recent set taken by the nurse, and note time.
General: Appearance and mental status of patient.
COR (coronary): No abnormalities.
Lungs: Clear, no cough.
ABD: Soft, no pain or masses. + bowel signs.
LEPE: Describe the dressing (dry and intact, or spotted with blood).
  Describe position of K-wire, if present.
  Position and function of drains, if present.
  Vascular: SPVPFT, pulses.
  Neurological: Sensation returned or absent.
Labs or post-op x-rays

A   1. Number of hours/p (name of procedure), doing well or complications.
    2. Any other problems the patient had or developed since surgery and status.

P   Anything and everything you are doing for the abovementioned problems.
  Discharge to home
  X-ray
  Gait or crutch training by physical therapy
  Meds to continue or discontinue
  Patient education

                                  Signature, degree
                                  Resident, degree
                                  Attending, degree

Post-op Orders (VANDILMAX)

DATE/TIME:
VITALS: q30 minutes
ACTIVITIES: Bed rest with bedside commode, bathroom privileges, NWB, bathroom privileges with use of crutches
NURSING: Elevate foot of bed, dressing changes, incentive spirometry, drain management
DIET: Regular, house, ADA diet, low sodium
I/O: IV, Foley catheter
LABS: Med levels; ABG/O_2: If COPD
MEDS: PRN for pain or nausea
ANCILLARY: Consults (infectious disease, PT to crutch train, social services)
X-RAY: Post-op x-rays

                                      SIGNATURE

SAMPLE H&PS

Lower Extremity H&P

Name: Age:
CC:
HPI:
PMH: Previous Sx
Meds:
All:
Family/Social Hx: EtOH, smoke
ROS: DM, HTN, lungs, heart, GI, kidney
Vitals: BP: Pulse: Resp:

Vascular

Dorsalis pedis pulse
Posterior tibial pulse
SPVPFT (normal 3 seconds)
Edema (pitting/nonpitting)
Pitting edema grading scale:

Grade +1 up to 2 mm depression
          rebounds immediately
Grade +2 3–4 mm of depression,
          rebounds in ≤15 seconds
Grade +3 5–6 mm of depression,
          rebounds in 60 seconds
Grade +4 8 mm of depression,
          rebounds in 2–3 minutes
Hair growth/varicosities/skin temp

Neurologic

Light touch
Vibratory
Proprioception
Sharp/dull
Temperature
Protective threshold (Semmes–
   Weinstein monofilament)
If the patient cannot feel a 5.07 monofil-
   ament, this means that they have lost
   protective sensation at that location
   and are at risk for developing an ul-
   cer. You need to list the level of loss.

Deep Tendon Reflexes

No response, always abnormal
1+ A slight but definitely present
    response, may or may not be normal
2+ A brisk response, normal

3+ A very brisk response, may or may
    not be normal
4+ A tap elicits a repeating reflex
    (clonus), always abnormal
Patellar (L-2, L-3, L-4)
Achilles (L-5, S-1, S-2)

Superficial Reflexes (Tests for UMN Lesions)

Babinski: The outer surface of the sole
   of the foot is vigorously stroked with
   a blunt instrument from the heel toward the small toe. Normal response
   is flexion of the toes; in upper motor
   neuron lesion, there is dorsiflexion of
   the hallux and fanning of the toes.
Chaddock: An instrument similar to
   that used for the Babinski is used to
   stimulate the lateral aspect of the foot
   below the malleolus from the heel forward to the small toe. A positive test
   results in dorsiflexion of the toes and
   is seen in upper motor neuron lesions.
Clonus: The foot is forcibly and quickly
   dorsiflexed, and slight pressure is
   maintained on the foot. If the test is
   positive, meaning an upper motor
   neuron lesion, a rhythmic flexion and
   extension of the foot continues.
Gordon sign: Dorsiflexion of the great toe
   or all the toes when the calf muscles
   are squeezed. A positive sign is dorsiflexion of the hallux. A positive test indicates an upper motor neuron lesion.
Oppenheim: Heavy pressure with the
   thumb applied to the anteromedial

tibia and stroking down from the infrapatellar region to the ankle. The response is a slow one and usually occurs at the end of stimulation. A positive sign is dorsiflexion of the hallux and indicates an upper motor neuron lesion.

Dermatologic

Skin (turgor, texture, temperature)
Nails (elongated, mycotic, incurved)
Callus (HD, HM, IPK)

Musculoskeletal

Bunions, hammertoes (reducible/nonreducible)
Joint ROM/crepitus
Muscle strength
(0 = no contraction, 1 = trace, 2 = poor, movement with gravity eliminated, 3 = fair, movement against gravity, but not against resistance, 4 = good, movement against gravity and some resistance, 5 = normal).
Gait

COMPLETE H&P

INTRODUCTION:
Name: Age:
Race: Sex: Occupation:
CHIEF COMPLAINT: In patients' own words
HISTORY OF PRESENT ILLNESS: Onset, duration, type of pain, trauma, radiating, provokes, relieves, quality, previous episodes, severity, previous Tx
PAST MEDICAL HISTORY: (OMAHI)
Operations
Medications
Allergies
Hospitalizations
Illnesses
Childhood Diseases (chicken pox, rheumatic fever, scarlet fever, measles, mumps, polio)
Chronic Disease and Systemic Disorders (hepatitis, TB, diabetes, cancer, arthritis, stroke, HTN, ulcers, seizures, heart, lung, or kidney disease)
SOCIAL HISTORY: Tobacco, EtOH, recreational drugs, type of work, marital status, children
FAMILY HISTORY: Diabetes, HTN, cancer, etc.
REVIEW OF SYSTEMS:
General: General health, weight change, fever, fatigue.
Skin: Patient denies Hx of changes in pigmentation, texture, eruptions, pruritus, bruising, hair loss, jaundice, and change in nails.

Lymph Nodes: Patient denies Hx of enlargement, pain, and drainage.
Ears: Patient denies changes in hearing, tinnitus, vertigo, discharge, recurrent infections, and pain.
Nose and Sinuses: Patient denies Hx of sinus infection, rhinitis, epistaxis, obstruction, drainage, or discharge.
Mouth and Teeth: Patient denies Hx of sores of mouth or tongue, bleeding gums, dentures, dental problems, or jaw pain.
Throat: Patient denies hoarseness and sore throat.
Neck: No history of goiter or enlarged nodes.
Breasts: No history of masses, lumps, pain, or discharge.
Respiration: Patient denies SOB, wheezing, dyspnea, cough, hemoptysis, pleurisy, bronchitis, TB, or asthma.
Cardiovascular: Patient denies Hx of palpitations, tachycardia, heart murmurs, irregular rhythm, chest pain, intermittent claudication, phlebitis, and cold extremities.
Gastrointestinal: Patient denies change in appetite and bowel habits. Patient denies nausea, vomiting, abdominal pain, ulcers, hematochezia, melena, diarrhea, constipation, and hemorrhoids.
Genitourinary: Patient denies dysuria, hematuria, oliguria, frequency, incontinence, stones, discharge, and

UTIs. Male—patient denies sores, discharge, testicular masses, or tenderness. Patient denies STDs. Female—menarche, length/flow of menses, or menopause. Patient denies dysmenorrhea, intermenstrual bleeding, dyspareunia, discharge, sores, pain, and STDs.

Hematopoietic: No Hx of bleeding disorders or anemia.

Endocrine: Patient denies Hx of goiter, polyuria, polyphagia, and dryness of skin or hair.

Musculoskeletal: Patient denies Hx of arthritis, joint pain, aches, loss of strength, gout, and RA.

Neurologic: Patient denies stroke, vertigo, syncope, sensory disturbance, numbness, tremors, paralysis, muscle weakness, and convulsions.

Psychiatric: Patient denies anxiety, nervousness, mood changes, depression, and hallucinations.

PHYSICAL EXAMINATION:
Vital Signs: Temp:
Pulse: Resp: BP:
Height: Weight:

General Appearance: The patient is a well-developed, well-nourished ___ years old who is alert, oriented, cooperative, and in no apparent distress.

Skin: Warm, dry, good color, turgor, and pigmentation with no lesions' scars or signs of cyanosis.

Head: Head is normocephalic with normal hair texture and distribution. Scalp shows no evidence of masses, scars, rashes, or scaling. Face is symmetrical with no signs of scars or edema.

Eyes: Visual acuity using the near card is 20/20, visual field is full B/L, EOMI, PERRLA, and the cornea and lens are clear. Sclera is clear, no conjunctival injection. Lashes and eyebrows show normal amount of hair with normal texture. Palpebral fissures are symmetrical.

Ears: Auricles have normal size, shape, symmetry, and location with no tenderness or tophi. External canals are patent and without erythema or exudates. Tympanic membranes are intact with good color and position. Weber midline, Rinne neg B/L.

Nose and Sinus: Septum is midline, mucous membrane pink and moist without erythema or exudates, and airways fully patent. No drainage noted; sinus is not tender to palpation.

Mouth and Throat: Gums are pink and moist; no bleeding is present. Tongue has normal color and good motility and is in midline. No noted swelling, erythema, exudate, or ulcerations. Uvula midline and elevates normally, gag reflex intact.

Neck: Neck is symmetrical and supple with no neck vein distention and full ROM; trachea midline; and freely moveable. Thyroid is smooth, not enlarged, and without nodules. There is no cervical lymphadenopathy. Palpation of the carotids reveals good upstroke. No carotid bruits were auscultated.

Lymphatics: No anterior, posterior, occipital, cervical, submaxillary, supraclavicular, axillary, epitrochlear, or inguinal lymphadenopathy.

Chest and Lungs: AP/transverse diameter (1:2). Breathing is unlabored. Thorax is symmetrical. Breath sounds are bilaterally clear to auscultation with no adventitious sounds, roles, rhonchi, wheezes, pleural friction rubs, or stridor. Respiratory excursion (3 to 5 cm).

Cardiovascular: Regular rate with no murmurs, gallops, rubs, or clicks appreciated. No S3/S4 noted. There are no heaves or other visible precordial movements. Apical impulse is palpable in the fifth left interspace in the midclavicular line. No neck venous distention at 30°.

Pulses: Carotid, radial, and femoral pulses are palpable; of good quality; and equal B/L at 3/4. The posterior tibial and dorsalis pedis are palpable 3/4.

Abdomen: Nontender and nondistended without scar or hernias present. Symmetric abdomen without aortic pulsations. Positive bowel sounds in all four quadrants. Percussion reveals normal variation between dullness and tympani. Palpation reveals no guarding or masses felt on superficial and deep palpation. Liver size percussed at ___ cm. Spleen was impalpable.

Extremities: There is no lower or upper extremity edema, ulcerations, tenderness, varicosities, erythema, tremor, or deformity. Toe and fingernails have good color and shape with no clubbing.

Breast: No discharge, retraction, asymmetry, tenderness, or masses noted.

Genitalia: No urethral discharge. B/L hernia examination was negative. Male—the penis is/is not circumcised. Testicles descended with no apparent atrophy. No masses or tenderness on palpation. No thickening or tenderness of epididymis. Female—external genitalia are without lesions, discharge, or erythema. Uterus and ovaries normal size and consistency.

Rectal: Good sphincter tone present with no pain on insertion of finger. No masses palpable and hemoccult was negative. Prostate without nodules or masses palpated.

Musculoskeletal: The patient ambulates without assistance. There is normal cervical, thoracic, and lumbar spine ROM. No scoliosis, lordosis, or kyphosis noted. No paravertebral muscular tenderness.

Neurological: Patient's behavior, level of consciousness, and emotional status appear normal. Cranial nerves II to XII are intact. Muscle size, tone, and strength are normal, and no involuntary movements are noted. Coordination is adequate. Sensory function appears intact. Reflexes are present and symmetrical.

SAMPLE DICTATIONS

Example 1

OPERATIVE REPORT (SAPPPPA HEMI)
PT. NAME: Spell it
PT MEDICAL RECORD#:
DATE:
SURGEON:
ASSISTANT:
PREOPERATIVE DIAGNOSIS:
POSTOPERATIVE DIAGNOSIS: Same
PROCEDURE:
PATHOLOGY:
ANESTHESIA: Local with monitored anesthesia care
HEMOSTASIS: Pneumatic ankle tourniquet
ESTIMATED BLOOD LOSS: Minimal
MATERIALS: Anything left in the body, screws/plates/pins
INJECTABLES: Back table meds
PROCEDURE IN DETAIL: Under mild sedation, the patient was brought into the operating room and placed on the operating table in the supine position. A pneumatic ankle tourniquet was then placed about the patient's R/L ankle. Following IV sedation, local anesthesia was obtained about the R/L ankle, utilizing ___ cc of a 1:1 mixture of 1% lidocaine plain and 0.5% Marcaine plain. The foot was then scrubbed, prepped, and draped in the usual aseptic manner. An Esmarch bandage was utilized to exsanguinate the patient's R/L foot, and the pneumatic ankle tourniquet was inflated.

Example 2

Bunionectomy (Kalish)

Attention was directed to the dorsal aspect of the 1st metatarsal head *R/L* foot where a 6-cm linear longitudinal incision was made medial and parallel to the tendon of the extensor hallucis longus and involved the contour of the deformity. The incision was deepened through the subcutaneous tissues, using sharp and blunt dissection. Care was taken to identify and retract all vital neural and vascular structures. All bleeders were ligated and cauterized as necessary.

At this time, a linear longitudinal capsulotomy was performed over the dorsal aspect of the 1st metatarsal phalangeal joint. The periosteal and capsular structures were then carefully dissected free of their osseous attachments and reflected medially and laterally, thus exposing the head of the 1st metatarsal at the operative site.

Next, utilizing an oscillating bone saw, the dorsal and medial prominences of the metatarsal head were resected and passed from the operative field. All rough edges were then smoothed with the bone rasp.

Attention was then directed to the first interspace via the original skin incision where the tendon of the extensor hallucis brevis was initially identified and tenectonized. The dissection was continued deep using blunt dissection down to the level of the fibular sesamoid, which was freed of its soft-tissue attachments proximally, laterally, and distally. The conjoint tendon of the adductor hallucis muscle was then identified and transected at its attachment to the base of the proximal phalanx of the hallux. At this time, the lateral contracture present on the hallux was noted to be reduced, and the sesamoid apparatus was noted to float into a more corrected medial position.

At this time, the hip was externally rotated and the knee was flexed to bring the medial surface of the foot superior to allow better access to the medial aspect of the metatarsal head for the osteotomy cuts. Attention was then redirected to the medial aspect of the 1st metatarsal head where a through and through V-type osteotomy was created in the metaphyseal region of this bone utilizing an oscillating bone saw. The apex of this osteotomy pointed distally, with the arms pointing proximo-plantarly and proximo-dorsally. The dorsal arm was made longer to accommodate internal fixation. Upon completion of the osteotomy, the capital fragment was distracted and shifted laterally into a more corrected position and impacted on the 1st metatarsal shaft.

At this time, two guide wires for a (*Stryker/Synthes/OsteoMed/ Arthrex/ Vilex/*etc.) cannulated screw set were driven from dorsal to plantar across the osteotomy site to serve as temporary fixation. A cannulated countersink was then placed over the guide wires to create a recess for the screw head. Next, the measuring guide was placed over the guide wires to establish appropriate screw lengths. Next, a 2.4 $\times$ ___ mm and a 2.4 $\times$ ___ mm cannulated cortical bone screws were placed over the guide wires and inserted in their place across the osteotomy site, with excellent compression noted.

Attention was then directed to the remaining medial bone shelf, which was resected utilizing the oscillating bone saw and passed from the operative site. Correction of the deformity was assessed at this time and noted to be excellent.

The wound was then flushed with copious amounts of sterile normal saline. The periosteal and capsular structures were reapproximated and coapted utilizing 3-0 Vicryl. Redundant capsular tissue was resected as necessary. The subcuticular tissues were then reapproximated and coapted utilizing 3-0 Vicryl, and the skin was reapproximated and coapted utilizing 5-0 Nylon in a continuous running interlocking suture technique.

Example 3

Hammertoe Arthroplasty

Attention was then directed to the ____ digit *R/L* foot where two converging 2-cm semielliptical longitudinal incisions were made over the dorsal aspect of this digit. The incisions were centered over the PIPJ and encompassed a dorsal callus present at the PIPJ. The incisions were deepened through the subcutaneous tissues, with care being taken to identify and retract all vital neural and vascular structures. The ellipse of skin was removed in toto using sharp dissection. All bleeders were cauterized and ligated as necessary.

At this time, a transverse tenotomy and capsulotomy were performed to the proximal interphalangeal joint of the ____ digit *R/L* foot. The head of the proximal phalanx was then freed of its capsular and ligamentous attachments. Next utilizing the oscillating bone saw, the head of the proximal phalanx was resected and passed from the operative site. The wound was then flushed with copious amounts of sterile normal saline. The extensor tendon was reapproximated and coapted utilizing 3-0 Vicryl, and the skin was reapproximated and coapted utilizing 5-0 Nylon using simple interrupted and horizontal mattress suture techniques.

Example 4

Hammertoe Arthrodesis

Attention was then directed to the ____ digit *R/L* foot where two converging 2-cm semielliptical longitudinal incisions were made over the dorsal aspect of this digit. The incisions were centered over the PIPJ and encompassed a dorsal callus present at the PIPJ. The incisions were deepened through the subcutaneous tissues, with care being taken to identify and retract all vital neural and vascular structures. The ellipse of skin was removed in toto using sharp dissection. All bleeders were cauterized and ligated as necessary.

At this time, a transverse tenotomy and capsulotomy were performed to the proximal interphalangeal joint of the ___ digit *R/L* foot. The head of the proximal phalanx was then freed of its capsular and ligamentous attachments. Next utilizing the oscillating bone saw, the head of the proximal phalanx was resected and passed from the operative site.

Attention was then directed to the base of the middle phalanx. The base was freed of its soft-tissue attachments. The articular cartilage was then resected utilizing an oscillating bone saw and passed from the operative site.

At this time, a 045 K-wire was driven through the proximal aspect of the base of the middle phalanx exiting the distal aspect if the ___ digit. The K-wire was then retrograded proximally through the remaining aspect of the proximal phalanx and into the metatarsal head. The K-wire extending out of the tip of the toe was bent 90° using a Kocher. The wire was then cut with a wire cutter, and a Jurgan Pin Ball was applied. Correction of the deformity was assessed at this time and noted to be excellent. The wound was then flushed with copious amounts of sterile normal saline. The extensor tendon was reapproximated and coapted utilizing 3-0 Vicryl, and the skin was reapproximated and coapted utilizing 5-0 Nylon using simple interrupted and horizontal mattress suture techniques.

Example 5

Hammertoe Correction Fifth Digit

Attention was then directed to the dorsal aspect of the 5th digit *R/L* foot where two converging 2-cm semielliptical incisions were created. The incisions were centered over the PIPJ and encompassed a dorsal callus present at the site. The incisions were obliquely oriented from distal medial to proximal lateral in an effort to both straighten and de-rotate the toe. The incisions were deepened through the subcutaneous tissues, with care being taken to identify and retract all vital neural and vascular structures. The ellipse of skin was removed in toto along with the callus using sharp dissection. All bleeders were cauterized and ligated as necessary.

At this time, a transverse tenotomy and capsulotomy were performed to the proximal interphalangeal joint of the digit. The head of the proximal phalanx was then freed of its capsular and ligamentous attachments. Next utilizing the *oscillating bone saw/bone cutting forceps*, the head of the proximal phalanx was resected and passed from the operative site.

Attention was then directed to the medial aspect of the middle and distal phalanx, which were cleared of their soft-tissue attachments using a 15 blade. At this time, using a Rongeur, a hemiphalangectomy of the middle and distal phalanx was performed.

The wound was then flushed with copious amounts of sterile normal saline. The extensor tendon was reapproximated and coapted utilizing 3-0 Vicryl, and the skin was reapproximated and coapted utilizing 5-0 Nylon using simple interrupted and horizontal mattress suture techniques.

Example 6

Metatarsophalangeal Joint Release

Attention was then directed to the ___ MPJ where a dorsal linear/transverse stab incision was made over this joint. Using blunt dissection, the incision was continued down to the long and short extensor tendons and capsular tissues. Utilizing a 15 blade, a tenotomy and capsulotomy were performed on the dorsal aspect of the ___ MPJ. Upon completion of the tenotomy and capsulotomy, the dorsal contractures were assessed and noted to be reduced.

Example 7

Neuroma

Attention was then directed to the *third/second* interspace of the *R/L* foot where a 3-cm linear longitudinal incision was made, beginning distally at the web space of the intermetatarsal area and extending proximally. The incision was deepened through the subcutaneous tissues being careful to identify and retract all vital neural and vascular structures, and all bleeders were cauterized and ligated as necessary. At this time, dissection was then continued down into the interspace using blunt dissection until the glistening soft white neural tissue mass of the ___ common plantar nerve was initially identified beneath the intermetatarsal ligament.

After initial identification, the hypertrophied soft-tissue neural mass was followed distally to the point of its bifurcation into the proper plantar digital nerves. The proper plantar digital nerves were tracked as far distally as possible and severed. The neural mass was then dissected as far proximally as possible, separated from its soft-tissue surroundings, and severed. At this time, the entire soft-tissue neural mass was resected and passed from the operative field in toto and sent to pathology. The wound was inspected for any remaining hypertrophied neural tissue, and it should be noted that none was found.

The wound was then flushed with copious amounts of sterile normal saline. The subcutaneous tissues were then reapproximated and coapted utilizing a 3-0 Vicryl, and the skin was reapproximated and coapted utilizing 5-0 Nylon in a continuous running interlocking suture technique.

Example 8

Endoscopic Plantar Fasciotomy

Attention was directed to the medial aspect of the *R/L* calcaneus where a 1.0-cm linear incision was made from superior to inferior ~4.0 cm anterior to the posterior aspect of the calcaneus and ~2 cm superior from the plantar surface of the calcaneus. The incision was then deepened through the subcutaneous tissues being careful to identify and retract all vital neural and vascular structures. All bleeders were cauterized and ligated as necessary.

At this time, a probe was inserted through the medial incision and directed laterally just plantar to the plantar fascia, which could be palpated with the probe. A plane was created between the plantar fascia and the plantar fat pad. The probe was then continued laterally until tenting was noted in the skin, over the lateral aspect of the heel.

At this time, the probe was removed and an obturator with a sliding cannula was inserted in its place through the medial incision and directed laterally in the plane between the plantar fascia and the plantar fat pad. Tenting was noted on the lateral aspect of the calcaneus, and a 15 blade was then used to make a second 1-cm incision over the tented skin on the lateral surface of the calcaneus. The obturator and sliding cannula were then continued laterally through the lateral incision. The obturator was removed, leaving the sliding cannula in place.

An endoscope was then inserted into the cannula through the medial incision, and a probe was used to identify the medial band of the plantar fascia through the lateral incision. The probe was removed and a retrograde knife was inserted through the lateral aspect of the cannula, and the medial 2/3 of the plantar fascia was incised from medial to lateral through and through under direct visualization. This required several swipes with the blade. The toes were then dorsiflexed to stretch the cut ends of the fascia away from one another. Upon doing this, the belly of the flexor digitorum brevis could be visualized through the scope.

The endoscope was then removed and reinserted through the lateral opening in the cannula, and the medial 2/3 of the plantar fascia were noted to be completely severed. The scope was then removed, and with the cannula in place, the wound was flushed with copious amounts of normal sterile saline. Next, the obturator was reinserted into the cannula, and the obturator and cannula were removed as one unit.

Both incisions were then reapproximated and coapted utilizing 4-0 Nylon, using simple interrupted suture technique.

Example 9

After the Procedure(s)

Upon completion of the procedure(s), a total of 1 cc of Decadron phosphate was infiltrated about the incision site. A postoperative block consisting of ___ cc of 0.5% Marcaine plain was also injected. The incision was dressed with Betadine-soaked *Adaptic/Xeroform* and covered with sterile compressive dressing consisting of 4 × 4′ and Kling. The pneumatic ankle tourniquet was then deflated, and a prompt hyperemic response was noted to all digits of the *R/L* foot. A posterior splint, Ace wrap, and post-op shoe were then applied.

The patient tolerated the procedure and anesthesia well. *They* were transferred to the recovery room, with VSS and vascular status intact to all toes of the *R/L* foot. Following a period of postoperative monitoring, the patient will be discharged home with the following written and oral postoperative instructions:

1. Keep dressing dry and intact.
2. Avoid excessive ambulation.
3. Ice and elevate *R/L* foot when at rest.
4. Wear surgical shoe at all times when ambulating.
5. Contact Dr. ____ for all postoperative follow-up care and if any problems arise.
6. Prescriptions were written for:

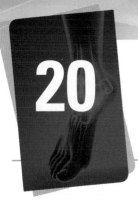

20

LABORATORY TESTS

URINE TESTS

A urinalysis is generally divided into two parts:

General: Includes macroscopic evaluation, specific gravity, and a dipstick segment

Microscopic evaluation: Quantitative assessment of cellular component

24-Hour Urine Creatinine

The 24-hour urine creatinine tests the amount of creatinine in urine over a 24-hour period. A 24-hour test is much more accurate than a single urine sample because urine creatinine varies throughout the day based on diet, exercise, and hydration levels. As kidney disease develops, urine creatinine levels will decrease and blood creatinine will increase.

Normal levels: 14 to 26 mg/kg of body mass for males
11 to 20 mg/kg of body mass for females

Albumin-to-Creatinine Ratio (ACR) (aka: Urine Albumin-to-Creatinine Ratio [UACR])

Albumin urine concentration is divided by creatinine concentration from a urine sample. This value increased as kidney disease increases.

ACR (microgram/mg)	Significance
<30	Normal
30–300	Moderately increased
>300	Severely increased

Albumin Urine Test/Protein Urine Test

Normal value: 0 to trace amounts
A healthy kidney does not let any albumin pass into the urine. Having albumin in the urine is called *albuminuria*. Albumin urine test and protein urine test are used interchangeably because most of the protein in the blood is albumin.
Increased in dysfunctional kidneys, dehydration, HTN, acute illness with fever, diabetes, stress, strenuous exercise, lupus
Bence Jones protein is a specific globulin protein, which, when found in urine, is suggestive of multiple myeloma.

Appearance

Normal: Clear
Cloudy urine indicates a UTI.

Bilirubin

Bilirubin is only found in the urine only when serum-conjugated bilirubin levels are high, indicating hepatobiliary disease.

Blood

Normal value: 0 to trace amounts
Blood in the urine is called *hematuria*. Causes are usually related to bladder or kidney problems.
  Gross hematuria: Hematuria observable through direct visual inspection of the urine. The most common causes of gross hematuria are UTI, bladder cancer, and ureteral stones.
  Microscopic hematuria: Hematuria only detectable by microscopic examination of the urine. The most common causes of microscopic hematuria are UTI, ureteral stones, exercise induced, benign prostate hyperplasia, and idiopathic.

Color

Normal: Yellow, straw colored, amber
In addition to the following, many medications and foods can alter urine color.

Red	Orange	Blue/Green or Black
Hemoglobinuria	Restricted fluid intake	Lysol poisoning
Hematuria	Concentrated urine	Melanin
Myoglobinuria	Urobilin	Bilirubin
Porphyrins	Fever	Methemoglobin
Menstrual	Porphyrin	Pseudomonas toxemia
Contamination		

Casts

Casts are tube-shaped particles made of up various types of cells depending on the condition. The absence of casts or the presence of a few hyaline casts is normal.

Fatty casts: Nephrotic syndrome

Granular casts: Cellular casts (e.g., RBC casts, WBC casts) break down to granular casts. They are nonspecific and associated with any form of nephritis.

RBC casts: Seen in many kidney diseases

WBC casts: Acute kidney infection and interstitial nephritis

Renal tubular epithelial cell casts: Reflects damage to tubule cells in the kidneys. Seen in renal tubular necrosis, viral dz, and kidney transplant rejection.

Waxy casts: Advanced kidney dz, chronic kidney failure

Crystals

Urine crystals are formed when there are excessive minerals in the urine. The presence can be a normal finding based on diet or dehydration. Some of the more common urine crystals include:

Struvite: Composed of phosphate, ammonium, magnesium, and calcium. Usually forms as a result of a UTI.

Uric acid crystals: Develop from highly acidic urine. Can be caused by kidney stones, gout, or chemotherapy.

Calcium oxalate crystals: Most common type. A common by-product of many foods that ends up in the urine. If a patient is dehydrated, they can form.

Cystine crystals: Caused from cystinuria, which is a genetic disorder

Epithelial Cells

Less than two cells per high-power field (hpf)

Increased epithelial cells in the urine can indicate yeast or UTI infection, kidney or liver dz, and certain kinds of cancer.

Glucose

Normal value: 0 to trace amounts

Glucose in the urine, known as *glucosuria*, usually occurs as a result of high blood sugar levels from diabetes.

Ketones (Acetone)

Normal value: 0 to trace amounts

Your body uses insulin to turn sugar into energy. When insulin is not available, as with diabetes, the body uses fat instead. Ketones are a byproduct of this fat metabolism. Keto diets also work on this principle. By depleting available sugar (low-carb diet), the body is forced to burn fat. Ketones are eliminated in the urine. In certain medical conditions such as diabetes, ketones can reach toxic levels in the blood and result in diabetic ketoacidosis.

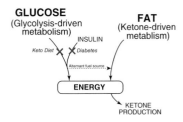

Ketonuria (ketones in the urine) occurs in: Uncontrolled diabetes, starvation, ketogenic diets, prolonged vomiting.

Leukocyte Esterase

Normal value: 0 to trace amounts
This test identifies white blood cells in the urine (pyuria), which can be a sign of a UTI.

Nitrite

Normal value: 0 to trace amounts
Nitrite in the urine (nitrituria) can indicate UTI. False negatives are not uncommon because not all bacteria convert nitrates to nitrites.

pH

Normal value: 4.6 to 8.0

Acidic (Low pH)	Basic (High pH)
Acidic foods (grains, fish, sodas, high-protein foods, sugar)	Alkaline foods (nuts, vegetables, most fruits)
Starvation	UTI
Diabetic ketoacidosis	Vomiting
COPD	Old urine specimen
Diarrhea	Kidney dz

RBCs

Normal values: Less than three cells per high-power field (hpf)
The RBC count tests for hematuria, similar to the blood in urine test, but is performed with direct visualization under a microscope as opposed to a dipstick.

RBCs indicate UTI or other problems with the urinary tract, kidneys, or bladder.

Smell

Fresh urine has an aromatic ammonia smell.
Sweet smell: Smell of acetone or a fruity smell indicates the presence of ketones and is a sign of diabetic ketosis.
Putrid smell: Presence of bacteria
Maple syrup smell: Due to a genetic disorder called *maple sugar urine disease.* An enzymatic defect (branched-chain keto acid decarboxylase) renders the children unable to break down branched-chain amino acids and they accumulate in the urine.

Specific Gravity

Normal value: 1.003 to 1.035
Measures the kidney's ability to concentrate urine; the higher the value, the more concentrated the urine.
Decreased in: Dehydration (excessive sweating/vomiting/diarrhea), diabetes mellitus, fever, CHF
Increased in: Diabetes insipidus, kidney dz, overhydration

Urobilinogen

Normal values: 0 to trace amounts
Urobilinogen is a byproduct of bilirubin, which is a yellowish compound processed by the liver. Bilirubin is responsible for breaking down RBCs. Any

condition that causes RBCs to be broken down (hemolysis) can result in an elevated urobilinogen level, bacterial infections, poisoning (lead), and parasite infections (malaria, sickle cell).

Other causes:

Pernicious anemia: Deficiency in folic acid and/or B_{12}, which are both necessary to produce RBCs. Insufficient amounts of these vitamins result in destruction of RBCs in the bone marrow.

Liver disease (hepatitis, cirrhosis): The liver processes bilirubin; when the liver is damaged, the levels of urobilinogen will build up.

WBCs

Normal values: Less than five cells per high-power field (hpf)

This test, like leukocyte esterase, tests for WBCs. Leukocyte esterase is performed with a chemical strip that is dipped in the urine as opposed to the WBC count, which is direct visualization of WBCs under microscope.

WBCs will increase with UTIs, pyelonephritis, and most renal disorders.

BLOOD TESTS

A_{1c}, HbA_{1c}, Glycosylated Hemoglobin

Normal (nondiabetic) value: 4.0% to 7.0%

Index of long-term glucose control. Reflects the average blood sugar level for the 2- to 3-month period before the test. Better method of monitoring a patient's diabetic control; blood sugar

levels alone are subject to instantaneous fluctuation based on diet. A patient with an A_{1c} between 6 and 7 may be classified as "prediabetic."

Albumin

Normal value: 3.5 to 5.5 g/dL

Albumin is produced in the liver and makes up about 60% of plasma protein. Albumin is used to transport substances such as hormones, vitamins, enzymes, and medications through the blood. Low levels of albumin may cause medications such as antibiotics, ASA, and sedative hypnotics to reach toxic levels. An albumin test is most commonly used as part of a liver or kidney function test. Low levels can mean either the liver is not making enough or the kidneys are allowing too much to leak into the urine. Albumin can also be measured in the urine.

Albumin is also responsible for keeping fluid in the blood vessels. Low levels can lead to ascites and edema.

Hyperalbuminemia	Hypoalbuminemia
Dehydration	Liver disease
	Malnutrition/ malabsorption
	Kidney disease
	Severe burns

Alkaline Phosphatase (ALP)

Normal value: 30 to 85 mU per mL

This enzyme is found mainly in the liver and bone and, to a lesser extent, the placenta and intestines. The test is used to help detect liver and bone disorders. To differentiate between bone and liver disease, this test can be run along with a GGT test.

Increased In	Decreased In
Obstructive biliary dz	Hypothyroidism
Liver dz	Malnutrition
Bone dz	Scurvy
Healing fx/bone growth	Pernicious anemia
Hyperparathyroidism	Placental insufficiency

Antinuclear Antibody (ANA)

Normal value: Negative
Used to detect connective tissue disease. ANAs are present in some apparent normal individuals.

Condition	% Testing Positive
Lupus	99
Scleroderma	73
RA	60
Sjögren	43
Dermatomyositis	33
Polyarteritis	22

Anti–dsDNA Antibody Test

Used to test for systemic lupus erythematosus

Aspartate Aminotransferase (AST) or SGOT

Normal: 10 to 50 mU per mL
Found in high concentrations in the heart and liver and in moderate amounts in skeletal muscle. Whenever there is heart or liver damage, AST spills into the blood and the amount in the blood is directly related to the number of damaged cells. AST is more specific for cardiac necrosis and less specific for liver necrosis. In EtOH liver disease, AST:ALT ratio is often >2:1.

Elevated In	Decreased In
MI	Pregnancy
Liver dz	Uncontrolled diabetes
Skeletal muscle necrosis	Beriberi

Alanine Aminotransferase (ALT) or SGPT

Normal: 10 to 50 mU per mL
This test is primarily used to diagnose liver disease and monitor drug effects of drugs on the liver. As the liver cells are damaged, ALT leaks into the blood and serum levels rise. ALT differentiates between hemolytic jaundice and jaundice due to liver disease. ALT is more liver specific than AST.
ELEVATED IN:
Same as AST, but will show very high elevation in acute (viral) hepatitis and hepatic necrosis

Bicarbonate (HCO_3)

Normal: 22 to 29 mEq/L
Bicarbonate is an electrolyte that is used to maintain the body's pH balance. It is a carbon dioxide containing waste product that develops from various metabolic processes. This test measures how much carbon dioxide is in your blood. Bicarbonate levels are controlled by the lungs and kidneys. The lungs exhale the bicarbonate as carbon dioxide,

and the kidneys can excrete, re-absorb, or make more bicarbonate to regulate pH.

Low levels (metabolic acidosis) are found in diabetic ketoacidosis, Addison dz, antifreeze (ethylene glycol) poisoning, and aspirin overdose.

High levels (metabolic alkalosis) are found in lung dz, COPD, dehydration (vomiting/diarrhea), and Cushing syndrome.

Bilirubin

Normal value: 0.2 to 1.3 mg/dL

Bilirubin is a brown and yellow substance that is a breakdown product of hemoglobin. Excessive breakdown of RBCs causes bilirubin levels to rise. Bilirubin is responsible for the yellow color in the skin and eyes in jaundice. Jaundice begins to occur when levels rise >3 mg/dL.

Albumin transports bilirubin to the liver where it is conjugated. Once conjugated, bilirubin becomes water soluble and is excreted into the intestines. Bilirubin in also what makes feces brown.

Most labs list separate values for conjugated and unconjugated bilirubin.

Conjugated bilirubin = DIRECT BILIRUBIN, indicates obstructive jaundice

Unconjugated bilirubin = INDIRECT BILIRUBIN, excessive destruction of RBCs

Conjugated + unconjugated = TOTAL BILIRUBIN

Bilirubin levels rise when there is an increase in RBC destruction or when the liver is unable to remove bilirubin from the blood as in cirrhosis.

Hyperbilirubinemia	Hypobilirubinemia
Bile duct obstruction	Caffeine
Hemolytic anemia	Penicillin
Liver damage	NSAIDs
	Barbiturates

Bleeding Time

Normal value: 2 to 9 minutes

Bleeding time measures the primary phase of hemostasis, the interaction of the platelets with the blood vessel wall, and the formation of a hemostatic plug. The test consists of a forearm scratch that is timed until a clot forms.

Bleeding time is increased in von Willebrand dz, thrombocytopenia, DIC, platelet dysfunction, and ASA or NSAID therapy.

Blood Urea Nitrogen (BUN)

Normal value: 7 to 20 mg/dL

Levels are higher in men due to increased muscle mass.

The liver produces ammonia as a byproduct of protein metabolism. Ammonia is too toxic to deliver through the bloodstream, so the liver converts it to urea nitrogen (BUN) for excreted by the kidneys. High levels of BUN indicate the kidneys are not functioning properly. BUN levels, alone, are not a reliable indicator of renal function. Levels can fluctuate based on how much fluid the patient drinks, age, gender, and body mass. BUN levels are also affected by the liver and the amount of protein intake. Another problem with evaluating BUN levels alone is that they only begin to rise after 50% renal damage. For this reason, creatinine levels should be evaluated alongside BUN. BUN and creatinine together provide a much better gauge of kidney function.

Azotemia is a condition characterized by abnormally high levels of nitrogen-containing compounds such as urea or creatinine. An elevated BUN is a type of azotemia. Azotemia can lead to uremia. Uremia is a type of acute kidney failure where there is urea in the blood.

BUN is a measure of liver function and kidney excretion.

BUN increases in conditions where there is an increased breakdown of protein, such as high-protein diet, steroids, tetracycline, GI bleeds (NSAIDs), burns, and compartment syndrome. BUN will also increase in cases where it cannot leave the body, such as renal failure. Dehydration will also cause a rise in BUN.

BUN will decrease if there is no protein available to break down such as malnutrition, or from liver damage where the liver cannot produce it. Overhydration (excessive IV fluids) will also cause a drop in BUN.

BUN/Creatinine Ratio

The ratio of BUN to creatinine (BUN:creatinine) gives much more information about the function of the kidneys than either test alone. Often reported without the second number, for example, 10:1 given as 10.
Normal value: 10:1 to 20:1 (optimum 15)

Low   Acute tubular necrosis
           Low protein intake
           Starvation
           Advanced liver dz

Certain meds: Trimethoprim, cimetidine, and triamterene cause increased SCr due to competitive inhibition of creatinine secretion, BUN will be normal.

High   CHF
          High-protein intake
          GI bleeding
          Dehydration
          Shock
          Kidney disease: Both BUN and SCr will be elevated.

Certain meds: Steroids and tetracyclines cause increased BUN. SCr will be normal.

C-Reactive Protein

Normal value: <0.8 mg per dL
Similar to ESR, in that it is a nonspecific indicator of inflammation and tissue trauma. This protein is virtually absent in healthy persons. May be more valuable than ESR because it becomes elevated sooner (6 to 10 hours after tissue trauma) and returns to normal sooner once the inflammatory process stops.

Calcium

Normal value: 8.5 to 11 mg%

Calcium levels are maintained by the kidneys and the parathyroid glands. As calcium levels drop, the parathyroid glands release parathyroid hormone (PTH), which causes calcium to be pulled from bone into the blood. The kidneys can also help increase calcium levels by converting vitamin D into its active form calcitriol, which caused calcium to be absorbed from the intestines.

Kidney function tests along with PTH levels should be reviewed along with calcium levels to help determine the cause of abnormal calcium levels.

The majority of the body's calcium reserves are in the bones and teeth. Calcium is required for muscular contractions, cardiac function, transmission of nerve impulses, and blood clotting. Serum calcium deficiency causes neuromuscular excitability, tetany, muscle twitching, and, eventually, convulsions. Increased serum calcium causes drowsiness, nausea, and cardiac arrhythmias.

Hypercalcemia	Hypocalcemia
Hyperparathyroidism (90%)	Hypoparathyroidism
Bone neoplasm	Malabsorption
Vitamin D overdose	Magnesium deficiency
	Kidney disease
	Low vitamin D levels

Carbon Dioxide

This is the same as a bicarbonate test.

Chloride

Normal value: 98 to 109 mEq/L

Chloride is the primary extracellular anion and plays a major role in water balance, acid–base balance, and osmolarity of body fluids. Chlorides are depleted anytime there is a massive loss of gastrointestinal fluids or urine.

Hyperchloremia	Hypochloremia
Dehydration	Vomiting
Eclampsia	Diarrhea
Excessive IV saline	Ulcerative colitis
	Severe burns
	Heat exhaustion

Cholesterol, Total

Normal value: <200 mg/dL

Total cholesterol consists of HDL, LDL, and the cholesterol portion of triglycerides. Although the total cholesterol value is the most recognized value, it is actually the least important number in a lipid panel. Cholesterol is necessary for making certain cell tissues and hormones. As the cholesterol blood levels rise, the risk of atherosclerosis and heart disease increases.

Increased In	Decreased In
Hypercholesterolemia	Malabsorption
Biliary obstruction	Anemias
Hypothyroidism	
Nephrosis	
Diabetes mellitus	

Chol/HDLC Ratio

This is your total cholesterol value divided by you HDL.

Normal value: <5

Creatine Phosphokinase (CPK), aka: Creatine Kinase (CK), CK Isoenzymes

Normal value: 6 to 30 U per mL

CK is found predominantly in skeletal muscle, heart muscle, and the brain. Anytime there is damage to these structures, CK can be elevated. CK levels can be further fractioned into isoenzymes (BB, MB, and MM) to determine whether the damage is to the brain, skeletal muscle, or heart. Normal CK values consist virtually entirely of MM isoenzymes due to skeletal muscles replacing and renewing dead cells. CK levels can also be elevated from strenuous workouts. Elevated CK levels may predispose a patient to malignant hyperthermia during anesthesia.

CPK Levels for an MI

CPK is elevated 4–8 hours after an MI, peaks at 12–24 hours, and returns to normal 4–6 days later. Also, SGOT will be elevated 6–12 hours after an MI and return to normal 5–7 days later. LDH will elevate 48 hours after an MI and return to normal 9 days later.

CK Isoenzymes and Their Associated Disease States

Serum Creatinine (SCr)

Normal: 0.6 to 1.6 mg/dL

Normal: Males: 0.6 to 1.2 mg/dL in adult males, males are higher due to higher muscle mass.
Females: 0.5 to 1.1 mg/dL in adult females

Creatinine is a byproduct of muscle metabolism; high levels indicate the kidneys are not functioning properly. SCr is used to estimate GFR. Creatinine levels can also be tested in the urine. As the kidneys begin to fail, serum creatinine levels rise and creatinine urine levels fall.

Creatinine levels are increased in renal failure, medications that block creatinine secretion (cimetidine, trimethoprim), and substances that interfere with creatinine assay (cefoxitin, flucytosine, acetoacetate).

Serum creatinine is used as an indicator of renal function and is a more sensitive indicator than BUN.

INCREASED IN:
Renal dz
Nephritis
Medications: Cimetidine, trimethoprim

CPK-BB (CK 1) (CNS)	CPK-MB (CK 2) (Cardiac Muscle)	CPK-MM (CK 3) (Skeletal Muscle)
CVA	MI	Muscular dystrophy
Brain injury	Angina	Crush injury
	Cardiac defibrillation	IM injection
	Heart surgery	Compartment syndrome

24-Hour Creatinine Clearance Test (CrCl)

The CrCl test compares the blood creatinine with the urine creatinine to determine the volume of blood cleared of creatinine per unit of time. CrCl is a useful in the diagnosis and prognosis of kidney disease. It requires both a blood and urine sample. This test is used to detect early-stage kidney disease or to adjust medication doses. CrCl has largely been replaced by serum creatinine levels for estimating GFR due to the hassle of collecting 24 hours of urine.

Creatinine Clearance (CCl) =

$$\frac{\text{Urine creatinine in mg/dL} \times \text{Total volume of urine}}{\text{Serum creatinine in mg/dL} \times 1440}$$

Normal values: Males: 125 mL/mt
                 Females: 115 mL/mt

Increased CrCl: Anemia

Decreased CrCl: Kidney damage or decreased blood flow to the kidneys

Cystine C

Cystine C is a protein produced by cells in the body that is cleared by the kidneys. When the kidneys are functioning properly, levels rise. Cystine C can be used to estimate GFR or can be added into the calculations of serum creatinine for improved eGFR accuracy. Cystine C is made by all nucleated cells, not just muscle as in creatinine. As a result, cystine C varies less than creatinine. Unlike BUN, cystine C is not affected by gender, age, race, or muscle mass.

Normal values: 0.6 to 1 mg/L

D-Dimer

D-Dimer is a venous blood test that measures the amount of a protein fragment that is made when a clot dissolves. It is a nonspecific test for a blood clot. Most commonly used to assist in the diagnosis of a DVT, PE, or DIC. False negatives may occur with recent surgery or trauma, MI, stroke, infections, DIC, pregnancy, collagen vascular dz, or cancer.

Normal levels are undetectable or very low.

Differential

A "differential" determines the relative amounts of each of the five types of WBCs, which is more diagnostically valuable than just the total number of WBCs alone.

Types	Normal Values	Significances of Increase
Neutrophils (total)	50%–70% (2,500–7,000/µL)	Bacterial infections
Segments	50%–65% (2,500–6,500/µL)	Right shift[a]—liver dz, some types of anemia

Types	Normal Values	Significances of Increase
Bands	0%–5% (0–500/μL)	Left shift[a]—acute bacterial infection
Eosinophils	1%–3% (100–300/μL)	Allergic and parasitic diseases
Basophils	0.4%–1.0% (40–100/μL)	Source of histamines—inflammation/allergies
Monocytes	4%–6% (200–600/μL)	Viral infection, TB, parasitic diseases, subacute bacterial endocarditis, monocytic leukemia, collagen dz
Lymphocytes	25%–35% (1,700–3,500/μL)	Viral infection, lymphocytic leukemia

[a]Normally, most circulating neutrophils are in their mature form, which the laboratory identifies by its segmented nucleus (segmented neutrophils). In contrast, the nucleus of less mature neutrophils is not yet segmented but still seen as a band (band neutrophils).
When lab reports were written by hand, the bands were written first on the left side of the page and the segments to the right, hence the terms *left shift* and *right shift*, respectively.

Enzyme-Linked Immunoabsorbent Assay (ELISA)

Normal value: Negative, nonreactive
Used to test for HIV

Erythrocyte Sedimentation Rate (ESR, Sed Rate)

Normal values: Varies by sex, age, and method
ESR measures the rate at which RBCs settle out of unclotted blood. Nonspecific test to follow the progression of disease. Sed rate increases with infections, inflammation, and malignancy.

GFR

The glomerular filtration rate (GFR) is the amount of blood filtered by the glomeruli per minute. GFR is the best test for measuring kidney function, and the GFR value is used to stage kidney disease. A true GFR test requires radionuclide assessment and is expensive and not widely available, so kidney function is usually assessed with an estimated GFR (eGFR).

eGFR

The eGFR is an estimate of the GFR using various methods. The most common of which uses blood creatinine levels (SCr). The SCr level is put into a formula that adjusts for age, muscle mass, gender, and ethnicity and arrives at an eGFR. There are several equations available for calculating eGFR:
MDRD (Modification of Diet in Renal Disease) also called the Levey formula
CKD-EPI (Chronic Kidney Disease Epidemiology Collaboration)
Crockoff–Gault Equation

eGFR Is Used to Stage Kidney DZ

Kidney Damage Stage (Chronic Kidney Dz [CKD])	Description	eGFR
CKD stage 1	Normal or minor kidney damage with normal GFR	90+
CKD stage 2	Mild reduced kidney function	60–89

(*continued*)

Kidney Damage Stage (Chronic Kidney Dz [CKD])	Description	eGFR
CKD stage 3A	Moderately reduced kidney function	45–59
CKD stage 3B	Moderate reduced kidney function	30–44
CKD stage 4	Severe reduced kidney function	15–29
CKD stage 5	Kidney failure	<15

Glucose: Fasting Blood Sugar (FBS)

Normal (fasting): 65 to 110 mg%

Used as an initial screening for diabetes. For borderline or slightly elevated blood glucose levels, a postprandial and/or a glucose tolerance test may be ordered.

Glucose spills over into the urine (glucosuria) at about 180 mg% or higher.

Hyperglycemia	Hypoglycemia
Diabetes (most common)	Excessive insulin administration
Cushing syndrome	Liver dz
Acute pancreatitis	Adrenal hypoactivity
Adrenal hyper-activity (stress, shock)	
Infection	

γ-Glutamyl Transferase (GGT)

Normal values: 0 to 51 IU/L

Elevated in liver damage or damage to the bile ducts. Best test for diagnosing bile duct obstruction. Also used to test for chronic EtOH abuse.

GGT can also be used to determine the source of elevated alkaline phosphatase (ALP). If ALT is elevated and GGT is normal, the ALP is elevated due to bone dz. If both ALP and GGT are elevated, the likely source of the elevated ALP is liver damage.

Oral Glucose Tolerance Test (OGTT)

Normal values:

Time	Glucose Level (mg/dL)
Fasting	65–110
0.5 h	<160
1 h	<170
2 h	<125
3 h	Fasting level

The patient is given a very sweet commercially available 100-g bottle of glucose to drink, and blood is drawn just before (fasting), and at 0.5, 1, 2, and 3 hours after drinking. The test can be extended up to 6 hours. Indicated when there is sugar in the urine or when the FBS or 2-hour PPBS is more than slightly elevated. Blood sugar levels for this test should peak around 0.5 to 1 hour and return to normal at 3 hours.

High-Density Lipoprotein (HDL)

Good cholesterol. HDL cholesterol functions to move excess cholesterol back to the liver so it can be processed and excreted. HDL is cholesterol that is not being deposited in your body but is on its way out. You want this number as high as possible. A high HDL does not make up for or cancel out a high LDL.

Normal values: >40 mg/dL

Hematocrit (Hct)

Average value is 45% (higher in males).

Hematocrit is the percentage volume of RBCs in a sample of anticoagulated whole blood. Hematocrit decreases in anemia and blood loss. Useful when evaluating a possible GI bleed or blood loss from trauma. The body reacts to blood loss by dumping more fluids into the vascular system to maintain BP. This excess fluid does not contain RBCs, and hematocrit decreases.

Hemoglobin (Hgb, Hg, Hb)

Normal value: (Average) male 16, female 14

Hemoglobin test measures the amount of hemoglobin in your blood. Hemoglobin is a protein in the red blood cells that carries oxygen. Decreased in anemia; increased in polycythemia.

HLA-B27

Normals are not applicable and require clinical correlation. Human leukocyte antigens (HLAs) are a major histocompatibility antigen found on all nucleated cells and play a major role in histocompatibility between donors and recipients for organ transplants. HLAs

are also used as part of a complete diagnosis for certain rheumatoid diseases, seronegative spondyloarthropathies in particular.

Ankylosing spondylitis

Reiter dz

Psoriatic arthritis

Ulcerative colitis

Regional enteritis

Ten percent of normal individual test false positive, HLA-B27 testing is best used as an adjunct to diagnosis and should not be regarded as diagnostic by itself.

Indices (RBC Indices)

Provide information about the size and hemoglobin content of red blood cells. Indices are a useful aid in differentiating anemias.

MCHC (mean corpuscular hemoglobin concentration)

Measures the proportion of each cell occupied by hemoglobin

Hyperchromia	Hypochromia
(abnormal increase in the Hb content of RBCs)	(abnormal decrease in the Hb content of RBCs)
Spherocytosis	Iron deficiency anemia
	Thalassemia

MCH (mean corpuscular hemoglobin)

Measures the average amount of hemoglobin in the RBCs

MCV (mean corpuscular volume)

Measures the average volume occupied by a single RBC

Microcytic Anemia	Normocytic Anemia	Macrocytic Anemia
(MCV < 80)	(MCV 80–100)	(MCV > 100)
Iron deficiency	Chronic dz	Folate acid deficiency
Thalassemia	Bone marrow failure	Vitamin B_{12} deficiency
Blood loss	Hemolysis	Liver disease
Lead poisoning		Drugs: Phenytoin, cytotoxic meds

International Normalized Ratio (INR)

Target INR range for Coumadin (warfarin) treatment is between 2.0 and 3.0.
Normal value when not treating with warfarin: 1
INR is a more accurate way of measuring the prothrombin time (PT). INR was developed to calibrate all the different labs and give a more standardized value for the PT. INR is most commonly used to monitor warfarin treatment.

Lactate Dehydrogenase (LDH, LD)

Normal: 90 to 200 mU per mL
LDH is an intracellular enzyme widely distributed in many tissues of the body, particularly the kidneys, heart, skeletal muscle, brain, liver, lungs, and RBCs. LDH is relatively nonspecific, but may be used to confirm MI or pulmonary infarction when viewed with other tests. LDH is elevated 12 to 24 hours after an MI, peaks at 2 to 5 days, and returns to normal at 6 to 12 days. LDH can be fractioned into isoenzymes for more specific diagnosis.
ELEVATED IN:
  MI
  Pulmonary infarction
  CVA
  Hepatitis
  CA
  Hemolytic anemia
  Skeletal muscle necrosis

LDH Isoenzymes

LDH can be fractioned into five isoenzymes by electrophoresis. Various diseases reveal abnormal patterns of isoenzymes.

Isoenzyme	Significance
LDH-1	MI[a]
LDH-2	
LDH-3	Pulmonary infarct
LDH-4	Liver dz
LDH-5	

[a]There is usually a prevalence of LDH-2 over LDH-1; however, after an MI, there is an LDH "flip" and LDH-1 predominates.

Low-Density Lipoprotein (LDL)

Bad cholesterol. This type of cholesterol circulates around in the blood and is used in cell development. When LDL levels gets too high, it begins to stick to the walls of the arteries, causing plaque. You want this number as low as possible.
Normal values: 90 to 130 mg/dL

Non-HDL Cholesterol

This number is your total cholesterol minus your HDL (good cholesterol). Your non-HDL includes LDL and other types of cholesterol such as very low-density lipoprotein (VLDL). This measures how much total bad cholesterol you have in your blood.
Normal value: <130 mg/dL

Parathyroid Hormone (PTH)

PTH levels are used to check for parathyroid disease, such as hyperparathyroidism or hypoparathyroidism. PTH also controls blood calcium levels. As calcium levels drop, PTH is released, which pulls calcium out of bone and into the bloodstream.

PTH levels can also help monitor kidney function. As kidney disease increases, so do PTH levels. This has to do with the kidney's role in maintaining blood calcium levels. Damaged kidneys cannot convert vitamin D into calcitriol. Calcitriol is the hormone responsible for absorbing calcium from the intestines. As a result, calcium levels drop, causing PTH levels to rise.

Phosphate (P)/Inorganic Phosphorus (PO₄)

Normal: 3 to 4.5 mg per dL
Phosphorus and calcium are both absorbed from the intestines and stored in bones in the form of hydroxyapatite. The kidneys are responsible for eliminating excess phosphorous. Patients with kidney disease cannot eliminate phosphorus and will have elevated phosphorous levels. When there is excess phosphorous in the blood,

parathyroid hormone (PTH) levels increase, which decreases phosphate levels and increases calcium levels. Phosphate levels are always evaluated in relation to calcium levels because there is an inverse relationship between the two, as one goes up and the other goes down. Calcitriol causes both serum calcium and phosphate to increase.

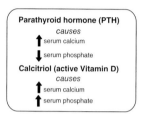

Hyperphosphatemia	Hypophosphatemia
Renal dz	Hyperparathyroidism
Hypoparathyroidism	Diabetes

Platelet Count

Normal value: 150,000 to 300,000
Spontaneous bleeding occurs <25,000 to 50,000.
Thrombocytopenia is a decrease in the number of platelets.
Thrombocytosis is an increase in the number of platelets.

Coagulation Factors	
Factors requiring vitamin K	II, VII, IX, X
Extrinsic pathway factors	III, VII
Intrinsic pathway factors	VIII, IX, XI, XII,
Common pathway factors	I, II, V, X, XIII

Potassium

Normal: 3.5 to 5.5 mEq per L

Potassium is the primary intracellular cation and is found in small amounts in the blood. Low blood potassium (hypokalemia) causes depression of the myocardial contractibility and can lead to arrhythmias (EKG signs include depressed or inverted T wave and a peaking P wave and prominent U wave). High blood potassium (hyperkalemia) causes cardiac excitability and can lead to fibrillations and death (EKG signs include elevated T wave, then flattening of the P wave and the PQ interval increases, and finally widening of QRS).

Treatment for hyperkalemia may include administering calcium, administering sodium bicarbonate, or administering a combination of insulin and glucose. In addition to cardiac problems, potassium deficiency causes leg cramps and weakness.

Increased In	Decreased In
(HYPERKALEMIA)	**(HYPOKALEMIA)**
Tissue trauma (hemolysis)	Vomiting/diarrhea
Burns	Diuretics
Renal failure	Starvation
Addison dz	

Protein

Normal: 6 to 8 mg per dL

Albumin is a protein formed in the liver that helps maintain normal distribution of water in the body (colloidal osmotic pressure); it also helps to transport many blood constituents and drugs.

Blood protein mostly refers to albumin because blood protein is 50% to 60% albumin. The nonalbumin portion of blood protein consists of globulins, and the albumin-to-globulin ratio (A/G ratio) is sometimes beneficial in diagnosing certain conditions such as multiple myeloma (Bence Jones protein is a globulin).

Increased In	Decreased In
Hyperproteinemia (rare)	Hypoproteinemia
Dehydration	Chronic liver dz
Vomiting/diarrhea	Malnutrition/ starvation
Multiple myeloma	Severe burns
Malignancies	

Prothrombin Time (PT, Pro Time)

Normal value: 10 to 12 seconds (varies according to lab)

Measures the integrity of the extrinsic pathway of the blood clotting cascade and common pathway

PT increases with vitamin K deficiency, biliary obstruction, liver dz, and warfarin (Coumadin) Tx. Therapeutic doses of Coumadin should maintain PT at two to three times normal.

Partial Thromboplastin Time (PTT)

Normal value: 60 to 70 seconds (varies according to lab)

Measures the integrity of the intrinsic pathway of the blood clotting cascade and common pathway

PTT increases with hemophilia A (factor VIII deficiency), hemophilia B, "Christmas disease" (factor IX deficiency), von Willebrand dz, DIC, liver dz, and heparin treatment. Therapeutic doses of heparin should maintain PTT at 1.5 to 2.5 normal or about 120 to 140 seconds.

Activated Partial Thromboplastin Time (APTT, aPTT)

Normal value: 30 to 40 seconds (varies according to lab)

aPTT is a PTT test with an activator (a) added to speed up the clotting time, which makes the normal range narrower and more accurate than PTT. aPTT is frequently used to monitor heparin therapy because it is a more sensitive than PTT.

Therapeutic heparin treatment should maintain PTT at 1.5 to 2.5 normal or about 60 to 80 seconds.

COAGULATION CASCADE

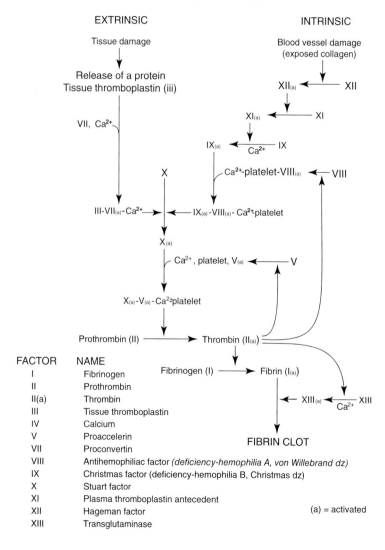

FACTOR	NAME
I	Fibrinogen
II	Prothrombin
II(a)	Thrombin
III	Tissue thromboplastin
IV	Calcium
V	Proaccelerin
VII	Proconvertin
VIII	Antihemophiliac factor *(deficiency-hemophilia A, von Willebrand dz)*
IX	Christmas factor (deficiency-hemophilia B, Christmas dz)
X	Stuart factor
XI	Plasma thromboplastin antecedent
XII	Hageman factor
XIII	Transglutaminase

(a) = activated

RA Factor (Rheumatoid Factor)

Absence of RA factor does not exclude the diagnosis of rheumatoid arthritis.

POSITIVE IN:
  Rheumatoid arthritis
  Systemic lupus erythematosus
  Scleroderma
  Dermatomyositis
  Sjögren syndrome
  Syphilis
  Sarcoidosis
  Liver dz

RBC

Normal value: Average 4,600,000 per μL (higher in males)
The average life span of a RBC is 120 days.
Decreased RBCs are found in anemia (for more specific diagnosis, evaluate Hct, Hb, and indices). Increase in RBCs is termed *polycythemia* and is associated with many factors that cause overproduction of RBCs or a decrease in plasma. Polycythemia is associated with many factors, including dehydration, acute poisoning, severe diarrhea, and pulmonary fibrosis.

Reticulocyte Count

Normal value: (Average) 0.5% to 1.5%
Percentage of immature RBCs
A reticulocyte is a young, immature, non-nucleated RBC formed in the bone marrow and, therefore, a reflection on bone marrow function. Reticulocyte count can be useful in determining whether an anemia is caused by bone marrow failure or by hemorrhage/hemolysis. It is also useful in evaluating the treatment of anemia.

Rapid Plasma Reagin (RPR)

Test for syphilis

Sodium

Normal: 135 to 145 mEq per L
Sodium is a major extracellular electrolyte that helps regulate fluid balance and hence blood pressure. Sodium is the most abundant cation in the blood, and its primary functions are maintaining osmotic pressure and acid–base balance and transmitting nerve impulses. Hyponatremia usually reflects a relative excess of body water rather than low total body sodium.

Hypernatremia	Hyponatremia
(Increased levels)	(Decreased levels)
Severe burns	Dehydration
Diarrhea/vomiting	Cushing dz
Excess IV (nonelectrolyte)	
Addison dz	
CHF	

Triglycerides

Triglycerides are only 20% cholesterol, the rest is mostly fat. That is why when you add up triglycerides + LDL + HDL, it does not equal the value of total cholesterol.
Normal values: <150 mg/dL (normal values vary widely)

Two-Hour Postprandial Blood Sugar (2-Hour PPBS)

Normal values: <120 mg per dL
This is a blood test taken 2 hours after eating a meal to screen for diabetes. For best results, eat a high-carbohydrate meal. A 2-hour PPBS >200 mL per dL is consistent with a diagnosis with diabetes.

Uric Acid

Normal: 1.5 to 7 mg per dL
Uric acid is a breakdown product of purines. Uric acid levels are used most commonly to evaluate renal failure, gout, and leukemia.
HYPERURICEMIA (Elevated)
   Renal failure
   Gout
   Leukemia
   Alcoholism
   Lead poisoning

Venereal Disease Research Laboratory (VDRL)

Test for syphilis

Very Low-Density Lipoprotein (VLDL)

VLDL is a type of LDL that carries triglycerides to the body's cells. LDL carries cholesterol. If VLDL levels increase they contribute to plaque buildup.
Normal value: <30 mL/dL

WBC

Normal value: 5,000 to 10,000 per µL
Measures the total number of circulating leukocytes

Leukopenia (<4,000/µL)	Leukocytosis (>10,000/µL)
Overwhelming infection	Bacterial infection
Viral infection	Inflammatory process
Hypersplenism	Tissue necrosis (MI, burns)
Bone marrow depression	Physical stress

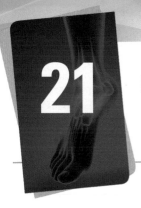

PRE-/PERI-/POSTOPERATIVE

PREOPERATIVE

Preoperative testing should be guided by the patient's clinical history, comorbidities, and physical examination. Some hospitals also have their own preoperative protocols. Common preoperative testing includes SMA 6, CBC, UA, PT/PTT, EKG, pregnancy test, and CXR. Aspirin and smoking should be discontinued 1 week before surgery. Patients should be NPO after midnight, or a minimum of 6 hours before surgery. Children (more prone to dehydration) may have clear liquids up to 4 hours before surgery.

American Society of Anesthesiologists Surgical Risk Classification

Class	Description
I	Healthy patient
II	Patient with mild systemic disease (i.e., essential HTN, NIDDM)
III	Patient with severe systemic disease that limits activity (i.e., angina, COPD)
IV	Patient with incapacitating systemic disease that is a constant threat to life
V	Moribund patient not expected to survive 24 hours with or without surgery
IV	Patient declared legally brain dead and awaiting organ harvesting

Adapted with permission from ©American Society of Anesthesiologists (ASA), All Rights Reserved. https://www.asahq.org/standards-and-guidelines/asa-physical-status-classification-system

When to Consider Cancelling Elective Surgery (General Guidelines)

Test	Cancel Elective Surgery
Hemoglobin	≤10 g/dL
Hematocrit	≤30%
WBC	<2,400/mm³ or >16,000/mm³
Neutropenia	≤1,000/mm
Platelets	<50,000–100,000 cells/mm³
A₁c	>8
Potassium	≤3 mEq/L (important cardiac electrolyte)
Glucose	≥200 (may adjust with sliding scale)
BUN	≥50 (R/O renal insufficiency)
Pregnancy test	Positive test
Creatinine	≥3.0 (R/O renal insufficiency)
Creatine kinase	Increased levels may indicate a threat of developing malignant hyperthermia

UA

Used to R/O infection, renal dz (proteinuria), and diabetes

Coagulation Studies

Important if patient is on blood thinners

EKG

Useful for identifying recent MIs, frequent premature ventricular contractures (PVCs). EKG is a poor indicator of ischemic heart disease.

CXR

Recommended for patients with a positive history of lung or heart disease and smokers

Antibiotic Prophylaxis

Prophylactic antibiotics are given IV 30 minutes before surgery. Conditions that warrant prophylactic antibiotics include surgery on dirty wounds, preexisting valvular heart disease, surgery >2 hours, blood transfusion, preexisting infection, and implants.

Cefazolin (Ancef)

Ancef is a first-generation cephalosporin used for prophylaxis against wound infections during surgery. Ancef is a popular choice because it provides good coverage against *Staphylococcus aureus* and *Streptococcus*, both of which are likely pathogens of infection whenever the skin is broken. This drug also has an appropriate long half-life. Dosage is 1 to 2 g IV pre-op.

Vancomycin

Vancomycin is used for prophylaxis against wound infections during surgery in penicillin-allergic patients. Vancomycin is the best choice for implant surgery because it covers *Staphylococcus epidermis*, which is a common pathogen in implant surgery. Dosage is 1 g IV.

Amoxicillin

Amoxicillin is used for prophylaxis against bacterial endocarditis. Dosage is 2 g PO or IV 1 hour before the procedure. For PCN allergies, use clindamycin 600 mg PO or IV.

Endocarditis prophylaxis

ABX	REGIMEN	
Amoxicillin	2 g PO IV	1 hr before procedure
Clindamycin (PCN allergic)	600 mg PO IV	1 hr before procedure

Clindamycin

Used for prophylaxis against bacterial endocarditis in penicillin-allergic patients. Dosage is 600 mg PO or IV 1 hour before procedure.

Erythromycin

Used for prophylaxis against bacterial endocarditis in penicillin-allergic patients. Dosage depends on the preparation.

Pregnancy Test

All female patients of childbearing age. All elective surgery should be postponed on pregnant women.

Pituitary–Adrenal Suppression

Patients on 7.5 mg of corticosteroids a day or more should be tested for endogenous cortisol suppression. Low plasma concentrations of cortisol and ACTH indicate suppression. Even if exogenous corticosteroids are discontinued, the pituitary–adrenal negative feedback can take up to a year to recover. Adrenal–pituitary axis suppression leaves patients unable to produce extra steroids in response to the stress of surgery. Patients on steroids often require increased dosing perioperatively and postoperatively. Steroids delay the wound healing process. This may be counteracted with the use of topical vitamin A. Usual dose is 1,000 U applied tid to the open wound bed for 7 to 10 days.

PERIOPERATIVE

Tourniquet

Inflate tourniquet 100 to 120 mm Hg above systolic blood pressure. Maximum tourniquet pressure is 250 mm Hg for the ankle and 500 mm Hg for the thigh. Tourniquet must be deflated after 2 hours for at least 15 to 20 minutes before reinflating.

Drains

Used in surgery where excessive bleeding is expected or there is a lot of dead space where fluid may accumulate. Most drains are removed at around 2 to 3 days.

Penrose Drain

A Penrose drain is a soft, flat, flexible tube made of latex. It is inserted into a wound to maintain an opening between the surgical site and outside the body. Although Penrose drains are a tube, the fluid is not intended to flow through the tube, but around it. Penrose drains are passive, meaning they provide no active suction or negative pressure to draw fluid out. They are merely intended to maintain patency at the surgical site to allow excess fluid to drain. The drainage is absorbed by the surgical dressing.

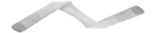

Jackson-Pratt Drain

Jackson-Pratt drains provide active drainage through negative pressure by way of a collapsible bulb reservoir. The collapsible bulb can be emptied by the patient at home and reused. Patients should be instructed to keep track of the amount of fluid that drains from the site and report the amount to their surgeon.

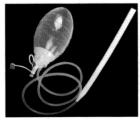

Hemovac Drain

Hemovac drains provide active drainage through negative pressure by way of a collapsible accordion-style reservoir. Patients should be instructed to keep track of the amount of fluid that drains from the site and report the amount to their surgeon.

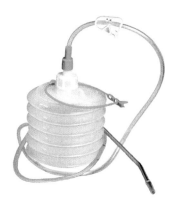

TLC Drain

TLC stands for tiny little sucker. Consists of a vacutainer as a reservoir that has a negative pressure to pull drainage from the surgical site. They are very compact and easily incorporated into a wound dressing.

Negative-Pressure Wound Therapy (NPWT)

Wound VACs are technically drains too, although they are more commonly associated with wound care as a type of dressing.

Diabetic

Diabetics are given early morning surgical preference to prevent extended periods NPO and in case post-op issues arise. Hyperglycemia (>200 mg per dL) impairs wound healing, and hypoglycemia can cause organic brain damage and death. Hypoglycemia is a more hazardous condition than hyperglycemia: "better sweet than sour." There is no standardized protocol for diabetic glucose control during the day of surgery while the patient is NPO, but a few general guidelines include the following:

Glucose Control on the Day of Surgery While Patient Is NPO

1. Plasma glucose levels should be maintained between 150 and 250 mg per dL. A little on the high side going into surgery is OK.

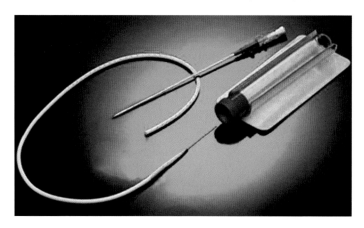

2. If surgery is delayed or patient expected to be NPO for many hours, start IV D5W to avoid hypoglycemia, and check glucose q2h to q3h.
3. NIDDM patients should not take their diabetic medication the day of surgery while they are NPO.
4. Have IDDM patients check their glucose level the morning of surgery before they arrive at the hospital; if it is elevated (>300 mg per dL), have them take half their normal morning dose, and check again once they reach the hospital.
5. Once the patient has reached the hospital, elevated glucose levels can be controlled with a sliding scale.
6. Exact values for insulin sliding scales vary depending on the doctor or hospital.

Insulin Sliding Scale	
<150	0 units
151–200	2 units
201–250	4 units
251–300	6 units
301–350	8 units
351–400	10 units
>400	12 units

Patients on Anticoagulants

When possible, discontinue anticoagulants 3 to 6 days before surgery and resume 24 hours post-op. Discontinue aspirin 7 days before surgery. If anticoagulants cannot be discontinued, bridging with heparin may be required.

Rheumatoid Patient

A cervical spine x-ray should be considered preoperatively with rheumatoid patients. Rheumatoid patients are predisposed to atlas/axis dislocation. They are also more prone to infection from the immunosuppressive medications they take.

Sickle Cell Patients (aka Hemoglobin S Disease)

A mutation in the β-chain gene resulting in a change in amino acid number 6 from glutamic acid to valine. On deoxygenation, hemoglobin S becomes relatively insoluble and aggregates into long strands of fibers, giving the RBC its distinctive "sickle" shape. Normal red blood cells are pliable and deform in shape to fit through small capillaries. Sickle cells cannot deform in shape to fit through the small capillaries. As a result, the capillaries become clogged, and the area becomes ischemia. In addition to ischemia, there is an anemia problem from the spleen destroying all the abnormal RBCs, which results in splenomegaly. Found almost exclusively in blacks. Hemoglobin SC is the heterozygous condition, in which usually the patient has fewer symptoms.

Diagnosis

Hemoglobin electrophoresis shows the presence of hemoglobin S.
Peripheral smear will show the characteristic sickle cells.

Signs/Symptoms

Long bone pain (e.g., pretibial) and hand and foot pain
Arthritis with fever
Avascular necrosis of the femoral head

Chronic punched-out lesions around the ankles

Abdominal pain with vomiting

Associated Crises

Aplastic crisis: During acute infections (especially viral), production of marrow RBCs slows.

Painful crises: Episodes of severe abdominal pain with vomiting that are usually associated with back and joint pain

Surgical Considerations

Sickle cell patients are prone to hypoxia due to the decreased oxygen-carrying capacity of the hemoglobin. Local anesthesia is preferred, and if possible, the use of a tourniquet should be avoided. With general anesthesia, extra precaution must be taken to avoid volume depletion and hypoxia.

There is an increase in postoperative complications with sickle cell disease. A high index of suspicion should be maintained for sepsis postoperatively. *Salmonella* is the most common organism isolated from sickle cell patients who develop osteomyelitis.

Cardiac Patients

Top factors that lead to post-op cardiac complications:

1. CHF	Manifested by S3 gallop or jugular venous distention
2. Rhythm	PACs, or >5 PVCs/min
3. Age	Over 70 years
4. Coronary dz	MI within past 6 months

Elective surgery should be postponed until at least 6 months after an MI.

Endocarditis prophylaxis should be given for patients with valvular heart disease, rheumatic murmur, and prosthetic valves.

Drug of choice for prophylaxis is IV PCN or first-generation cephalosporin (Ancef). If PCN allergic, clindamycin 300 mg pre-op and 150 mg post-op.

HTN (diastolic pressure > 110) increases the chances of intraoperative and postoperative MI or stroke.

Patients on diuretics—check K^+

Most heart medications should be continued up to and through the day of surgery.

POST-OP MANAGEMENT/ COMPLICATIONS

Fever

Intraoperative
  Transfusion reaction
  Malignant hyperthermia
  Preexisting sepsis
Post-op

0 to 6 Hours

Pain

Rebound from cold operating room

Anesthesia reaction

Endocrine cause (thyroid crisis, adrenal insufficiency)

24 to 48 Hours

Atelectasis

Aspiration pneumonia (after general)

Dehydration

Constipation

72 Hours or Greater

Infection (3 to 7 days)
DVT
Thrombophlebitis from IV
UTI (especially if catheterized)
Drug allergy

Five "W"s

5 W's
DDx for post-op fever

Wind	Atelectasis, aspiration pneumonia, PE
Wound	Infection, thrombophlebitis (IV site), pain
Water	UTI, dehydration, constipation
Walking	DVT
Wonder drugs	Any drug can cause fever (Patient appears less ill than fever suggests)

DVT

Phlegmasia cerulea dolens (PCD): An uncommon but severe form of DVT resulting from extensive thrombotic occlusion. Most common in the upper leg it presents with edema and severe cyanosis of the limb. It is considered a medical emergency.

Surgical patients have additional risk factors for DVTs.
Bed rest
Tourniquet
Surgical trauma
Infection
Dehydration (due to NPO status)
Change in medication (i.e., d/c ASA)
Thrombolytics
IVC filters: Greenfield vena cava filters

Post-Op Infection

Occurs 3 to 7 days post-op (group A strep may occur earlier)
Symptoms:
Increased throbbing pain
Edema
Drainage
Dehydration
Erythema
Fever

Treatment for post-op ischemic toe conditions

WHITE TOE Arterial problem	BLUE TOE Venous problem
Place foot in dependent position Loosen bandages Twist the K-wire Apply head to small of back PT block Remove K-wire Remove dressing Consider reopening wound	Elevate foot Loosen bandages Remove K-wire Remove dressing Consider reopening wound

If systemic symptoms are present (fever/chills), consider admitting to hospital.

Factors increasing the chances of a surgical infection:

Surgery > 2 hours
Blood transfusion
Preexisting infection
Implants

Pain

Post-op pain unresponsive to narcotic analgesics usually indicates one of the following three things:

Infection
Hematoma
Dressing pressure
Severe pain within 48 hours post-op:
Sutures too tight
Dressing too tight
Hematoma
Edema (foot in dependent position)
Vasospasm (from K-wire)
Compartment syndrome

Hematoma

A hematoma is a collection of blood within a closed tissue space. Hematomas can lead to infection and may result in long-term swelling and disability. Often mimics an infection with intense pain and inflammation, but occurs sooner than one would expect with infection (occurs within the first 24 hours after surgery).

Etiology

Traumatic surgical dissection
Poor hemostasis
Creating a dead space and not using a drain
Exposed cancellous bone
Anticoagulants
Hypertension
Improper bandaging

Fate of an Untreated Hematoma

1. A hematoma that has walled itself off from surrounding tissue from pressure will ultimately clot and undergo fibroplasia into a dense scar.
2. A hematoma that is more diffusely located within the tissue will tend to resorb itself.

Treatment

EARLY (before all the hematoma has clotted)
   Extravasation: Pop a stitch or two, and squeeze out the fluid.
   Aspiration: Aspirate the hematoma using a large-bore needle.
   Steroid injection: Decrease inflammation and pain, and interfere with fibroplasia and clotting.
   Wound reentry: The patient is taken back to the OR and the wound is reopened, drained, and irrigated; ligate bleeders; and insert a drain.
LATE
   Gentle heat: In an attempt to accelerate enzymatic degradation of the hematoma
   Physical therapy: Exercise, ROM, massage, and ultrasound. All serve to break up the hematoma and encourage resorption.

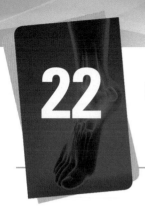

22 INSTRUMENTS

BLADE HANDLES

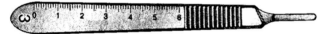

Bard Parker Blade Handle #3
(for blades 9–15, 17)

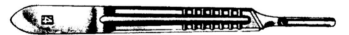

Bard Parker Blade Handle #4
(for blades 20–25)

Beaver Handle
(for blades 61–88, 312–316)

BLADE

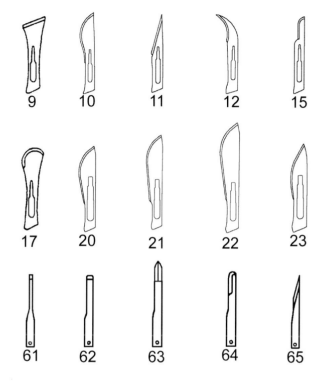

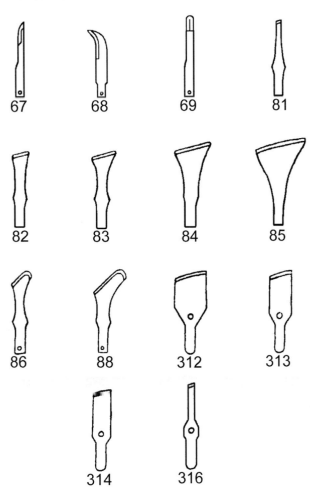

67   68   69   81

82   83   84   85

86   88   312   313

314   316

INSTRUMENTS

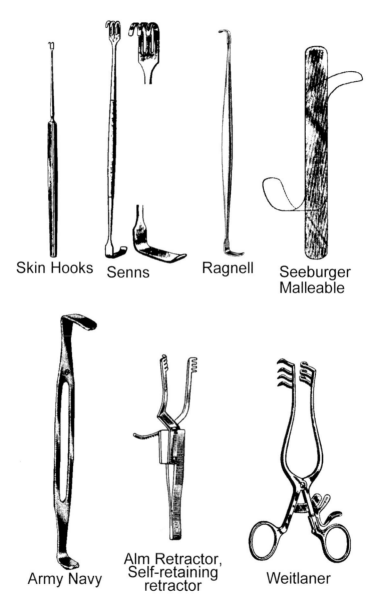

Skin Hooks   Senns   Ragnell   Seeburger Malleable

Army Navy   Alm Retractor, Self-retaining retractor   Weitlaner

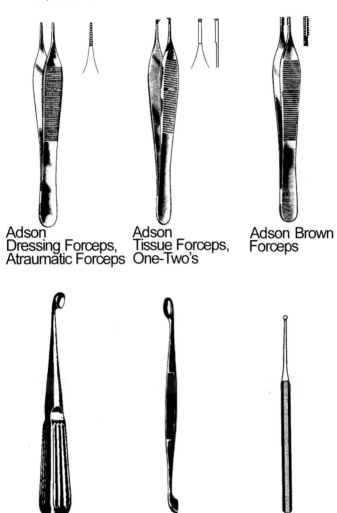

Adson
Dressing Forceps,
Atraumatic Forceps

Adson
Tissue Forceps,
One-Two's

Adson Brown
Forceps

Brun (Spratt)
Curette

Volkmann
Curette

Nail Curette

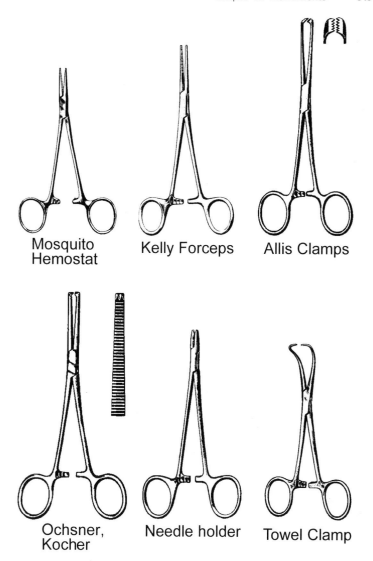

Mosquito
Hemostat

Kelly Forceps

Allis Clamps

Ochsner,
Kocher

Needle holder

Towel Clamp

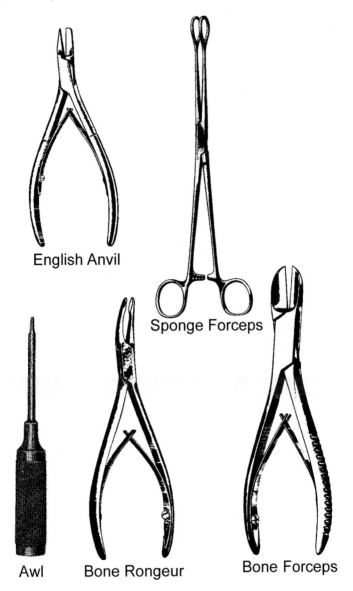

English Anvil

Sponge Forceps

Awl

Bone Rongeur

Bone Forceps

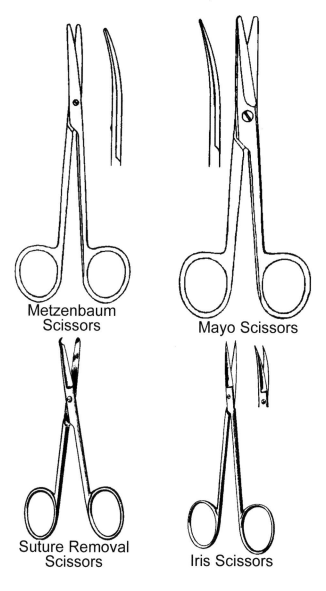

Metzenbaum
Scissors

Mayo Scissors

Suture Removal
Scissors

Iris Scissors

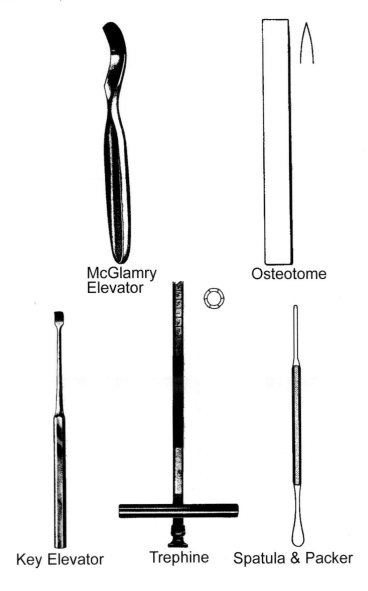

McGlamry
Elevator

Osteotome

Key Elevator

Trephine

Spatula & Packer

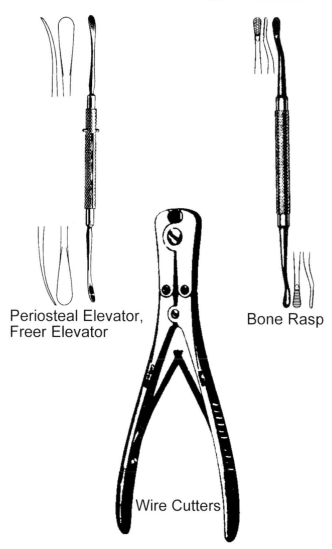

Periosteal Elevator,
Freer Elevator

Bone Rasp

Wire Cutters

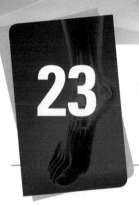

23 SUTURE

NEEDLE SHAPE

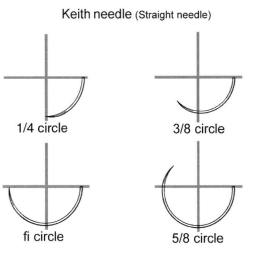

Keith needle (Straight needle)

1/4 circle

3/8 circle

fi circle

5/8 circle

Point Configuration

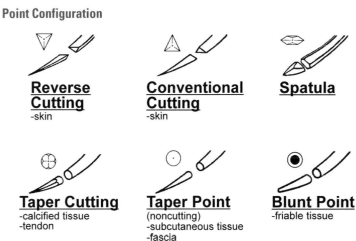

Reverse Cutting
-skin

Conventional Cutting
-skin

Spatula

Taper Cutting
-calcified tissue
-tendon

Taper Point
(noncutting)
-subcutaneous tissue
-fascia

Blunt Point
-friable tissue

TYPES OF SUTURE

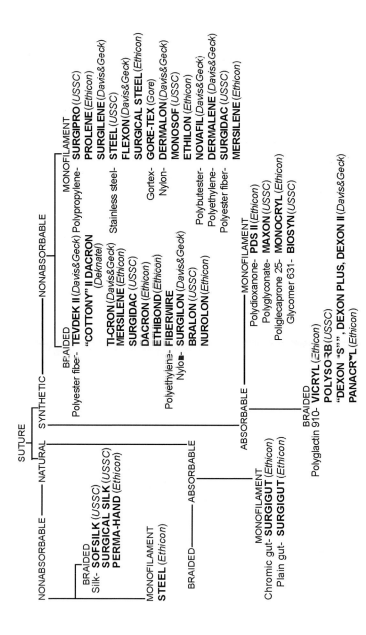

SUTURE

NONABSORBABLE

NATURAL

BRAIDED
Silk- **SOFSILK** (USSC)
SURGICAL SILK (USSC)
PERMA-HAND (Ethicon)

MONOFILAMENT
STEEL (Ethicon)

SYNTHETIC

NONABSORBABLE

BRAIDED
Polyester fiber- **TEVDEK II** (Davis&Geck) Polypropylene-
"COTTONY" II DACRON
(Deknatel)
TI-CRON (Davis&Geck)
MERSILENE (Ethicon)
SURGIDAC (USSC)
DACRON (Ethicon)
ETHIBOND (Ethicon)
Polyethylene- **FIBERWIRE**
Nylon- **SURGILON** (Davis&Geck)
BRALON (USSC)
NUROLON (Ethicon)

Stainless steel-

Gortex-
Nylon-

Polybutester-
Polyethylene-
Polyester fiber-

MONOFILAMENT
SURGIPRO (USSC)
PROLENE (Ethicon)
SURGILENE (Davis&Geck)
STEEL (USSC)
FLEXON (Davis&Geck)
SURGICAL STEEL (Ethicon)
GORE-TEX (Gore)
DERMALON (Davis&Geck)
MONOSOF (USSC)
ETHILON (Ethicon)
NOVAFIL (Davis&Geck)
DERMALENE (Davis&Geck)
SURGIDAC (USSC)
MERSILENE (Ethicon)

ABSORBABLE

MONOFILAMENT
Polydioxanone- **PDS II** (Ethicon)
Polyglyconate- **MAXON** (USSC)
Poliglecaprone 25- **MONOCRYL** (Ethicon)
Glycomer 631- **BIOSYN** (USSC)

BRAIDED
Polyglactin 910- **VICRYL** (Ethicon)
POLYSORB (USSC)
"DEXON "S"", DEXON PLUS, DEXON II (Davis&Geck)
PANACRYL (Ethicon)

NONABSORBABLE

MONOFILAMENT
Chromic gut- **SURGIGUT** (Ethicon)
Plain gut- **SURGIGUT** (Ethicon)

BRAIDED

ABSORBABLE

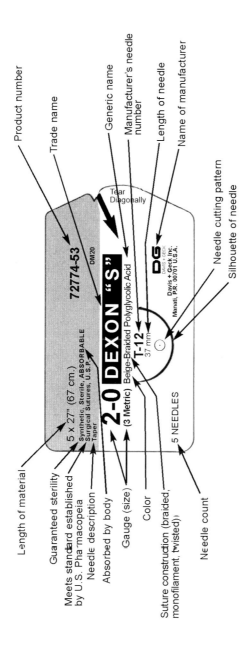

Product number
Trade name
Generic name
Manufacturer's needle number
Length of needle
Name of manufacturer

Length of material
Guaranteed sterility
Meets standard established by U.S. Pharmacopeia
Needle description
Absorbed by body
Gauge (size)
Color
Suture construction (braided, monofilament, twisted)
Needle count

Needle cutting pattern
Silhouette of needle

72774-53
DM20
5 x 27" (67 cm.)
Synthetic, Sterile, ABSORBABLE
Surgical Sutures, U.S.P.
Taper
2-0 DEXON "S"
(3 Metric) Beige-Braided Polyglycolic Acid
T-12
37 mm
5 NEEDLES
Tear Diagonally
DG DAVIS + GECK
Davis + Geck Inc.
Manati, P.R. 00701 U.S.A.

ABSORBABLE SUTURE: TENSILE STRENGTH AND ABSORPTION TIME

Suture	50% Tensile Strength	Completely Absorbed	Reactivity
Gut	7–10 d	70 d	+++
Chromic gut	21–28 d	90 d	+++
Monocryl	2 wk	90–120 d	+
Maxon	3 wk	90–120 d	+
Biosyn	3 wk	90–110 d	+
Vicryl	3 wk	56–70 d	++
Polysorb	3 wk	56–70 d	++
Dexon II	3 wk	56–70 d	++
PDS II	4 wk	180–210 d	+
Panacryl	4 months	1–1.5 y	++

+ = slightly reactive, ++ = moderately reactive, +++ = highly reactive.

Suture Sizes

Suture is sized by diameter stated as a number of zeros. The more the zeros, the smaller the suture (i.e., 5-0 suture is smaller than 2-0 suture).

Suture "Tracks"

May result from sutures being too tight or from sutures being left in too long

Gut vs. Chromic gut

Chromic gut is soaked in chromium salts, which causes it to be resistant to break down and less irritating to tissue.

Pop-Off, Control Release, and D-Tach

All terms used to describe needle–suture combinations. The needle is released with a straight tug of the needle holder without cutting the suture.

Swagged

A term to describe the technique. A suture strand is mounted on a needle. The suture is inserted into the hollowed out proximal end of the needle and then closed or "swagged" around the suture.

Suture Removal

Skin incisions reach 35% of their original strength around the 14th day. At this point, the tensile strength of the incision equals the strength of the sutures, so sutures can be removed.

KNOTS

Simple Interrupted

Simple (Continuous) Running

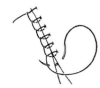

SUTURE

Vertical Mattress (aka Donati Suture)

Far-far, near-near

Used for difficult-to-approximate skin edges
Everts tissue well

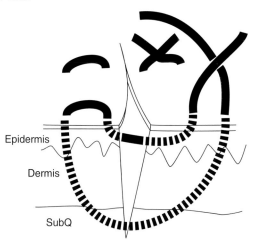

Allgöwer–Donati Suture

A modification of the vertical mattress. Subcutaneous suture on one side and intracutaneous on the other. It maintains better microcirculation at the wound edges. Offers improved incision perfusion and may decrease wound complications after ORIF. This suture technique is recommended with incisions commonly associated with dehiscence such as the extensile incision used in calcaneal fractures or pilon fracture repair.

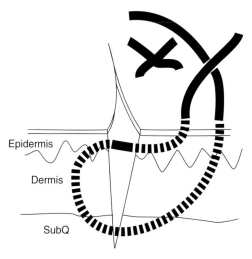

Horizontal Mattress

Good for everting skin edges

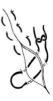

Subcutaneous Stitch

A stitch, usually running, placed in the dermis

Often used in conjunction with Steri-Strips for a more pleasing scar

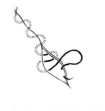

Purse String Suture

Often used to interpose soft tissue between two bones (i.e., Keller)

Retention Stitch

Far-near, near-far

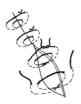

Buried Knot

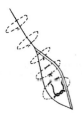

Whip Stitch

Used to anchor suture to tendon for purposes of a tendon transfer

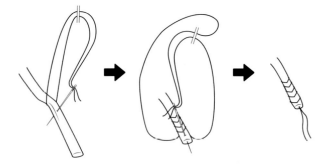

TWO HAND TIE

May be used to tie off small vessels

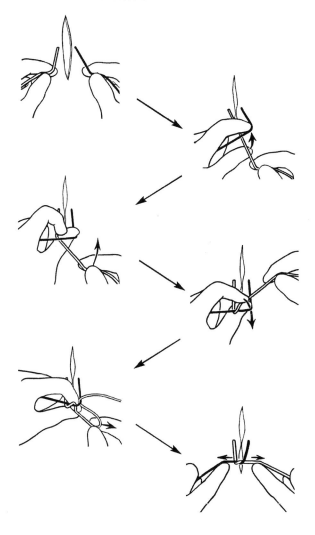

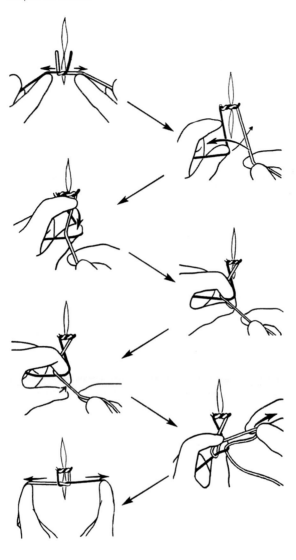

STAPLES

Advantage of staples is speed. An incision can be closed much quicker with staples. The disadvantage is that they leave a more noticeable scar compared with sutures and they require two people to properly apply. The skin edges should be grasped with forceps, pulled together, and everted, while a second surgeon applies the staples. Another potential disadvantage with staples is that they require a special staple remover to remove the staples. Skin edges should be everted.

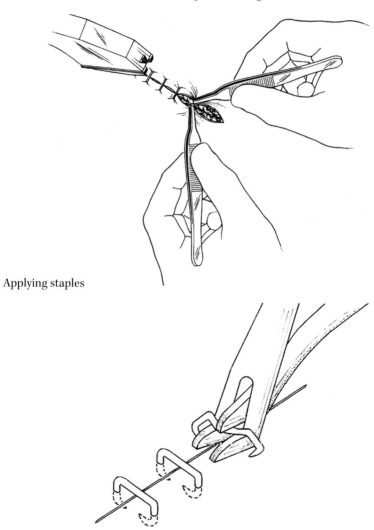

Applying staples

Removing staples

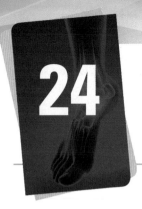

24 FIXATION

SCREWS

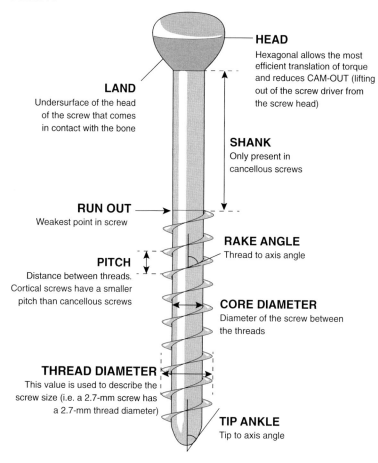

HEAD
Hexagonal allows the most efficient translation of torque and reduces CAM-OUT (lifting out of the screw driver from the screw head)

LAND
Undersurface of the head of the screw that comes in contact with the bone

SHANK
Only present in cancellous screws

RUN OUT
Weakest point in screw

RAKE ANGLE
Thread to axis angle

PITCH
Distance between threads. Cortical screws have a smaller pitch than cancellous screws

CORE DIAMETER
Diameter of the screw between the threads

THREAD DIAMETER
This value is used to describe the screw size (i.e. a 2.7-mm screw has a 2.7-mm thread diameter)

TIP ANKLE
Tip to axis angle

Interfrag screw: A screw placed across a fracture or osteotomy site in order to provide compression

Absolute stability—primary (haversian) healing
Relative stability—heal with enchondral healing (bone callus)

Instrument Sizes for Respective Screws

Screw (mm)	Thread Hole (mm)	Glide Hole (mm)	Tap (mm)	Surgical Set
1.5 Cortical	1.1	1.5	1.5	Mini fragment
2.0 Cortical	1.5	2.0	2.0	
2.7 Cortical	2.0	2.7	2.7	
3.5 Cortical	2.5	3.5	3.5	Small fragment
4.0 Cancellous	2.0 or 2.5	None	3.5	
Partially threaded				
Fully threaded				
4.5 Cortical	3.2	4.5	4.5	Standard fragment
4.5 Malleolar	3.2	None	4.5	
6.5 Cancellous	3.2	None (4.0 in hard bone)	6.5	

Cortical screws are fully threaded (historically). Tend to have fine threads with a small pitch that are designed to anchor to cortical bone.

Cancellous screws are partially threaded (historically), allowing them to be used as lag screws. The threads are coarser with a higher pitch intended to engage medullary bone.

Self-tapping screws should be advanced an extra 2 mm because the cutting flute decreases the overall surface area of bone–screw interface.

Insertional torque is 65% higher using a star driver vs. hexagonal driver.

Lag Technique

A lag screw allows compression across a fracture or osteotomy site. The head of the screw pushes down on the near fragment, and the threads pull up on the far fragment.

Example: Inserting a 2.7-mm cortical bone screw
1. *Drill thread hole* (2.0-mm drill bit)—near and far cortex
2. *Drill glide hole* (2.7-mm drill bit)—near cortex
3. Counter sink
4. Measure
5. *Tap* (2.7-mm tap)
6. Flush
7. *Insert 2.7-mm screw* (two fingers' tightness)

Shannon Burr

A Shannon burr is a side cutting burr used in minimally invasive surgery (MIS).

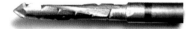

PINS

Trochar

Diamond

Kirschner Wires (K-Wires)

Sizes (inches): 0.028, 0.035, 0.045, 0.062

Available smooth and threaded

Steinmann Pin

Larger than K-wires (usually used for rearfoot)

Sizes (inches): 5/64, 3/32, 7/64, 1/8, 9/64, 5/32, 3/16

Available smooth and threaded

Rush Pin/Nail/Rod

Used for intramedullary fixation

Solid, circular in cross section, straight, with sharp beveled tips and a hook at the driving end. Intended for fractures of diaphyseal or metaphyseal fractures of long bones like femur, tibia, fibula, humerus, radius, and ulna. Pointed tip facilitates easy insertion. Curve at top prevents rotation and stabilizes fracture. Rush pins have largely been replaced by plates and nails due to their superior fixation qualities.

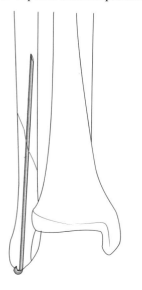

WIRES

Cerclage Wire (Monofilament Wire)

Sizes: For podiatric forefoot cases, usually range between 26 and 28 gauge

Tension-Band Fixation

Tension-band fixation is used when there is asymmetrical distraction at a fracture site due to muscle or ligamentous pull. Tension banding converts distractive forces into compressive forces.

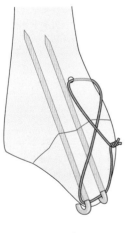

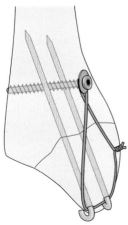

Cerclage wire is placed on the tension side of a fracture, which prevents distraction and causes a corresponding compression on the opposite side of the wire.

Tension-band fixation is accomplished by inserting a K-wire through the fracture line. A second K-wire is inserted parallel to the first to prevent fragment rotation.

Cerclage wire is then applied in the form of a figure 8 and united by twisting.

Common lower extremity uses of tension-band fixation include the medial or lateral malleolar fractures and styloid process fractures. Tension-band wiring is preferred to tension-band plating when the fracture fragments are small or the bone is osteoporotic.

MATERIALS
Stainless Steel

Stainless steel is an alloy, meaning it is composed of several different metals. Iron (~70%), chromium (~18%), nickel (~16%). Chromium is what makes stainless steel "stainless," it prevents rust and corrosion. It also allows the steel to withstand greater temperature changes. Chromium, however, makes steel weak, so nickel is added to increase strength. Unfortunately, nickel is the most common causes of metal allergies. Stainless steel is relatively cheap but has a Young modulus 10 times stronger than bone, which can lead to stress shielding. Stainless steel's Young modulus makes it a good choice for a bridge plate where you want the plate to bear all the weight. Stainless steel plates can be bent to conform to bone. Uses include plates, screws, IM nails, external fixators.

> **Stress shielding**
>
> Bones have the ability to bend somewhat based on the amount of force place on them. This subtle bending is quantified with the Young's modulus, which measures stress and strain of materials. The ideal implant has a Young's modulus similar to bone. Implants that are too stiff (high Young's modulus) protect the surrounding bone to the point of shielding it from normal levels of mechanical loading. As a result, as per Wolff law, the bone resorbs.

Titanium (Ti)

Titanium is also an alloy but contains mostly titanium. There are minor amounts of other elements such as aluminum and vanadium. Allergies and immune reactions from corrosion are much less common with titanium. Titanium is stronger and lighter than stainless steel, but it is more brittle. This means that titanium plates cannot (should not) be bent. Titanium has a Young's modulus of elasticity that most closely approximates cortical bone, which decreases the amount of stress on the surrounding bone.

This also means they make great neutralization plates and IM nails and some very slight physiologic loading may be desired. Uses include internal fixators, plates, vertebral spacers, and IM nails. When using a titanium locking plate system, screws should not be tightened as much as with stainless steel because the screw and plate can become cold welded together, making later removal difficult.

Cobalt Chrome (CoCr)

Cobalt chrome contains primarily cobalt (30% to 60%). Chromium (20% to 30%) is added to improve corrosion resistance. Minor amounts of carbon, nickel, and molybdenum are added. Cobalt chrome is extremely hard and can be finished with a surface polish that is very smooth. This makes it the perfect choice for joint implants, hips, knees, ankles, and metal-on-metal devices. It is more expensive than stainless steel or titanium. It has an elastic Young modulus similar to, but slightly less than, stainless steel.

Nitinol

Nitinol is an acronym for
nickel-**ti**tanium alloy discovered at the **N**aval **O**rdinance **L**aboratory. It is composed of nickel and titanium in approximately equal proportions and has the unique property of shape memory and pseudoelasticity. Nitinol can be bent into a deforming shape and hold that shape until heat is applied, at which time it becomes elastic and reverts back to its original shape.

Plastics

Polyetheretherketone (PEEK) biomaterial commonly used in place of metal. PEEK has advantages over metal in that it does not show up on radiographs and so it does not obscure areas of importance. PEEK is a type of plastic, it is nonmagnetic, and there are no artifacts with MRIs.

ABSORBABLE MATERIALS

There are two main products on the market used for bioabsorbable fixation devices: PGA and PLA. PGA absorbs faster than PLA. A concern with rapidly resorbing implants is osteolysis and bone cyst formation. Absorbable materials are used for screws, anchors, and interference screws. They are nonradiopaque, so their placement is difficult to evaluate by postoperative radiographs. They tend to splinter if cut with wire or bone cutters, so absorbable devices should be cut with an oscillating saw, Bovie, or scalpel.

PGA and PLA are often combined with composite materials, such as hydroxyapatite (HA) and β-tricalcium phosphate (β-TCP). These composite materials are osteoconductive and help bone form in the dead space as the implant dissolves. In addition, the composite materials act as a buffer to minimize the decrease in pH associated with the resorption of these materials. The by-product of PGA and PLA degradation is lactic acid, which is acidic.

PGA

Includes several forms:

PGA (polyglycolic acid)
PLGA (poly lactic-co-glycolic acid)

PLA

Includes several forms:

PLA (poly lactic acid)
PLLA (poly-L-lactic acid)
PLDLA (poly-L-lactide, L-lactic acid)
PLDLLA (poly-L-lactide-co-D, L-lactic acid)

BONE PLATES

Regardless of their length, thickness, geometry, configuration, or types of hole, all plates can be classified into five groups based on their function: compression plate, neutralization plate, bridge plate, buttress plate, or a tension-band plate. Plates can function in more than one of these classification group at the same time.

PLATE CLASSIFICATION (FUNCTIONAL)

Compression Plate

Compression plating provides rigid fixation and absolute stability. Compression plating is useful in transverse fractures, where lag screw placement is not possible. Compression plating can be accomplished by prebending the plate, use of an articulated tension device, plate design (dynamic compression plate), or any combination of these techniques.

Prebending the Plate

Prebending a plate will produce compression at the fracture site due to the memory of the metal plate. The screws lag the plate to the bone, straightening the plate and causing axial compression across the fracture site. As the plate is lagged to the bone, the plate retains some memory and causes compression.

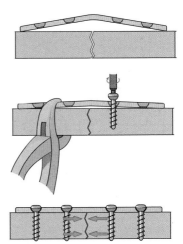

Articulated Tension Device

An articulated tension device is a device that attaches to a plate and applies distraction of the plate and corresponding compression of the bone beneath it. Once the screws are inserted, the device is removed. These devices are somewhat antiquated because they require an extra-long incision and placement of an additional screw.

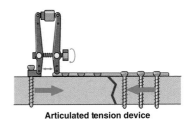

Articulated tension device

Dynamic Compression Plate (DCP)

Dynamic compression plates compress due to the special geometry of their screw holes. They have a slope built into one side of their screw holes. Effect occurs according to Newton's third law (action–reaction).

Application of a Dynamic Compression Plate

Application of a dynamic compression plate begins with applying an anchor screw that is placed concentrically. Next, screw 2 is applied on the other side of the fracture, eccentrically in the screw hole away from the fracture site. As screw 2 engages the plate, the screw and underlying bone are forced toward the fracture line due to the design of the plate that causes compression.

Added compression can be applied by inserting screw 3 eccentrically away from the fracture. Once screw 3 has engaged the bone, but before the screw head reaches the plate, loosen the original screw (screw 1). Then tighten screw 3, which will cause additional compression from the other side of the fracture. Screw 1 is then retightened, and any additional screws are inserted concentrically for added fixation.

Dynamic compression plate

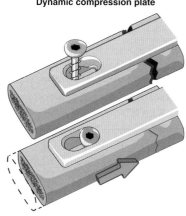

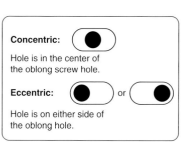

Concentric: ●
Hole is in the center of the oblong screw hole.

Eccentric: ● or ●
Hole is on either side of the oblong hole.

Dynamic compression plate

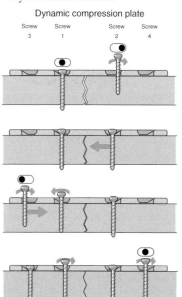

| Screw 3 | Screw 1 | Screw 2 | Screw 4 |

STATIC COMPRESSION VS. DYNAMIC COMPRESSION

Static compression is compression that remains constant, whether the limb is at rest or functioning. Dynamic compression is a phenomenon by which a plate transfers or modifies functional physiologic force into compression force at the fracture site.

"Dynamic compression plate" is a misnomer; once the screws are tightened, static compression is being applied.

A dynamic compression plate can provide dynamic compression, but it would be functioning as a buttress plate or tension-band plate.

Buttress plates and tension-band plates provide dynamic compression because compression increases with movement. External fixators and IM nails can also be "dynamized" at which point they are also providing dynamic compression.

Dynamic compression

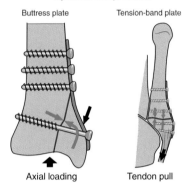

Buttress plate

Tension-band plate

Axial loading

Tendon pull

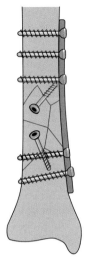

Neutralization (Protection) Plate

Neutralization plates are "protection plates" placed over other hardware to "neutralize" other forces on the fracture site. The plate bridges the fracture and protects the lag screws. Neutralization plates protect the primary repair by neutralizing shearing, bending, and torsional forces across a fracture that may disrupt the primary fixation. The lag screws can be part of the plate construct or independent.

The most common clinical application of the neutralization plate is to protect the screw fixation of a short oblique fracture, a butterfly fragment or mild comminuted fracture of a long bone, or for the fixation of a segmental bone defect in combination with bone graft.

With neutralization plates, the bone provides some support as opposed to a bridge plate that bears all the load.

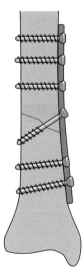

Bridge Plate

A bridge plate provides relative stability. Mechanical link between healthy segment of bone above and below fracture. There is no compression at the fracture site, it acts as a "bridge." Intended to maintain length and alignment often used with comminuted fractures. With a bridge plate, the plate bears all the load. A bridge plate used in combination with lag screws for fixating fracture fragments becomes a neutralization plate.

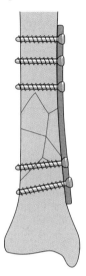

Buttress Plate

Buttress plates are plates applied to the metaphyseal/epiphyseal area of an intra-articular fracture to prevent a bone fragment from sliding off the shaft. Antiglide plates are the same as buttress plates, but application is to the shaft (diaphysis) vs. the metaphysis/epiphysis. Both plates reduce an oblique fracture indirectly through interference between the plate and the undisplaced main fragment. The tip of the distal fragment becomes wedged between the plate and the proximal fragment, preventing it from sliding during axial loading. The plate must be well contoured to the bone to provide this effect. The plate can be slightly under bent

as a way to increase the force with which the plate pushed against the sliding fragment. Antiglide plates are commonly used for fibula fractures, and buttress plates are commonly used on the tibia.

Fixation of a buttress plate to the bone should begin in the middle of the plate, closest to the fracture site on the shaft. This screw will ensure good bone plate contact, especially if the bone has been purposely under bent. Subsequent screws should be applied one after the other toward both ends of the plate. Buttress plates and antiglide plates can be used with or without interfragmental lag screws. Buttress plates provide dynamic compression.

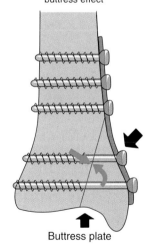

The top three screws provide the basis for the buttress effect

Buttress plate

Tension-Band Plate

Tension-band plating takes advantage of asymmetrical biomechanical distraction forces across a fracture site and converts them into compressive forces.

Tension banding shifts the neutral axis of the bending force from the center of the bone to the plate, allowing compression across the entire length of the fracture.

Plate must be placed on the convex (tension) side of the bone to counteract distraction forces, and the cortex on the opposite side of the bone must be relatively intact. Tension-band plates provide dynamic compression.

Tension-band plate

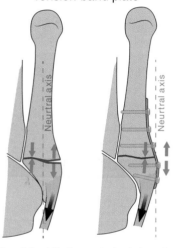

The plate shifts the neutral axis from the center of the bone to the plate, causing compression along the entire fracture

SPECIALTY PLATE FEATURES

Locking Plates

Locking plates are "internal fixators" that have screws that secure to the plate, preventing toggle and providing a more stable fixation. They do not require bicortical fixation of screws, and they are indicated in osteopenic bone. Locking plate screws do not lag the plate down to bone. Plate-to-bone contact is not critical as with nonlocking plates. This diminished contact between bone and plate causes less damage to the periosteum and improves blood supply to help healing. Some locking plates allow up to 15° angulation of screw called polyaxial or variable axial or variable pitch locking screws.

Limited Contact Plates (LC)

Limited contact plates have scalloped undercuts on the bottom of the plate that reduce the area of contact between the bone and the plate. These limited contact plates crush less periosteum underneath the plate and thus improve healing. This scalloped undersurface has other advantages, including decrease stress at the screw holes, bend distribution over entire plate rather than screw holes, and uniform strength along the entire plate.

Plate footprint on bone in red

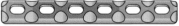

Blade plate: A blade plate is a plate with a long "blade" that sticks out at various angles. They provide good stability and compression and may be used when an IM rod is not indicated. A chisel is used to make the hole for the blade. Blade plates are most commonly used in the hip for intertrochanteric fractures. In podiatry, they are only used on the tibia. Lower extremity applications include pilon fractures, ankle fusions, and pantalar fusions.

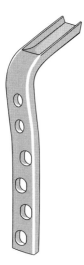

Spoon plate: Used anteriorly in distal intra-articular tibial fractures where the comminution is anterior

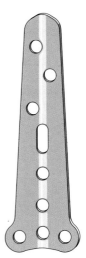

Cloverleaf plate: Used for distal intra-articular tibial fractures. They are used as a buttress plate over the medial malleolus to prevent varus collapse in a pilon fracture. Cloverleaf plates are anatomically designed to fit the contour of the medial malleolus.

Hook plate: Used for malleolar fractures and Jones fractures

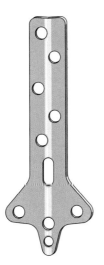

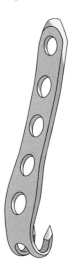

STAPLES

Staples provide more stable fixation than screws in osteopenic bone. They are also useful when fixation is required, and the only access to the fracture/osteotomy is perpendicular to the fracture/osteotomy line. Frequently used for fixation of the large cancellous bones of the midfoot and rearfoot.

INTRAMEDULLARY NAIL

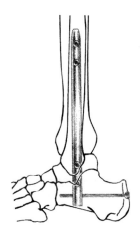

Intramedullary nails or IM nails are used in the foot as a way of fixating a tibiotalocalcaneal arthrodesis or pantalar fusion. IM nails have the advantage of minimal disruption of soft tissue relative to large plates. IM nails are indicated for failed ankle implant, marked ankle and STJ instability, severe rheumatoid or post traumatic arthritis, AVN of the talus, and fixation following a talectomy (tibial–calcaneal arthrodesis).

IM nails function as an internal splint to resist bending, and the locking screws attached to the nail function to resist rotation and shortening. Compression is also possible with these devices. Fixation should begin with the ankle joint and then the STJ.

Indications

Charcot arthropathy
End-stage PTTD
Failed ankle implant
Talar AVN
Post traumatic arthritis

Positioning Foot

The sole of the foot should be plantigrade.
The foot should be 90° to tibia in sagittal plane.
The foot should be 0° to 5° of valgus, as with triple arthrodesis; varus position of the foot should be avoided.
There should also be 10° to 15° of external rotation of the foot so the 2nd ray aligns with the tibial crest.

SUTURE ANCHORS

Suture anchors, also called *bone anchors*, are fixation devices for fixating tendons, ligaments, and other soft tissues to bone. They consist of an anchor that is screwed or tapped into bone and sutures that come off the device to secure the soft tissues. They were first developed for and are most commonly used for arthroscopic procedures.

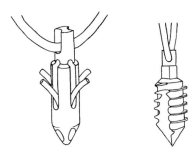

INTERFERENCE SCREWS/ TENODESIS SCREWS

Interference screws, also called *tenodesis screws*, are fixation devices, designed to attach tendons to bone. The procedure is performed by drilling a hole in the bone and pulling the end of the tendon into the hole. The interference screw is then screwed or tapped into the same hole, pinning the tendon between the device and the surrounding bone. Interference screws are commonly used in tendon transfers.

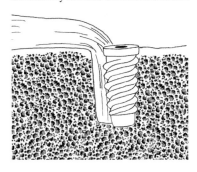

EXTERNAL FIXATORS

General

External fixation is a surgical technique used to immobilize bone at a distance from the operative site using pins and screws anchored in bone extending outside the body and held together by an external bar or frame.

Advantages of external fixation:

Decreased soft-tissue dissection
In cases of large bone defects, skeletal architecture can be maintained.
Can be used with infection
Allows for adjustment to be made post-op (angular corrections, distraction, compression)
Early ROM and early WB

The external fixation apparatus should be applied at least 2 to 3 cm off the skin to accommodate post-op swelling. If a pin or wire is painful, it is most likely either loose or infected.

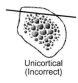
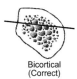

Unicortical (Incorrect)   Bicortical (Correct)

Terminology

Dynamization

Before the x-fix is removed, the patient should go through a period of dynamization, whereby all wires and pins are loosened and the patient is allowed to weight bearing. This allows for axial forces without distraction, which strengthens the bone and decreases the potential of fractures when the x-fix is removed.

Ligamentotaxis

The natural tendency of bone fragments to realign into their correct position when the extremity is distracted

Pins/Wires

Pins

Half pins have a greater diameter than wires and can be bicortical or unicortical.

The strongest double half pin configuration is divergent pins, followed by convergent and then parallel.

Wires

Wires are thinner than half pins but 1.5 to 2 times stronger due to tensioning. The level of tension applied to the wires varies with clinical circumstances and individual preference. Typically, forces of 100 to 130 kg are used in the leg and 60 to 90 kg in the foot. For wires used on open rings or on posts, tensioning should be kept <90 kg. When inserting wires through muscle, ideally, the muscle should be stretched (extended).

How to Enhance the Stability of an Ilizarov Frame

Increase diameter of wires and half pins

Decrease ring size (distance between ring and bone)

Use olive wires/drop wires

Additional wires or pins

Cross wires or half pins at 90°

Increase wire tension

Place central two rings closer to each side of the fracture

Reduce space between adjacent rings

Olive Wires

Olive wires have an enlarged "olive" in their midshaft, which is used to realign bone. As the wire is drilled through bone, the olive engages the near cortex and can be used to push or pull the bone to correct translational deformities.

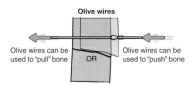

Olive wires

Olive wires can be used to "pull" bone | OR | Olive wires can be used to "push" bone

Callus Distraction

Callus distraction is a surgical technique used to lengthen bone. The bone is cut, and as the bone callus develops to repair itself, the bone fragments are slowly pulled apart from one another using an external fixation device, causing elongation of the bone.

Technique

Preserve periosteum when cutting the bone. Apply pins and as much frame as possible before cutting bone to maintain position and alignment. The optimal rate of distraction is 1 mm per day by 0.25 mm intervals qid. Compress site for 7 days before distraction to give time for the bone callus to start to develop. Ideally, the osteotomy is performed at proximal metaphyseal/diaphyseal junction. Osteoblastic activity occurs proximally and distally to the center of growth zone during Ilizarov distraction.

FRAMES GENERAL

Uniplanar (Unilateral or Bilateral)

Unilateral-uniplanar: All fixation pins and connecting frame occupy a single plane.

Bilateral-uniplanar: Transfixion pins

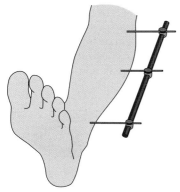

Uniplanar-unilateral

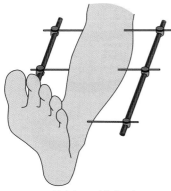

Uniplanar-bilateral

Biplanar (Unilateral or Bilateral)

Bilateral-biplanar: Indicated mainly for the tibia, provides great torsional stability. Pins placed ~90° to each other.

Generally refers to any construct without rings. A-fames and delta frames are types of Hoffmann constructs. Monolateral or bilateral

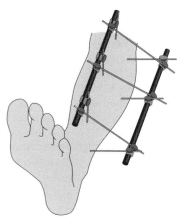

Biplanar-unilateral

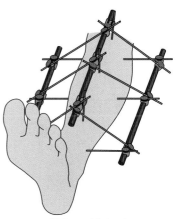

Biplanar-bilateral

SPANNING ANKLE EXTERNAL FIXATOR

Spanning fixators are used to maintain limb length in pilon fractures and lower leg fractures. They involve a transcalcaneal pin inserted through the calcaneus from medial to lateral. This pin is them secured medially and laterally to two rods that come together at the upper tibia where they are attached to pins in the tibia above the fracture site. Manual traction is applied to the transcalcaneal pin, while an assistant tightens the fixator. There may be other bars added to the construct to further stabilize the foot and leg. There are many variations of this construct. In their simples form, they form a triangle or delta and are often referred to as *delta frames*. Sometimes, a cross bar is attached for extra stability or for translational deformities. These constructs are sometimes referred to as an "A" frame.

Where the bars come together at the upper tibial, the lateral bar should be placed anterior than the medial bar. This allows clearance of the soft-tissue envelope of the anterior compartment.

ILIZAROV EXTERNAL FIXATOR

An Ilizarov external fixator is a circular fixator that allows not only stability of bone fragments but also triplanar reconstructions possible. Uses half pins and/or transfixion wires.

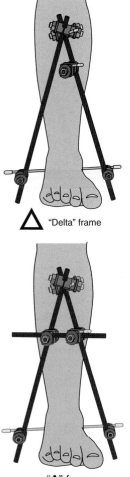

"Delta" frame

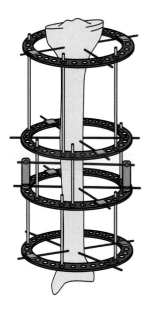

"**A**" frame

TAYLOR SPATIAL FRAME, "HEXAPOD EXTERNAL FIXATOR"

ANATOMY AND SAFE ZONES FOR FIXATION IN THE LEG

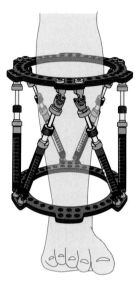

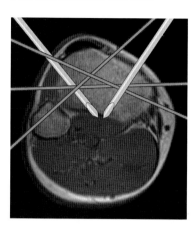

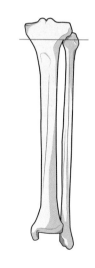

A Taylor spatial frame or hexapod external fixator is a modified Ilizarov device consisting of two rings connected by six struts with a ball joint at each end that can be independently lengthened or shortened to correct deformities in any plane. The Taylor spatial frame provides more freedom with regard to angular, translational, and lengthening corrections without the need for a complicated frame. It allows rings to be positioned in any orientation within their respective limb segment. It is not necessary that the rings be parallel with respect to the long axis of the bone. For optimal use, the Taylor spatial frame comes with computer software, which interfaces with digital x-rays to calculate strut lengths to achieve the desired limb alignment.

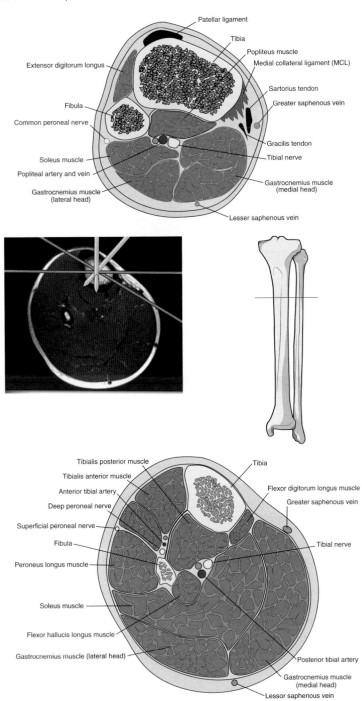

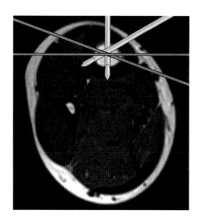

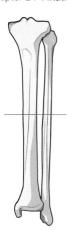

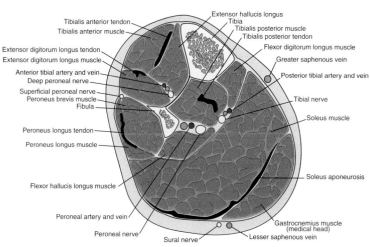

Tibialis anterior tendon
Tibialis anterior muscle
Extensor digitorum longus tendon
Extensor digitorum longus muscle
Anterior tibial artery and vein
Deep peroneal nerve
Superficial peroneal nerve
Peroneus brevis muscle
Fibula
Peroneus longus tendon
Peroneus longus muscle
Flexor hallucis longus muscle
Peroneal artery and vein
Peroneal nerve
Sural nerve
Extensor hallucis longus
Tibia
Tibialis posterior muscle
Tibialis posterior tendon
Flexor digitorum longus muscle
Greater saphenous vein
Posterior tibial artery and vein
Tibial nerve
Soleus muscle
Soleus aponeurosis
Gastrocnemius muscle (medial head)
Lesser saphenous vein

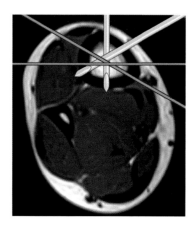

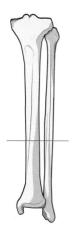

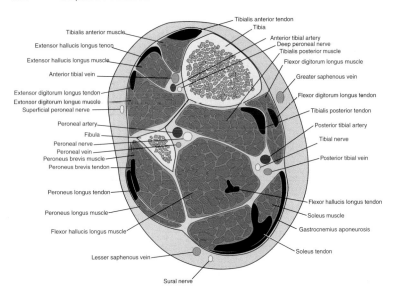

Tibialis anterior tendon
Tibia
Tibialis anterior muscle
Anterior tibial artery
Extensor hallucis longus tendon
Deep peroneal nerve
Tibialis posterior muscle
Extensor hallucis longus muscle
Flexor digitorum longus muscle
Anterior tibial vein
Greater saphenous vein
Extensor digitorum longus tendon
Flexor digitorum longus tendon
Extensor digitorum longus muscle
Superficial peroneal nerve
Tibialis posterior tendon
Peroneal artery
Posterior tibial artery
Fibula
Tibial nerve
Peroneal nerve
Peroneal vein
Peroneus brevis muscle
Posterior tibial vein
Peroneus brevis tendon
Peroneus longus tendon
Flexor hallucis longus tendon
Peroneus longus muscle
Soleus muscle
Flexor hallucis longus muscle
Gastrocnemius aponeurosis
Soleus tendon
Lesser saphenous vein
Sural nerve

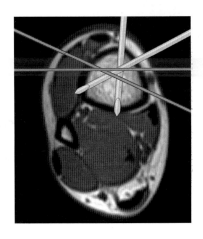

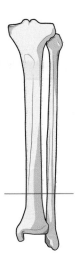

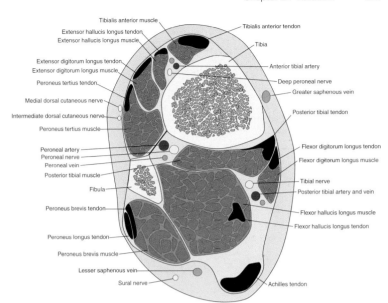

Tibialis anterior muscle
Extensor hallucis longus tendon
Extensor hallucis longus muscle

Extensor digitorum longus tendon
Extensor digitorum longus muscle

Peroneus tertius tendon

Medial dorsal cutaneous nerve

Intermediate dorsal cutaneous nerve

Peroneus tertius muscle

Peroneal artery
Peroneal nerve
Peroneal vein
Posterior tibial muscle

Fibula

Peroneus brevis tendon

Peroneus longus tendon

Peroneus brevis muscle

Lesser saphenous vein

Sural nerve

Tibialis anterior tendon

Tibia

Anterior tibial artery

Deep peroneal nerve

Greater saphenous vein

Posterior tibial tendon

Flexor digitorum longus tendon

Flexor digitorum longus muscle

Tibial nerve

Posterior tibial artery and vein

Flexor hallucis longus muscle

Flexor hallucis longus tendon

Achilles tendon

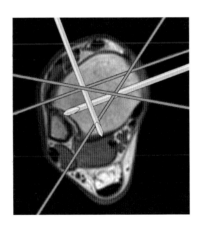

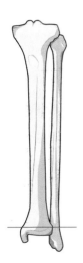

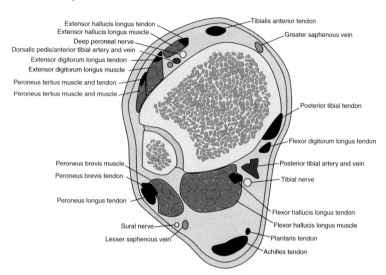

INTRAMEDULLARY (IM) NAILS

IM nails are the fixation method of
choice for extra-articular long bone
fractures, including diaphyseal and
selected metaphyseal fractures.
Fractures that are too distal (within
1 to 2 cm of the joint) may not be
appropriate for an IM nail. Special
nails have been developed for pantalar fusions in the foot as well as
beaming nails for repair of a col-
lapsed Charcot foot.

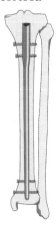

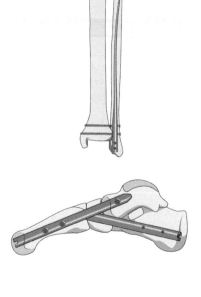

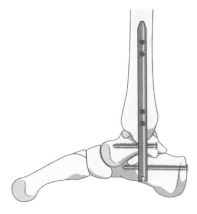

IM nails act as an internal splint and provides relative stability, allowing some micromotion to occur.

POLLER SCREWS (BLOCKING SCREWS)

Screws can be inserted into the bone to help correct deviations of the fractured bone. These screws are called *Poller screws* or *blocking screws*. Poller screws are used to prevent malalignment during nail insertion. Poller screws functionally narrow the IM canal. Poller screws are placed from anterior to posterior for frontal plane deformities and medial to lateral for sagittal deformities. They can be left in for stability or removed after nail insertion.

Proximal Tibial Fractures

Tibial fractures that occur in the proximal 1/3 of the bone tend to be valgus and procurvatum due to the pull of the patellar tendon. By using a Poller screw from medial to lateral and posterior to where the nail will be inserted, procurvatum is corrected. A second Poller screw placed anterior to posterior, lateral to where the nail will be place will prevent valgus deformity.

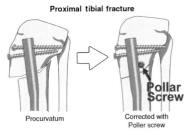

Proximal tibial fracture

Procurvatum

Corrected with Poller screw

Poller Screw

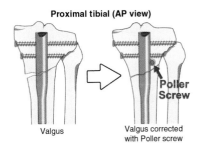

Proximal tibial (AP view)

Valgus

Valgus corrected with Poller screw

Poller Screw

Distal Tibial Fractures

Tibial fractures that occur in the distal 1/3 of the bone tend to deviate into either varus or valgus. For varus deformities, a proximal Poller screw should be placed medially and a distal Poller screw should be placed laterally. Conversely, for valgus deformity a proximal Poller screw is placed laterally and a distal Poller screw is placed medially.

Correcting valgus/varus with poller screws

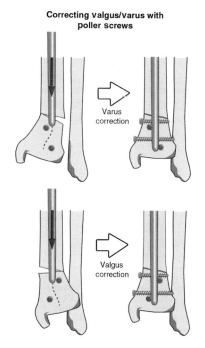

Varus correction

Valgus correction

REAMING

Reaming is performed to drill out the medullary canal to make room for the nail. Reaming is performed in 0.5-mm increments until the canal is 0.5 to 1.5 mm larger than the nail diameter.

Reaming allows insertion of a larger diameter nail, which provides more rigidity in bending and torsion. Some disadvantages of reaming include possible damage to endosteal blood supply and the potential risk of fat necrosis.

INSERTIONS POINT

Insertion point of a tibial nail is through a longitudinal incision just above the patella (transquadriceps approach). In the AP radiograph view, the entry point is in line with axis of the medullary canal and with the lateral tuberical of the interchondular eminence. Angle the pin distally at 15° in the sagittal plane to the axis of the tibial shaft.

NAIL LENGTH

Nail length may be determined intraoperatively with a radiographic ruler or by using the intact opposite tibia as a guide.

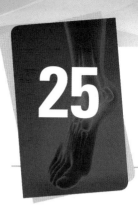

25 IMPLANTS

IMPLANTS

The most common pathogen to cause infection during implant surgery is *Staphylococcus epidermis*. Vancomycin is the drug of choice for antibiotic prophylaxis during implant surgery. Most metal joint implants are made of cobalt-chromium due to its high strength and smooth-polished finish. The smooth-polished finish is less destructive on cartilage. These same implants may have stems and undersurfaces that are coated with titanium plasma spray to encourage osseous integration.

FIRST METATARSOPHALANGEAL JOINT IMPLANTS

Hemi Implants (Base of Proximal Phalanx Implants)

Hemi implants are indicated for hallux limitus and hallux rigidus in the 1st ray and advanced arthritis in the lesser MPJs. They are used to replace the base of the proximal phalanx. On the 1st ray, minimal bone resection is important to preserve the insertion of the flexor hallucis brevis tendon. These implants require an adequate articular surface on the metatarsal head.

AnaToemic Hemi-Prosthesis

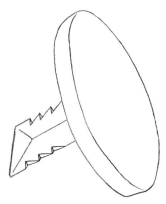

Made of cobalt-chromium with
   grit-blasted phalangeal surface
   and stem
Arthrex

Vilex Cannulated Hemi Implant

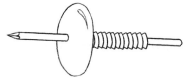

Cobalt-chrome
Cannulated
Implant screws into the bone
Cannot be used at the same joint
   with the Vilex Cannulated Hemi
   Implant

Wright Hemi Phalangeal Implant (HPI)

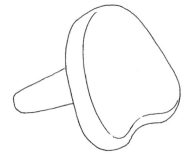

Cobalt-chromium
Trapezoidal shape matches the
   shape of the phalanx.
Recessed central plantar area to
   avoid irritation of the flexor
   tendons
Partial, plasma-sprayed, titanium
   stem and undersurface coating
   for osseous integration
Includes optional suture holes for
   flexor tendon attachment

BioPro First MPJ Hemi Implant

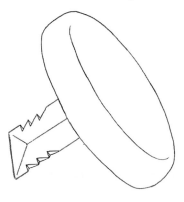

Cobalt-chromium
Available in porous and
   nonporous-coated stems

BioPro Lesser MPJ Hemi Implant

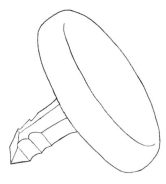

Cobalt-chromium
Indicated for the lesser MPJs
Different stem design to accommo-
date the smaller phalanges
Available in a cannulated version

OsteoMed Hemi Great Toe Implant

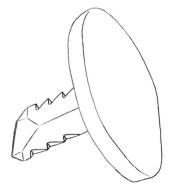

Cobalt-chromium
Plantar surface of the implant is
flat to avoid irritation of the
flexor tendons.

Metal Hemi Toe (MHT)

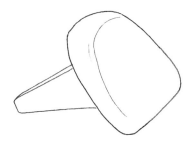

Cobalt-chromium with a titanium
plasma–sprayed stem
Trapezoidal articular surface and
stem better match the geometry
of the proximal phalanx.
Fifteen-degree angle between the
articular surface and the stem in
the sagittal plane to accommodate for the metatarsal declination angle

Stem becomes thicker going from
the tip toward the base to better conform to the shape of the
medullary canal of the proximal
phalanx.
Integra LifeSciences Corp.

Low-Profile Toe (LPT) 2 Great Toe Implant

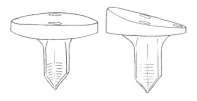

Titanium
Available in straight or angled op-
tions for increased PASA
Angled option comes in two sizes:
size 1 is 18° and size 2 is 16°.
Only difference between the LPT and
the LPT 2 is the instrumentation.
Cruciate stem
Two perforating holes to secure
FHB, angled version has a third
hole, placed medially to prevent
lateral subluxation
Wright Medical Technology Inc.

K2 Hemi Implant

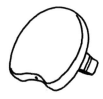

Cobalt-chromium with titanium
plasma–coated stem
Perforating hole plantarly to secure
FHL to the base of the phalanx
and implant, preventing a hallux
hammertoe
Integra LifeSciences Corp.

3S Hemi Toe

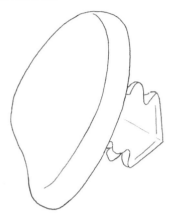

Cobalt-chromium
Low-profile head with plantar sur-
face of the implant is flat to avoid
irritation of the flexor tendons.
Tri-spade stem
Trilliant

Metatarsal Resurfacing Implants (Metatarsal Head Implants)

Metatarsal Decompression Implant (MDI)

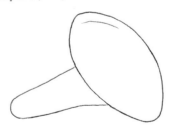

Cobalt-chromium with
plasma-sprayed titanium coating on stem
Head is angled to avoid interference with the weight-bearing
surface and provide progressive
decompression through dorsiflexory ROM.
Wright Medical Technology Inc.

Lesser Metatarsal Head Implant (LMH)

Same as MDI but made for lesser
metatarsals
Wright Medical Technology Inc.

Arthrosurface HemiCAP Toe Implant

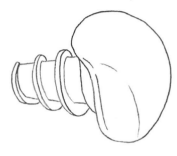

Consists of two components, a cap
(cobalt-chrome) and a screw in
stem (titanium), that fit together

EnCompass Metatarsal Resurfacing Implant

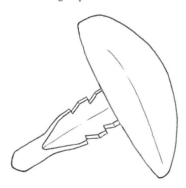

Cobalt-chromium with titanium
plasma– and hydroxyapatite-
coated undersurface
Osteomed

Vilex Cannulated Metatarsal Head Implant

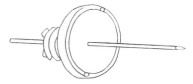

Cobalt-chromium
Cannulated
Implant screws into the bone
Cannot be used in the same joint with the Vilex Cannulated Metatarsal Head Implant

Cartiva

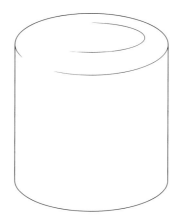

Made of 40% polyvinyl alcohol and 60% saline
Same material as contact lens

Total One Piece Hinged Implants

Swanson Flexible Toe Implant

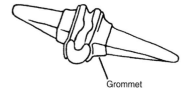

Grommet

Silicone
Two stem sizes, standard and small
Midsection of the implant is U shaped; opening of "U" can be directed dorsally or plantarly.
The two stems are in the same plane and perpendicular to the hinge.
Stems are rectangular in cross section.
Available with grommets; grommets are titanium shields contoured to fit over the base of the stems. They are designed to protect the implant from shearing forces and sharp bone edges.
Grommets are available only for implant sizes 0 to 5.
Wright Medical Technology Inc.

Swanson Double-Stemmed Hinged Implant

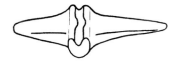

Smaller version of the Swanson 1st MPJ implant made for lesser MPJs
Not available with grommets
Wright Medical Technology Inc.

Swanson Flexible Toe Implant

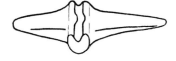

One stem size
Smaller version of the Swanson 1st MPJ implant made for IPJs
Not available with grommets

Primus Flexible Great Toe Implant (FGT)

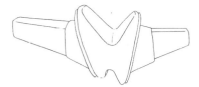

Made of UltraSIL, a medical grade high-performance silicone elastomer

Shorter distal stem that is trapezoidal to match the shape of the phalanx

Distal stem angles 10° for metatarsal declination angle.

The bone cuts are angled toward the joint from dorsal to plantar to preserve integrity of sesamoid apparatus or FHB insertion.

Hinge designed with greater ROM (95°)

Available with grommets

Integra LifeSciences Corp.

Classic Flexible Great Toe (CGT)

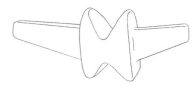

Made of UltraSIL, a medical grade high-performance silicone elastomer

Intended more for salvage-type procedures and redo's vs. the FGT

Bone cuts are made parallel to each other; does not preserve integrity of sesamoid apparatus or FHB insertion.

Does not come with grommets

Integra LifeSciences Corp.

Lesser Metatarsal Phalangeal (LMP)

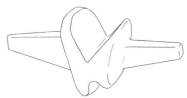

Made of UltraSIL, a medical grade high-performance silicone elastomer

Designed for lesser metatarsal phalangeal joints

Integra LifeSciences Corp.

Great Toe Arthroplasty Implant Technique (GAIT)

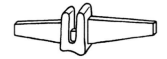

Silicone

Stems are rectangular in cross section.

U-shaped hinge, opening of "U" can be directed dorsally or plantarly.

The two stems are in the same plane and perpendicular to the hinge.

Proximal collar and stem are larger than distal collar and stem.

Sgarlato Labs, Inc.

Reference Toe System (RTS)

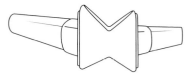

Silicone

Disposable instrumentation

Broachless system

In2Bones

RTS Lesser

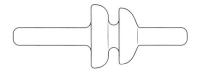

Silicone
Indicated for lesser MTP joints
Disposable instrumentation
In2Bones

Two-Component Implants

The Kinetik Great Toe Implant

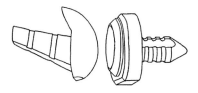

Metatarsal component made of
  cobalt-chromium, phalangeal
  component made of
  titanium-backed polyethylene
Notched stem for more secure fit
Metatarsal component has flattened surface to avoid sesamoid
  disruption.
Metatarsal stem angled 10° in the
  sagittal plane.
Metatarsal component has an
  extended dorsal curvature for
  implant articulation upon maximum dorsiflexion.
Integra LifeSciences Corp.

Reflexion Toe

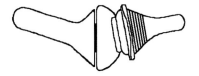

Metatarsal component made of titanium with a cobalt-chromium
  head
Phalangeal component made of
  titanium-backed polyethylene
Three-piece implant, the metatarsal component is composed of
  two pieces. The head is applied
  after the stem is inserted.
Proximal stem is angled 17°.
Osteomed

Integra Movement Great Toe

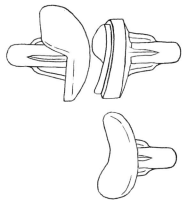

Cobalt-chromium with titanium
  plasma spray on under surface
The phalangeal component has a
  polyethylene cap for articulation
  with the metatarsal component.
Metatarsal component has a dorsal
  flange for full ROM.
Phalangeal component contains
  suture holes for when the flexor
  hallucis brevis is compromised.
Both pieces can be used independently of each other as
  hemi's, but in this situation, the
  proximal phalanx component
  is different. The head is thinner,
  and there is no polyethylene cap.

Arthrosurface ToeMotion System

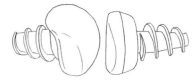

Consists of a HemiCAP implant
for the metatarsal head and a
titanium phalangeal component
with a polyethylene head for articulation with HemiCAP
The HemiCAP metatarsal component can be used alone as
a resurfacing implant.
Integra LifeSciences Corp.

Bio-Action Great Toe Implant

Available in two sizes and in neutral, right, or left configurations

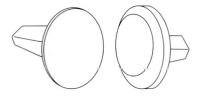

Toefit-Plus

Modular components that can be
used for either hemi joint or total joint
Stems are titanium, bearing surfaces are cobalt-chrome.

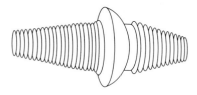

The phalangeal bearing surface is
available in cobalt-chrome or
polyethylene.
Smith & Nephew

Moje MTP Joint Replacement

Press fit ceramic implant
Coated with Bioverit 1 to increase biocompatibility and
osteo-integration

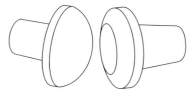

Roto-Glide Great Toe System

Implants International
Three-piece implant
Includes a sliding and rotating
meniscus

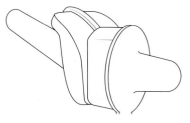

DIGITAL IMPLANTS

Weil-Type Swanson Design Hammertoe Implant

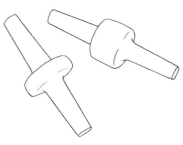

Silicone
No hinge
Cylindrical midsection comes in
two sizes and preserves length
of digit.

Cylindrical stems
Indicated for the PIPJs
Wright Medical Technology Inc.

Sgarlato Hammertoe Implant Prosthesis (SHIP)

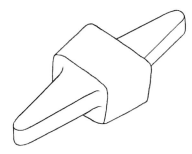

Silicone
No hinge
Rectangular tapered stem
Tapered rectangular midsection;
    narrow end goes distally
Indicated for the PIPJs
Sgarlato Labs, Inc.

Long SHIP

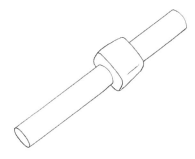

Silicone
No hinge
Indicated for the PIPJ or the DIPJ
Sgarlato Labs, Inc.

SHIP—Shaw Rod Hammertoe Implant

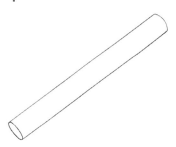

Silicone
Indicated for the PIPJ or the DIPJ
Provides a flexible stable joint and
    maintains length
Available in varying stiffnesses (2.0
    mm—flexible, 2.3 mm—regular,
    2.5 mm—stiff)
Sgarlato Labs, Inc.

Flexible Digital Implants (FDI)

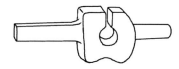

Silicone
Designed for the PIPJ of digits 2
    through 5
Proximal stem is square; distal
    stem is cylindrical.
Midsection of the implant is U
    shaped; opening of "U" is to be
    directed dorsally.
Integra LifeSciences Corp.

InterPhlex

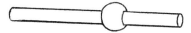

Silicone

Indicated for both MPJs and PIPJs of digits 2 through 5

Cylindrical stem with a spherical spacer

Sphere comes in four sizes: 4.0, 4.5, 8.0, and 10 mm.

Osteomed

ANKLE IMPLANTS

Total ankle replacements (TARs) were initially two-component implants cemented into the bone. These early models proved unstable and had a high rate of failure. Today, the use of three-component ankle implants with cementless fixation has become more standard. The three components consist of a metal piece that attaches to the tibia, a metal piece that attaches to the talus, and a third piece made of a special high-grade surgical polyethylene that acts as a bearing or meniscus. This bearing allows for shock absorption as well as up-and-down motion, side-to-side motion, and axial rotation.

Common ankle joint implant complication includes subsidence (the gradual caving in or sinking of the implant into the bone), loosening, and malleolar fractures.

Ankle implants are classified according to several factors:

Fixation

Cement
Cementless

Number of Components

Two components
Three components

Constraint

Constrained: With constrained type implants, the talar and tibial components are mechanically coupled around an axis of motion, allowing more stability *(constraint)* in the device.

Semiconstrained: Semiconstrained implants lie somewhere in between constrained and nonconstrained.

Nonconstrained: Nonconstrained implants have no mechanical link between the talar and tibial components and rely on the surrounding musculotendinous structures for stability.

Bearing

Fixed bearing: With fixed bearing, the polyethylene spacer is fixed to either the tibial or talar implant component.

Mobile bearing: Mobile-bearing implants have a polyethylene spacer that is not attached to either the talar or tibial component and floats between the two. This allows for some varus/valgus tilt and axial rotation, and there is less stress on the metal–bone interface. Mobile-bearing devices are all considered three-piece designs, the "third piece" being the mobile polyethylene spacer.

SECOND-GENERATION ANKLE IMPLANTS

Agility Ankle

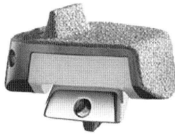

FDA approved in 1992
Two-component implant
Approved with cement
Semiconstrained
Fixed bearing
The Agility device requires an arthrodesis of the distal tibiofibular syndesmosis.
Tibial component is composed of titanium with a polyethylene element secured inferiorly to articulate with the talar component. The talar component is cobalt-chromium.
DePuy Orthopaedics

Buechel–Pappas Implant

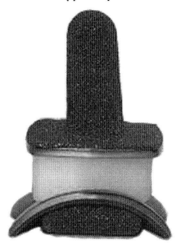

Not FDA approved
Three components
Cementless
<u>Mobile bearing</u>
Has had many different designs through the years and is often referenced for historical purposes
Talar component has a central trochlear groove.
Uses a tibial stem for stabilization
Not available in the United States

Scandinavian Total Ankle Replacement (STAR)

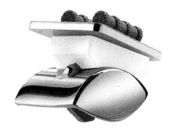

FDA approved in 2009
Three components
Cementless
Nonconstrained
<u>Mobile bearing</u>
Tibial and talar components are made of cobalt-chromium with a polyethylene disc between them.
The talar surface has a central rib running anterior to posterior with a corresponding groove in the polyethylene disk.
DonJoy Global

THIRD-GENERATION ANKLE IMPLANTS

Inbone and Inbone II Total Ankle Systems

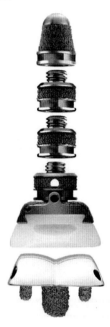

Inbone was FDA approved in 2005; Inbone II was FDA approved in 2010.

Two components

Approved with cement in the United States and Canada; outside the United States and Canada approved with or without cement

Semiconstrained

Fixed bearing

Tibial stem component consists of a long modular intramedullary stem. Interconnecting pieces are assembled in situ to minimize dissection and eliminate the need for windowing of the anterior tibia. This long customizable tibial component also provides better support and stress sharing, decreasing the incident of subsidence. The polyethylene component is fixed on the tibial tray. The Inbone II differs from the Inbone in that it has a talar sulcus, allowing more biomechanically stable articulation between the polyethylene insert and the talar component.

The Inbone ankle replacement is a preferred system for previously failed ankle replacement.

Wright Medical Technology

Hintegra

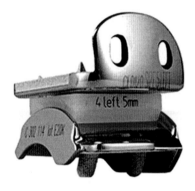

Three components

Unconstrained

Mobile bearing

Tibial and talar components are made of cobalt-chrome alloy with hydroxyapatite coating.

Relies on minimal bone resection for placement in cancellous subchondral bone

Tibial and talar components have ventral shields for screw placement.

Anterior tibial flange reduces post-op heterotropic ossification and soft-tissue adherence.

Not available in the United States; only cleared for Canada and international use
Integra LifeSciences Corp.

Salto Talaris Anatomic Ankle Prosthesis

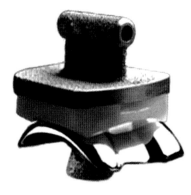

FDA approved in 2006
Two components
Semiconstrained
Fixed bearing (Note: There is a Salto mobile-bearing device available in Europe.)
Stability is provided by a hollow fixation plug in tibia.
Titanium plasma spray on tibial and talar components
Tibial surface covered with poly-ethylene flat that fits congruent surface of talar component with a sulcus that allows varus–valgus motion
Medial impingement is prevented by medial metallic tibial rim polyethylene Implant on fibular replaces the talofibular joint.
Integra LifeSciences Corp.

Eclipse Total Ankle

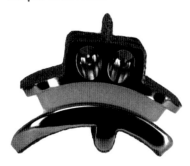

FDA approved in 2006
Two components
Fixed bearing
Implanted from a medial or lat-eral approach via a malleolar osteotomy
Not currently commercially available
Integra LifeSciences Corp.

Trabecular Metal Total Ankle

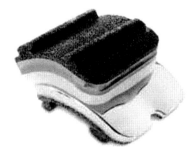

FDA approved in 2012
Two components
Approved with cement
Semiconstrained
Fixed bearing
<u>Implanted through a lateral approach</u>
Approved with cement
Zimmer/Biomet

Infinity Total Ankle System

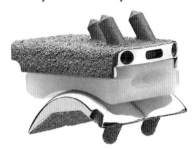

FDA approved in 2013

Two components

Approved with cement in the United States and Canada; outside the United States and Canada approved with or without cement

Semiconstrained

Fixed bearing

Designed to give surgeons a non-stemmed option

The talar component has the same sulcus articular geometry as Inbone II and is interchangeable with the Inbone II tibial component.

The talar component is more of a resurfacing implant vs. the Inbone II talar component.

Stryker

Mobility Total Ankle System

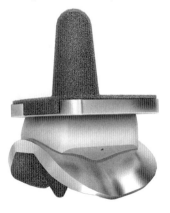

Three components

Cementless

Unconstrained

Mobile bearing

Buechel–Pappas type prosthetic

DePuy started a clinical trial for mobility but abandoned it early on due to poor device performance outside the United States.

Integra LifeSciences Corp.

Cadence Total Ankle Flat Cut Talar Dome

Two components

Fixed bearing

Minimal tibial and talar resection required.

Biased polyethylene insert allows correction in both the sagittal and frontal planes.

Smith & Nephew

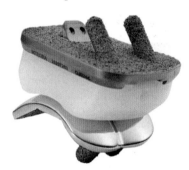

Vantage Total Ankle System

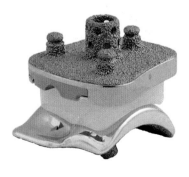

Minimal tibial and talar resection required.

Talar component extends onto the talar neck to prevent subsidence.

The tibial component does not violate the anterior cortex.

Exactech, Inc.

Quantum Total Ankle

Cruciate shaped vertical stem in the tibial component

A two-component prosthesis. The polyethylene bearing is fixed to the titanium tibial base. The talar component is made of cobalt-chromium.

Comes with a web-based 3D software to help position implant components

In2Bones

Apex 3D

Fixed bearing

The polyethylene component is vitamin E infused to expedite healing.

Paragon 28

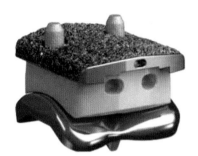

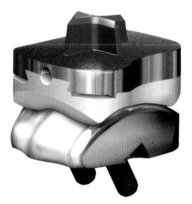

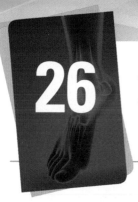

26

TENDONS AND TENDON TRANSFERS

TENDON ANATOMY

1. Epitenon: The outer covering of a tendon within its sheath. Most important structure in the tendon repair process.
2. Endotenon: A loose acellular tissue carrying blood vessels that surrounds small bundles of collagen fibers throughout the tendon
3. Paratenon: The loose elastic areolar tissue surrounding the entire tendon, which allows the tendon to slide. It supplies the blood supply to the tendon and should be reapproximated after tendon surgery. Supplies the majority of a tendon's blood supply.

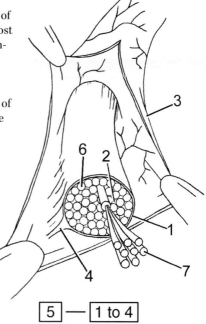

5 — 1 to 4

4. Mesotenon: A delicate connective tissue sheath attaching a tendon to its fibrous sheath. A part of the paratenon that attaches the paratenon to the epitenon, which can stretch several centimeters and allows a blood supply to be transferred from the paratenon to the tendon. The point at which it attaches to the epitenon is called the *hilus*.

5. Peritenon: All the connective tissues associated with a tendon (epitenon, endotenon, paratenon, mesotenon)

6. Fascicles: A group of collagen fibers bundled together and surrounded by an endotenon

7. Collagen fibers: Formed from a polymer of tropocollagen, which is the basic molecular unit of a tendon. Healthy tendon is mostly composed of type I collagen fibers.

Collagen

The main collagens found in connective tissue are types I, II, and III. These collagens form fibers that give tensile strength to tissues.

Type I	Most abundant, found in skin, **ligaments, tendon, fibrocartilage**, bone
Type II	Found in articular cartilage **(hyaline cartilage)**
Type III	Skin, vessels, lymphatics, granulation tissue, **tendinosis**

Tendonitis vs. Tendinosis

Tendonitis	Tendinosis
Inflammation	Degenerative
Caused by acute overloading	Caused by chronic over use
Tendon appears white, glistening, and firm	Tendon appear gray, dull, soft (lipid or mucoid degeneration)
Composed of type I (normal) collagen fibers	Composed of type III (abnormal) collagen fibers
Treatment takes days to weeks	Treatment takes months
	Disrupted collagen fibers, increased cellularity, neovascularization (angiofibroblastic hyperplasia)
	Increased bulk, decreased strength
Treatment: anti-inflammatory modalities, RICE, NSAIDs	Treatment: break the cycle of injury, reduce ground substance, pathologic vascularization, and subsequent tendon thickening. Optimizes collagen production and maturation so the tendon regains strength. Rest, braces, inserts, stretching, ice, eccentric strengthening, massage

TENDON REPAIR

End-to-end anastomosis

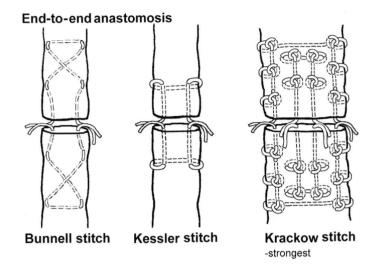

Bunnell stitch   **Kessler stitch**   **Krackow stitch**
-strongest

Anchoring Tendon to Bone

Trephine Plug

- A round cortical plug is removed with a trephine, the tendon is inserted, and the plug is replaced.

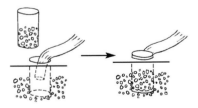

Three-Hole Suture

- The tendon is anchored to a piece of suture, the tendon is then inserted in a hole in the bone, and the two suture ends exit the bone through two additional holes and are tied.

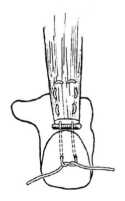

Buttress and Button Anchor

- The tendon is anchored to a piece of suture, the tendon is then inserted in a hole in the bone, and the suture ends continue through the bone and exit the skin on the other side of the foot and are fixated with a button.

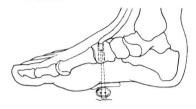

Tunnel With Sling

- A hole is drilled through the entire bone; the tendon is then passed through the bone and sutured back on itself.

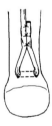

Tendon With Bony Insertion

- A portion of bone is removed with the tendon and reinserted into a preformed hole of similar size and shape.

Mason–Allen Stitch

- Tendon-to-bone technique often used in rotator-cuff repair

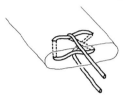

Screw and Washer Bone Anchor

Screw and washer

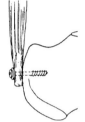

Bone anchor

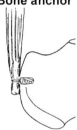

Bone Anchors/Suture Anchors

See Chapter 24

Interference Screws/Tenodesis Screws

See Chapter 24

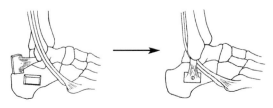

Passing Tendon Through Bone

Chinese Finger Trap Technique

Suture is wrapped around the tendon from proximal to distal in a crisscross manner. The ends of the suture are then tied in a knot. A second piece of suture is then wrapped around the tendon in an identical manner but out of phase with the first piece of suture.

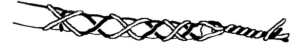

Whip Stitch Technique

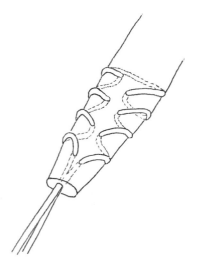

Tubularization

Tubularization is a tendon repair technique most commonly associated with the peroneal tendons. The most common pattern of peroneal tendon damage is a longitudinal split tear that occurs as the tendon rounds the fibula. Surgical repair involved cutting out the damaged portion of the tendon. The tendon is often left shredded, splayed out, and flattened in this area. Tubularization is aimed at making the tendon more functional as a solid round structure.

TENDON LENGTHENING PROCEDURES

Accordion-type lengthening. Cuts are made no <51% of the way through the tendon, and the tendon ends are distracted away from one another, allowing the central fibers to slide past one another.

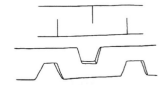

TENDON TRANSFERS

■ During tendon transposition, the paratenon should be preserved to allow gliding of the tendon and preserve blood supply.
■ With tendon transfers, the involved muscle loses grade 1 of strength.
■ To qualify for a tendon transfer, a muscle must be of grade 4 or higher.
■ CVA patients should not have tendon transfers for at least 6 months following the CVA.

Phase Conversion

■ Muscles are divided into two phases depending on their use: swing phase and stance phase.

- A muscle transferred from one phase to be used in the other phase is said to be *transferred out of phase*.
- It is easier to retrain a muscle transferred within the same phase.
- Muscles transferred out of phase often never regain their activity but can still be beneficial by acting as a sling and eliminating the need for bracing.

Swing-Phase Muscles	Stance-Phase Muscles
Anterior tibialis	Gastrocnemius
EHL	Soleus
EDL	FHL
Peroneus tertius	FDL
Peroneus longus	
Peroneus brevis	
All intrinsics	

Tendon Healing and Post-Op Care

- After a tendon has been transferred, the patient should be casted NWB for 4 weeks.
- Gentle passive ROM and/or isometric exercises inside the cast may be started at 3 weeks to prevent adhesions.
- At 4 weeks, active mobilization should begin, but maximum contracture should be postponed for several more weeks.

Types of Transfers

Adductor Tendon Transfer

- The adductor tendon is transected at its attachment to the lateral sesamoid and the lateral base of the proximal phalanx and rerouted over the metatarsal head and attached to the medial capsule.
- Performed with hallux abductovalgus surgery to help realign the sesamoid apparatus under the metatarsal head

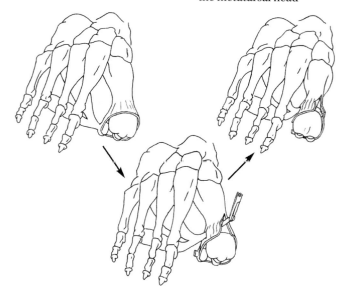

Flexor Tendon Transfer

- The flexor digitorum longus tendon is transected close to its insertion on the distal phalanx, split longitudinally to the base of the proximal phalanx, wrapped around the proximal phalanx, and sutured together.
- Also known as *Girdlestone procedure*

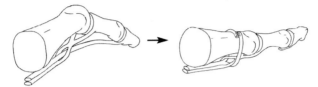

Jones Tenosuspension

- EHL tendon is transected and rerouted medial to lateral through the head of the 1st metatarsal and sewed back on itself. Kirk modification passes tendon from top to bottom (dorsal to plantar); this technique requires less tendon.
- The distal stump of the EHL is then attached to the EHB to maintain some extensor function of the hallux.
- Arthrodesis the 1st IPJ to prevent overpowering of the EHL and hammering
- Performed for pressure problems under the 1st metatarsal head
- Indications: Flexible cavus foot, flexible plantarflexed 1st ray

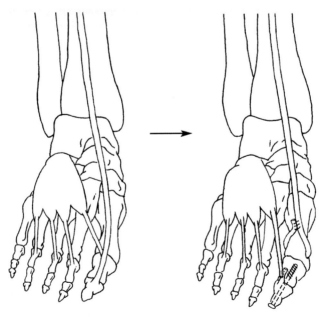

Hibbs Tenosuspension

- The EDL tendon slips are detached from their insertion, combined, and reattached to the 3rd cuneiform or the base of the 3rd metatarsal.
- The EDB tendons are transected and reattached to the stump of the corresponding EDL tendon; the 4th and 5th longus slips are both attached to the 4th EDB slip.
- Releases the buckling force at the MPJs and elevates the forefoot
- Indications: Equinus with or without claw toes

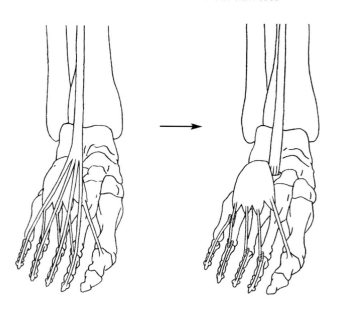

Split Tibialis Anterior Tendon Transfer (Statt)

- Tibialis anterior is split from its insertion up just proximal to the superior extensor retinaculum.
- The lateral fibers are passed through the peroneus tertius sheath and sutured to the tendon or attached to the cuboid.
- The procedure increases dorsiflexion of the foot and balances the force laterally.
- Indications: Flexible rearfoot varus, excessive supination, dorsiflexory weakness

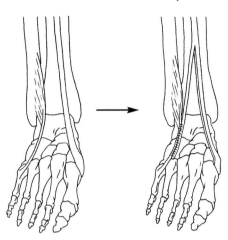

Peroneus Longus Tendon Transfer

- Peroneus longus is released at the level of the cuboid and transferred through the intermuscular septum down the EDL sheath and inserted into the lesser tarsus or base of the 3rd metatarsal.
- Peroneus longus may also be split, and half is anastomosed to the tibialis anterior at its insertion and the other half to peroneus tertius.
- Indications: Drop foot, pes cavus

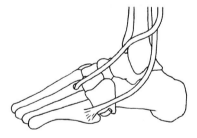

Heyman Procedure

- Transfer of all long extensor tendons to their respective metatarsal heads

Tibialis Anterior Tendon Transfer (Tatt)

- Tibialis anterior tendon is transferred to the 3rd cuneiform through the EDL tendon sheath.

- Acts to reduce supination and increase dorsiflexion
- Indications: Drop foot, recurrent clubfoot, flexible forefoot equinus

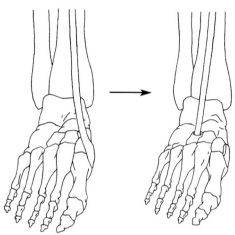

Tibialis Posterior Tendon Transfer

- The tibialis posterior tendon is transferred through the interosseus membrane and fixated to the 3rd cuneiform.
- This is an out-of-phase tendon transfer.
- Indication: Drop foot, recurrent clubfoot

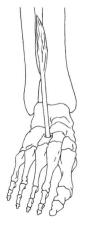

Anchovy Procedure

The anchovy procedure is a tendon interposition arthroplasty. It involves rolling up a tendon graft from end to end like an anchovy and inserting it into a damaged or resected joint. A convex reamer can be used to create two opposing concave surfaces to better hold the anchovy. The capsule is closed to hold the interposing tendon in place. A percutaneous K-wire may be placed across the joint and through the graft for 6 weeks to hold the structures in place.

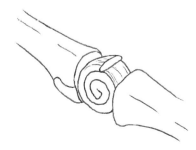

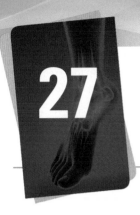

FIRST RAY SURGERY

27

BUNION EVALUATION

Stage I	Subclinical subluxation of the 1st metatarsal joint
Stage II	Development of clinical hallux abduction deformity
Stage III	Development of metatarsus primus adductus deformity
Stage IV	Clinical subluxation/dislocation of the 1st MPJ

Watkins Bunion Classification

Type 1

1st metatarsal congruent with sesamoids, no frontal plane rotation

Type 2

Sesamoids dislocated laterally, no frontal plane rotation of the 1st metatarsal

WATKINS BUNION CLASSIFICATION

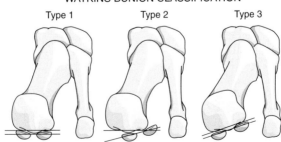

Type 1   Type 2   Type 3

Type 3

1st metatarsal and sesamoids both rotated in the frontal plane but remain congruent

1st Metatarsal Position in a Bunion

Sagittal plane: dorsiflexion
Transverse plane: medial deviation, adduction
Frontal plane: bunion frontal plane rotation may be described as pronation, eversion, valgus, or external rotation. All of these terms are used interchangeably and are describing the same thing.

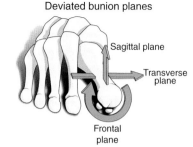

Deviated bunion planes

Sagittal plane

Transverse plane

Frontal plane

Tracking and Track Bound

Tracking and *track bound* are terms used during the clinical assessment of a bunion. They help determine whether the sesamoids are dislocated and/or if there is a frontal plane deformity of the metatarsal head.

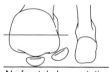

No frontal plane rotation
Dislocated sesamoids

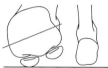

Frontal plane rotation
No sesamoid dislocation

TRACKING/TRACK BOUND

Both scenarios to the left look identical on radiograph. Assessing for tracking or track bound will help differentiate the two.
In the lower example, when the hallux is manually reduced, the sesamoids will dislocate from the valgus metatarsal head resulting in decreased ROM and stiffness. This example will demonstrate tracking or be track bound.
In the upper example, reducing the hallux will relocate the sesamoids and ROM will improve.

If the hallux glides through its range of motion in the pathologic abducted position but does not move (or has limited motion) through its range of motion when manually reduced in the rectus position, it is said to be track bound or tracking. In this situation, there is a frontal plane deformity. The metatarsal head and sesamoids are congruent with one another, but they are rotated in a valgus position. By mechanically reducing the bunion deformity, you are essentially dislocating the sesamoids.

If there is stiff, limited, or crepitation in the pathologic abducted position but increased motion with less stiffness when the bunion is manually reduced, there is likely no significant frontal plane deformity because by manually reducing the deformity, in this scenario, you are relocating the sesamoids.

Center of Rotation Angulation (CORA)

CORA is the intersection of the proximal and distal anatomic axes of a deformity. A line passing through the CORA that bisects the angle formed by the proximal and distal angle is called the <u>bisector</u>. CORA is a universal concept used for all bony deformities, but in podiatry, it is mostly discussed in the context of bunion corrections.

The CORA is the optimal location for a surgeon to perform an angular correction, be it an osteotomy or arthrodesis. This site, where the deformity is corrected, is called the <u>angulation correction axis</u> (ACA). Ideally, the ACA is performed at the CORA. If the correction of angulation (ACA) is performed at a site other than the CORA, an iatrogenic translation deformity may result.

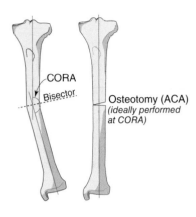

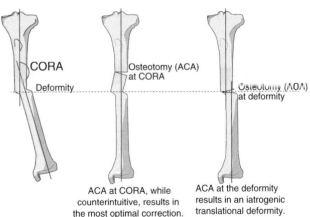

ACA at CORA, while counterintuitive, results in the most optimal correction.

ACA at the deformity results in an iatrogenic translational deformity.

Bunion deformities usually have a CORA located at the 1st metatarsal–medial cuneiform joint. This makes a Lapidus procedure, in theory, the most logical choice for correction. A Lapidus places the ACA at the CORA. Other procedures may be less optimal because they create a translational deformity.

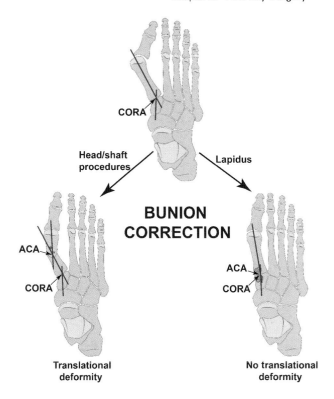

CORA

Head/shaft procedures

Lapidus

BUNION CORRECTION

ACA

CORA

Translational deformity

ACA

CORA

No translational deformity

Sesamoidal Rotation Angle

Angle the sesamoids make with the ground

Must be a weight-bearing x-ray

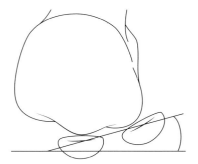

Metatarsal Head Rotation Angle

The angle of the plantar surface of the metatarsal head in relation to the ground

Must be a weight-bearing x-ray

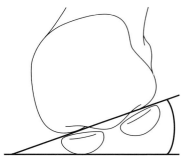

Metatarsus Adductus Angle

Normal is 15°.
Values <15° represent a rectus
    foot.
At birth, MTA is around 30°.
At 1 year (begin walking), it is
    around 20°.
By age 4 years, the MTA reaches its
    adult normal value of 15°.

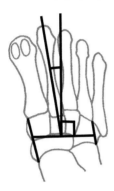

Intermetatarsal Angle

Also known as *metatarsus primus
    adductus angle*, metatarsus pri-
    mus varus
Normal is 8° to 12° in a rectus foot
    and 8° to 10° in an adductus foot.
Base wedge osteotomies are indi-
    cated in feet with an IM angle of
    ≥15° in a rectus foot or ≥12° in
    an adducted foot.
When metatarsus adductus is pres-
    ent, the foot functions as if the
    IM angle is larger. The formula
    to account for this metatarsus
    adductus and find the "true IM
    angle" is as follows:
True IM angle = IM angle +
    (metatarsus adductus angle
    − 15°)

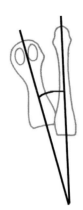

Hallux Abductus Angle

Also known as *hallux valgus angle*

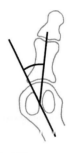

Normal 0° to 15°

PROXIMAL ARTICULAR SET ANGLE (PASA)

Also known as *distal metatarsal
    articular angle* (DMAA)

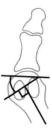

Normal 7.5° to 12°

DISTAL ARTICULAR SET ANGLE (DASA)

Normal 7.5°

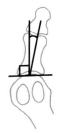

Hallux Abductus Interphalangeus Angle

Normal 10°

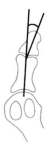

Metatarsal Protrusion Distance

Normal (+ or −) 2 mm

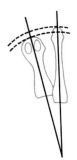

Tibial Sesamoid Position

Normal 1 to 3

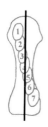

BUNIONECTOMIES

Head Procedures

Austin

Corrects IM angle
Chevron osteotomy with a 60°
    angle
Can incorporate wedge (bicorrec-
    tional) to correct PASA

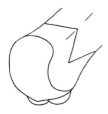

Youngswick Modification

A modification of the Austin de-
    signed to shorten and plantar-
    flex the metatarsal head
Indicated in metatarsus elevates

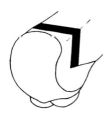

Reverdin

Closing lateral wedge
Corrects PASA
Lateral cortex remains intact.

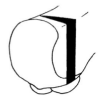

Reverdin–Green

Closing lateral wedge
Corrects PASA
"L-shaped" cut preserves the integrity of the sesamoid articulation.
Lateral cortex remains intact.

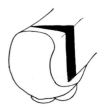

Reverdin–Laird

Corrects PASA and IM
Same as Reverdin–Green with completion of the osteotomy through the lateral cortex to allow IM correction

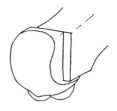

Reverdin–Todd

Corrects PASA and IM and allows plantarflexion of the metatarsal head
Same as Reverdin–Laird with penetration of the plantar cortex to allow sagittal plane correction

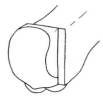

Watermann

Removal of dorsal wedge
Indicated in hallux limitus
Plantar cortex is left intact.

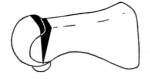

Green–Watermann

Indicated in hallux limitus
Watermann procedure reserves the sesamoid articulation.

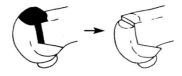

Neck Procedures

Peabody

Similar to the Reverdin but the osteotomy is made more proximal to avoid the sesamoids

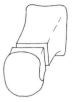

Hohmann

Corrects IM angle (capital fragment shifted laterally)
Corrects PASA (medial wedge resected)
Corrects metatarsus elevatus (capital fragment plantarflexed)

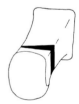

Wilson

Shortens and laterally displaces head

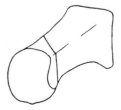

Derotational Abductory Transpositional Osteotomy (DRATO)

Metatarsal head can be manipulated at any angle in any plane.
Wedge resection can be incorporated.
Very unstable osteotomy

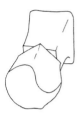

Mitchell

Corrects IM angle
Procedure shortens, plantarflexes, and laterally displaces metatarsal head

Shaft Procedures

Kalish

Modified (long arm) Austin
Does not correct PASA

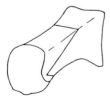

Scarf

Corrects IM angle

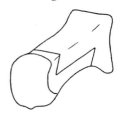

Ludloff

Dorsal-proximal to plantar-distal osteotomy; capital fragment is rotated to correct IM angle.

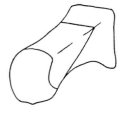

MAU

Dorsal-distal to plantar-proximal osteotomy; capital fragment is rotated to correct IM angle.

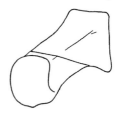

Lambrinudi

Closing plantarflexory base wedge
Corrects metatarsus primus elevates

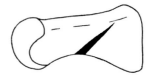

Base Procedures

Crescentic

Corrects IM angle
May be fixated slightly dorsiflexed or plantarflexed
Advantage is that it does not shorten the metatarsal.

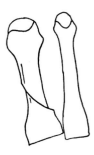

Trethowan

Opening base wedge

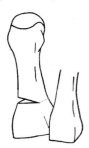

Juvara

Closing oblique base wedge osteotomy
Juvara type A: Wedge removed, medial cortex preserved (transverse correction)
Juvara type B: Wedge removed, medial cortex not preserved
Juvara type B1: Transverse and sagittal correction
Juvara type B2: Transverse and sagittal correction and corrects for long or short metatarsal

Juvara type C: No wedge resected
    Juvara type C1: Sagittal correction only
    Juvara type C2: Sagittal correction and corrects for long or short metatarsal

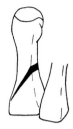

Loison–Balacescu

Laterally closing base wedge
Corrects IM angle

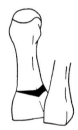

Logroscino

This is a Reverdin plus a
    Loison–Balacescu.
Corrects IM angle and PASA
An opening Logroscino may be
    performed by taking the wedge
    from the Reverdin and inserting
    it into an opening abductory
    wedge at the base.

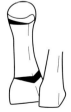

Arthroplasties

Indicated in older patients with
    hallux rigidus/limitus and severe
    DJD
Capsular tissue is sutured across
    the joint space (purse string) to
    prevent bone contact.
Usually performed with an extensor hallucis longus lengthening

Keller

Metatarsal head is remodeled, and
1/2 to 1/3 of the proximal phalanx
is resected.

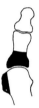

Mayo–Hueter

Excision of approximately two-thirds of the metatarsal head; the remaining portion is rounded off.

    A soft-tissue flap is used to prevent bone-on-bone contact at the joint.

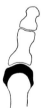

Stone

Oblique resection of the metatarsal
    head
The weight-bearing portion of the
    head articulating with the sesamoids is left intact.

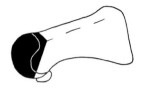

Valenti

Resect 1/2 to 2/3 of the dorsal aspect of the joint

Preserves plantar intrinsic musculature

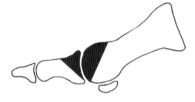

Arthrodesis

Lapidus

Fusion of the 1st metatarsal–medial cuneiform joint

Indicated for moderate-to-severe bunions with a concurrent ligamentous laxity or instability at the 1st TMT joint

Lapidus procedure can address frontal plane deformities.

Lapidus procedures correct the deformity at the CORA.

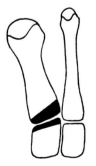

McKeever

Fusion of the 1st MPJ

Performed with 15° to 20° extension in males and up to 40° in females depending on the type of shoes worn

Fixation techniques vary but generally involve spearing the head of the metatarsal into the base of the proximal phalanx.

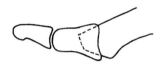

Miscellaneous

Silver

Medial bumpectomy

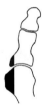

Cheilectomy

Dorsal bumpectomy indicated in hallux limitus

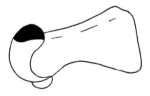

Kessel–Bonney

Closing wedge osteotomy
Indicated in hallux limitus

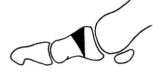

McBride

Similar to a Silver but may be performed with an adductor tendon transfer and a fibular sesamoid excision

Akin

Proximal Akin corrects DASA.
Distal Akin corrects IPJ.

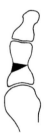

Hiss

Similar to a McBride bunionectomy with dorsal transfer, and advancement of the abductor hallucis tendon in an attempt to reestablish joint medial balance

Regnauld (Mexican Hat Procedure)

Similar to a peg-in-hole procedure
Indicated in hallux limitus

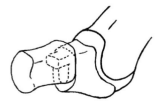

Fowler

Medial cuneiform opening wedge
Bone graft is inserted into the opening wedge.

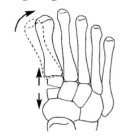

CAPSULOTOMIES

Mediovertical

More capsules are resected plantarly.

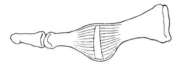

Medial "U"

Transverse plane correction
Good exposure of medial aspect of the 1st metatarsal head
Enables removal of redundant medial capsule

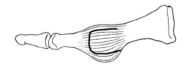

Medial "H"

Transverse plane correction
Good exposure of medial aspect of the 1st metatarsal head
Enables removal of redundant medial capsule

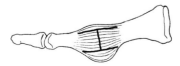

Medial "T"

Transverse plane correction
Good exposure of medial aspect of
the 1st metatarsal head
Enables removal of redundant medial capsule

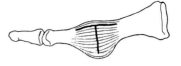

Inverted "L"

Transverse plane correction
Good exposure of medial aspect of
the 1st metatarsal head
Enables removal of redundant medial capsule

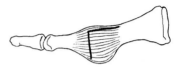

Lenticular

Allows both transverse and frontal
plane correction
Good exposure of medial aspect of
the 1st metatarsal head
Enables removal of redundant medial capsule

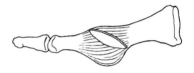

Washington Monument

Allows both transverse and frontal
plane correction

Good exposure of medial aspect of
the 1st metatarsal head
Strengthens the medial capsule

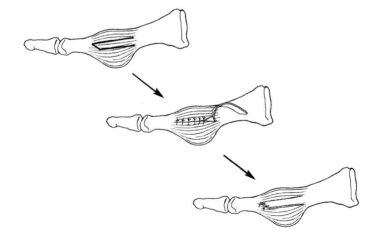

HALLUX LIMITUS AND HALLUX RIGIDUS

A condition in which the 1st MPJ has a decreased ROM or absent ROM

Radiographically, there is joint narrowing, flattening of the 1st metatarsal head with subchondral sclerosing, and loose bodies.

Hallux Limitus

Decreased ROM at the 1st MPJ
Approximately 50° to 60° of dorsiflexion are necessary for normal functional gait.

Hallux Rigidus

Absence of ROM at the 1st MPJ
The end result of hallux limitus

Classification

Grade I: Functional limitus
    No DJD
    Pain at the end of ROM
    Hyperextension of the IPJ
    ROM WNL
Grade II: Joint adaptation
    Pain at the end of ROM
    Flattening of metatarsal head
    Passive ROM limited
    Small dorsal exostosis and periarticular lipping
Grade III: Joint destruction/arthritis
    Continued DJD and osteophytic formation
    Crepitus on ROM
    Pain on full ROM
Grade IV: Ankylosis
    Less than 10° ROM
    Obliteration of joint space
    Loss of majority of articular cartilage

Cause

Metatarsus primus elevates
Hypermobile 1st ray
Immobile 1st ray
Long 1st ray
DJD
Neoplasm
Trauma
Septic joint
Iatrogenic
Neuromuscular dz
Arthritis (RA, psoriatic, gout)

Functional vs. Structural

Functional Hallux Limitus

Hallux dorsiflexion decreases only when the forefoot is loaded.
Responds well to orthotics by keeping the foot in neutral position and allowing the hallux to dorsiflex

Structural Hallux Limitus

Hallux dorsiflexion decreases whether forefoot is loaded or unloaded.
Orthotics do not help this condition.

Signs/Symptoms

Gradual onset pain and decreased ROM at the 1st MPJ
Pain tends to be on the dorsal aspect of the 1st MPJ.
Dorsal bony prominence
Plantar callus at the IPJ due to hyperextension of the IPJ
Hallux tends to be rectus with possible spastic EHL.
Joint narrowing
Flattening of the 1st metatarsal head with subchondral sclerosing

Osteophytic proliferation on the 1st metatarsal head and base of the proximal phalanx

Loose bodies

Treatment

Conservative

Shoe with a stiff sole

Rocker-bottom shoe

Intra-articular corticosteroid injections

Surgical

Bunionectomy

Removal osteophytic proliferation and loose body excision (cleanup joint)

Shorten and/or plantarflex the 1st metatarsal

CPM or early passive ROM exercises

HALLUX VARUS

An adductus and/or varus deviation of the hallux at the 1st MPJ

Cause

Iatrogenic (failed bunionectomy)

Resection of fibular sesamoid

Trauma

Congenital

Treatment

Conservative

Strapping, splinting

Surgical (Stepwise Approach)

1. Total soft-tissue release of the 1st MPJ

2. Medial capsulotomy

3. Tibial sesamoidectomy (if 30% to 50% of the tibial sesamoid is exposed medially)

4. Release EHL and transfer it to the plantar lateral aspect of the proximal phalanx (IPJ must be fused)

5. Osteotomy (if the IM angle is negative, a reverse Austin may be indicated)

6. Joint destructive procedure (arthroplasty or implant)

7. Arthrodesis

METATARSUS PRIMUS ELEVATUS

Metatarsus primus elevatus is a condition in which the 1st metatarsal is dorsally deviated in the sagittal plane relative to the lesser metatarsals. This causes "jamming" of the joint and usually results in hallux limitus or hallux rigidus. Normal ROM is 10 mm.

Causes

Excessively long or short 1st metatarsal

Hypermobile medial column

Uncompensated forefoot varus

DJD

Iatrogenic (failed base wedge osteotomy)

Symptoms

IPK sub 2nd metatarsal head

Hallux limitus/hallux rigidus

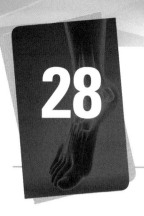

28

TAILOR'S BUNION (BUNIONETTE)

TAILOR'S BUNION (BUNIONETTE)

Description

Enlargement of, or prominence of, the 5th metatarsal head

Evaluation

IM Angle

Two Methods

1. Traditional method
   The angle between the bisection of the 4th metatarsal and the bisection of the 5th metatarsal
   Average normal value is 7°; higher values (8° to 10°) indicate an abnormality.
2. Fallat and Buckholz
   The angle between the bisection of the 4th metatarsal and the medial cortical margin of the proximal portion of the 5th metatarsal
   Average normal value is 7°; higher values (8° to 10°) indicate an abnormality.

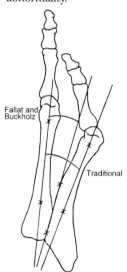

Lateral Deviation Angle

Bisection of the 5th metatarsal head and neck in relation to the medial cortical margin of the proximal portion of shaft

Average normal value is 3°; higher values (8°) indicate an abnormality.

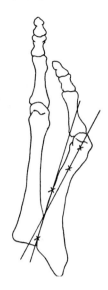

Classification

Type I	Type II	Type III

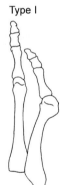 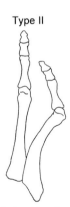 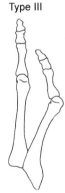

Enlarged head   Lateral bowing   Enlarged 4th and 5th IM angle

Causes

Enlarged 5th metatarsal head or hypertrophied plantar condyles

Lateral bowing of the 5th metatarsal shaft

Increased 4th IM angle

Biomechanical
    Cavus foot
    Uncompensated rearfoot varus
    Uncompensated forefoot varus
    Splay foot
    Metatarsus adductus
    Forefoot valgus

Treatment

Conservative treatment
    Padding
    Wider shoes
    NSAIDs
    Steroid injections
    Reduce callus
Surgical treatment

Exostoses

Davis

Removal of the lateral eminence
    (reverse Silver)

Dickson and Dively

Same as Davis but includes removal of an inflamed bursa

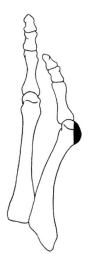

DeVries

Technically, it is the removal of the
lateral plantar condyle. Because the
5th metatarsal is often rotated medially, the lateral plantar condyle
is often the most lateral structure,

thus making the procedure the
same as the Davis.

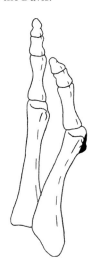

Amberry

Same as Davis plus removal of the
laterally prominent base of the
proximal phalanx

Arthroplasties

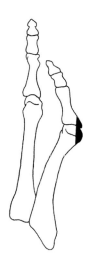

Head Resection

To prevent a callus beneath the stump of the metatarsal, make the cut oblique from distal/medial/dorsal to proximal/lateral/plantar. Toe retraction makes the 5th toe appear shorter.

Modifications to Prevent Toe Retraction

Addonte and Petrich and Dull

Recommended a Silastic interpositional sphere (Calnan–Nicole implant) to prevent retraction. The force vectors at this joint make stemmed implants unsuccessful.

Kelikian

Recommended syndactylizing the 4th and 5th toes to prevent retraction

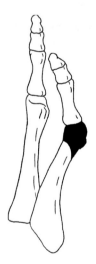

McKeever

Resection of ½ to ⅔ of the 5th metatarsal

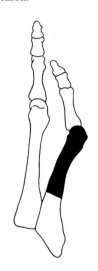

Brown

Resection of the entire 5th ray and toe

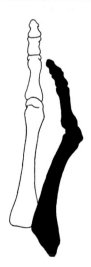

Osteotomies

Hohmann

Simple transverse osteotomy in neck

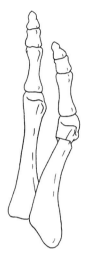

Sponsel or Keating

Reverse Wilson
Oblique osteotomy in neck
Shortens metatarsal

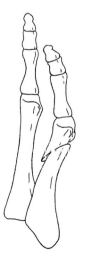

Yu

Distal oblique closing wedge
Intermedullary tension band
  K-wire fixation

Mann

Proximal oblique osteotomy

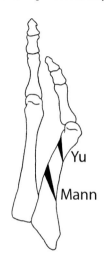

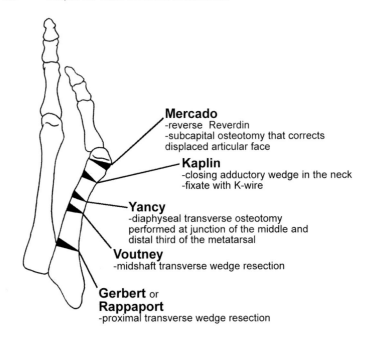

Mercado
-reverse Reverdin
-subcapital osteotomy that corrects
displaced articular face

Kaplin
-closing adductory wedge in the neck
-fixate with K-wire

Yancy
-diaphyseal transverse osteotomy
performed at junction of the middle and
distal third of the metatarsal

Voutney
-midshaft transverse wedge resection

Gerbert or
Rappaport
-proximal transverse wedge resection

Haber and Kraft

Distal crescentic osteotomy

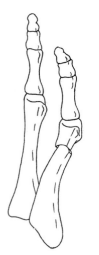

*Throckmorton and Brandless or
Campbell or Johnson*

Reverse Austin

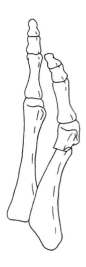

Leach and Igou

Reverse Mitchell

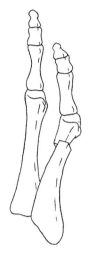

Leventen

Metatarsal head is staked on the shaft.

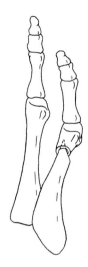

Thomasen

Peg in hole

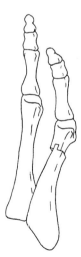

Diebold and Bejjani

Proximal Austin
Fixated to the 4th metatarsal with Steinmann pins

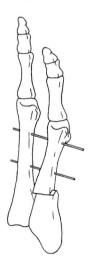

Bishop

Opening base wedge osteotomy
   with bone graft

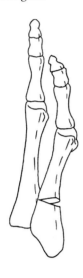

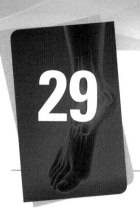

APGAR

APGAR is an acronym for a scoring system to evaluate perinatal asphyxia. It is not an indicator of long-term outcome, but rather an indicator of immediate needs. The score is the sum of points gained on assessment of the following five signs.

Sign	0	1	2
Appearance	Blue/pale	Body pink/blue extremities	Pink
Pulse	Absent	<100	>100
Grimace	No response	Grimace	Cry
Activity	Limp	Some flexion	Active motion
Respiratory effort	Absent	Some/irregular	Good/crying

Score: Add the scores from all five signs to assess infant.

0–2	Serious asphyxia
3–4	Moderate asphyxia
5–7	Mild asphyxia
8–10	Normal

DEVELOPMENTAL LANDMARKS

3 months	Lifts head up when prone
6 months	Rolls over
9 months	Sits up
12 months	Stands/cruises
14 months	Walks
15–18 months	Uses words
18–21 months	Combines words
21–24 months	Three-word sentences
36 months	Child develops a propulsive gait

CHILDHOOD IMMUNIZATION SCHEDULE

Childhood Immunization Schedule

Vaccine	Birth	1	2	4	6	12	15	18	19–23	4–6	11–12	16
				MONTHS							YEARS	
HepB	1st dose	2nd dose				3rd dose						
Rotavirus			1st dose	2nd dose	3rd dose#							
Diphtheria, tetanus, & pertussis (DTaP)			1st dose	2nd dose	3rd dose		4th dose			5th dose		
Haemophilus influenzae type b (Hib)			1st dose	2nd dose	3rd dose	4th dose						
Pneumococcal (PCV13)			1st dose	2nd dose	3rd dose	4th dose						
Inactivated polio (IPV)			1st dose	2nd dose		3rd dose				4th dose		
Influenza					Annually - – – – – – – ► (NOTE: First flu shot at age 6 is given twice, 2nd dose given 1 month after the 1st)							
Measles, mumps, rubella (MMR)						1st dose				2nd dose		
Varicella (VAR)						1st dose				2nd dose		
HepA						2nd dose series, 1st dose 12–23 months, 2nd dose 6–18 months later						
Human papillomavirus (HPV)											2 dose series, 1st dose 11–12 years, 2nd dose 6–12 months later**	
Meningitis (Serogroup A, C, W, and Y)											1st dose	2nd dose
Meningitis B												2 dose series, 1st dose 16–23 years, 2nd dose 6 months later**
Tdap											1st dose (repeat every 10 years with Tdap or Td)	

May be a 3 dose series depending on brand   # Some brands are only 2 doses
** Depending on brand, 2nd dose may be 1 month later   * Depending on brand, there is also a 3 dose series, 3rd (and final) dose given 12–15 years

SPLINTS AND BRACES

Splints and braces are used between 3 months and 3 years. When sizing a splint with a bar, measure from one ASIS to the other plus 1 inch. Splints used to abduct the foot are best used with triplanar varus wedge to prevent subluxation of the MTJ, and braces that have a rigid bar connecting the feet should have a 15° to 20° varus bend to prevent subluxation of STJ or MTJ. Splints and braces are best used on positional abnormalities, which are soft-tissue problems (i.e., internal and external femoral rotation), as opposed to bony abnormalities or torsional problems (i.e., tibial torsion). Splints and braces should be worn as much as possible at night, during naps, and as much as tolerated during the day. If splints follow serial plaster immobilization, wear splint for twice as long as total casting time.

Ganley Splint

First splint to treat combination foot and leg disorders

Same indications as Denis–Browne bar but also allows FF to RF control

If treating internal rotational problems, torque bar is placed between the rearfoot plates, and if treating an external rotational problem, the torque bar is placed between the two forefoot plates.

Adjustments are made by simply bending the aluminum bars.

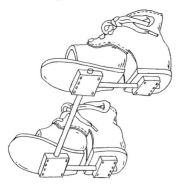

Denis–Browne Bar

Has been used to treat metatarsus adductus, convex pes planovalgus, and positional abnormalities of the leg

Originally designed to treat clubfoot

The bar is screwed or riveted on the child's shoes.

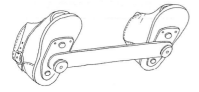

Fillauer Bar

Same as Denis–Browne bar, except it clamps to soles of patient's shoes

Requires rigid soled shoes for attachment

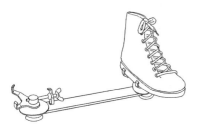

Unibar

Same as the Denis–Browne bar, except it has a ball and socket joint beneath each foot, which can be tightened into a varus position (preventing STJ and MTJ subluxation) eliminating the need to bend the bar.

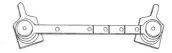

Counter Rotation System (Langer)

Designed to correct torsional abnormalities of the leg

Functionally the same as the Denis–Browne bar, but several hinges allow greater freedom of motion

Best tolerated splint; allows unencumbered crawling

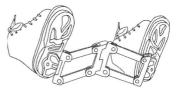

Bebax Shoe

Used to treat forefoot to rearfoot abnormalities, such as metatarsus adductus

Recommended for use after serial casting of metatarsus adductus, but not for primary correction

Also available is the Clubax, a device designed for rearfoot or leg deformities, specifically clubfoot

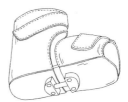

Standard AFO

Ankle set at 90°

Used in various neuromuscular disorders that may cause equinus (CP, muscular dystrophy [MD])

Also used to treat drop foot

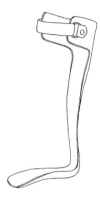

Wheaton Brace

Used for metatarsus adductus

Designed as an alternative to serial casting for metatarsus adductus

Similar in appearance to an AFO, with a medial flare to abduct the forefoot

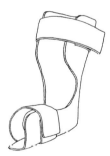

Wheaton Brace System

This additional AK piece is designed to lock into the BK component.

The knee is fixed at 90°, preventing twisting of the femur or hip and allowing isolated unilateral treatment of tibial torsion.

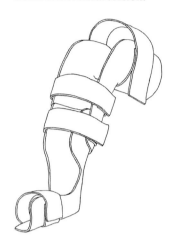

Twister Cables

Belt (around waist) cables (inside pant leg course down to shoe)

Controls the degree of abduction at heel contact

Used to treat scissors gait of CP patients

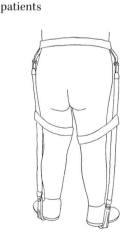

Friedman Counter Splint or Flexosplint

A dynamic splint consisting of a belt around the posterior heels, allowing motion in all planes, except internal rotation
Indicated for internal tibial torsion

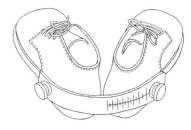

IPOS Shoe

Anti-adductus orthosis type 2
Indicated for metatarsus adductus
Functions by the use of varied correctional elastic tension bands (formerly springs were used)

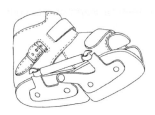

OSTEOCHONDROSIS (EPIPHYSEAL ISCHEMIC NECROSIS)

A disease of the growth or ossification center in children, which begins as a degeneration or necrosis and is followed by regeneration or recalcification

Blount Disease

Osteochondrosis of the medial portion of the proximal epiphyseal ossification center in the tibia causing bowing of the leg or legs. Symptoms include limping and lateral bowing of the leg. Radiographic evaluation reveals sclerotic medial cortex with spurring.

Infantile Type

Occurs before age 6 years
Caused by early walking and obesity

Adolescent Type

Occurs at 8 to 15 years
Caused by trauma and infection

Freiberg Infraction

Osteochondrosis of the metatarsal head. The 2nd metatarsal head is most frequently involved followed by the 3rd, 4th, and then 5th. The condition is more common in girls and usually occurs between ages 10 and 18 years. The condition can occur in adults. Radiographic evaluation reveals sclerosis and fragmentation of the metatarsal head with flattening of the articular surface.

Symptoms

Pain on ROM of the affected MPJ
Local tenderness and swelling
Generalized thickening at the MPJ

Treatment

Conservative care involves metatarsal pads, short leg casts, and stiff post-op shoe.
Surgical treatment is aimed at removing any bony lipping from the perimeter of the metatarsal head; when DJD is severe, an implant may be indicated.

Köhler Disease

Osteochondrosis of the navicular (tarsal scaphoid). The condition is more common in boys and occurs between ages 3 and 6 years.

Symptoms

Often asymptomatic but may present with pain and swelling
Navicular becomes sclerotic and flattened (coin on edge, or silver dollar sign).
Köhler disease is self-limiting, and recovery usually takes from 2 to 4 years. The navicular ultimately resumes normal shape and density.

Legg–Calvé–Perthes Disease

Osteochondrosis of the femoral head occurring primarily in males (5:1) between ages 3 and 12 years. Ten percent of cases are bilateral, and a history of trauma precedes 30% of cases. Legg–Calvé–Perthes is the most common form of osteochondrosis; the younger the child; the better the prognosis.

Symptoms

Insidious in onset
Limping
Generalized groin pain
Referred pain to the knee is common.

Osgood–Schlatter Disease

Osteochondrosis of the tibial tuberosity. More common in boys and occurs between ages 10 and 15 years. Caused by excessive traction on the patellar ligament. Symptoms include local pain and swelling with tenderness on palpation. The condition is self-limiting, and treatment is symptomatic.

Sever Disease

Osteochondrosis of the calcaneus (apophysis) caused by excessive traction of the Achilles tendon
Occurs between ages 6 and 12 years and is more common in patients with equinus. Radiographic diagnosis is difficult because the normal epiphysis can have multiple ossification centers and irregular borders and is often sclerotic.

Treatment

RICE
NSAIDs
Elimination of sports
Heel lifts
Achilles stretching exercises

Other Less Common Osteochondrosis

Buschke dz
Osteochondrosis involving the cuneiforms

Diaz or Mouchet dz
Osteochondrosis involving the talar body (usually associated with trauma)

Thiemann dz
Osteochondrosis involving the epiphyseal ossification centers in the phalanges

Iselin dz
Osteochondrosis involving the 5th metatarsal base

Lewin dz
Osteochondrosis involving the distal tibia

Ritter dz
Osteochondrosis involving the fibular head proximally

Treves dz
Osteochondrosis involving the fibular sesamoid

Renandier dz
Osteochondrosis involving the tibia sesamoid

Lance dz
Osteochondrosis involving the cuboid

Assmann dz
Osteochondrosis involving the head of the 1st metatarsal

CONGENITAL DISLOCATED HIP

Occurrence is 0.1%.
Sixty percent are on left side, 20% to 30% B/L.
Increased incident in:

1. Females (5 to 8 times greater)
2. Children with older sibling with a dislocated hip (10 times more likely)
3. Breech presentation
4. Joint laxity
5. First born

Classical signs in older children include limited abduction, asymmetric thigh folds, relative femoral shortening, a limp, positive Trendelenburg test, externally rotated foot, and waddling gait.
Best position for the hips to prevent dislocation is flexed and abducted.
When a dislocation occurs, the femoral head is usually posterior and superior to the acetabulum.

Most dislocations occur during the first 2 weeks after birth.
It is commonly associated with oligohydramnios, torticollis, metatarsus adductus, and calcaneal valgus.

Etiology

Ligamentous laxity
Acetabular dysplasia
Malpositioning
  a. In utero (i.e., breech)
  b. Postnatal (carrying babies with hips adducted and extended)

Clinical Diagnostic Studies

Ortolani Sign

With the baby supine, hips and knees are flexed to 90°. The hips are examined one at a time by grasping the baby's thigh with the middle finger over the greater trochanter and lifting and abducting the thigh while stabilizing the pelvis and opposite leg with the other hand. The test is positive when a palpable click is felt as the femoral head is made to enter the acetabulum.

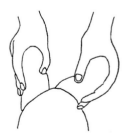

Barlow Sign

With the baby supine, the hips and knees are flexed. With the thumb on the lesser trochanter in the groin and the middle finger of the same hand on the greater trochanter laterally, gently apply pressure down on the knee while simultaneously applying lateral pressure with the thumb. The dislocatable hip then becomes displaced with a palpable clunk as the head slips over the posterior aspect of the acetabulum. This is a provocative test, which actively dislocates an unstable hip.

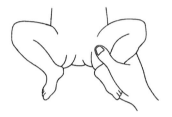

Anchor Sign

With the baby prone, legs are adducted and extended. Look for asymmetry of thigh and gluteal folds. There will be more folds on the dislocated side.

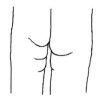

Galeazzi Sign

Also known as Allis sign. While the hips and knees are flexed, a dislocated hip results in a lower knee position on the affected side. May be false positive in B/L cases.

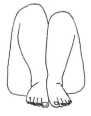

Abduction Test

With the baby supine, hips and knees are flexed to 90°. Abduct the knees to resistance. A dislocated hip will have limitation of abduction on the affected side.

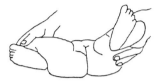

Nelaton Line

Particularly useful in children with B/L dislocations. An imaginary line is drawn connecting the anterior iliac spine and the tuberosity of the ischium. If the tip of the greater trochanter is palpable distal to this line, the hip is dislocated.

Radiographic Diagnostic Studies

Hilgenreiner line (Y line): A line connecting the most inferior portion of the acetabulum on both sides
Ombrédanne line (Perkins vertical line): Draw a line perpendicular to Hilgenreiner line at the outer most aspect of the acetabulum.

Quadrant System

After drawing the Hilgenreiner and Ombrédanne lines, the normal position of the developing femoral head should be in the lower medial quadrant. A dislocated hip will show at least part of the femoral head in the outer upper quadrant.

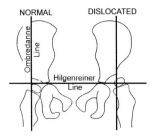

Acetabular Index

Draw a line extending through the most medial and lateral aspect of the acetabulum. The angle created between this line and Hilgenreiner line is the acetabular index. This value should be between 27° and 30° at birth and decrease to 20° by age 2. An angle >30° indicates a dislocated hip.

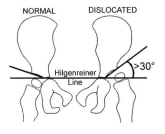

Shenton Curved Line (Menard Curved Line)

Draw a line up the medial side of the femoral neck to continue up into the obturator foramen. This should be a continuous arc; with a hip dislocation, the obturator foramen is too low.

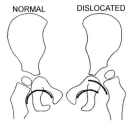

Von Rosen Sign (Frog Leg View)

An A/P radiograph is taken with the hips extended and the thighs abducted 45° and medially rotated. A line is drawn through the long axis of the femur. In a normal hip, this line should extend through the lateral corner of the acetabulum. In a dislocated hip, the line will bisect the ASIS.

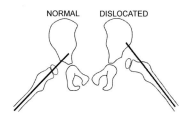

Von Rosen Method

Draw the Hilgenreiner line and then draw a parallel line passing through the upper margin of the pubic symphysis. In a dislocated hip, the femur will extend up between these lines.

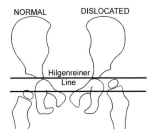

Wiberg CE Angle

Based on the assumption that if the femoral head is inadequately covered by the acetabulum, it will develop DJD. This test shows how much is covered. Draw a line connecting the center of the femoral head (C) with the lateral most aspect of the acetabulum (E). Measure the angle created by this line and Ombrédanne line. If this angle is <20° in a child over 5 years, there is an increased likelihood of developing DJD.

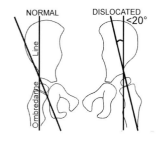

Treatment

Treatment is aimed at aligning the femoral head in the acetabulum and holding it there, by keeping the hips in a flexed and abducted position. With early detection, this may be accomplished by specific pillow arrangement in the crib, double or triple diapering, a Pavlik harness, or a Spica cast. As the child grows, traction plus closed reduction is required. If undiagnosed by age 6 or 7, open reduction and eventually a hip implant may be required due to permanent arthritic changes.

IN-TOEING

Normal rotational profile of the leg varies wildly during childhood and, in most instances, is not a pathologic condition. All infants start out in-toed. This benign rotational position will improve over time, a progressive deformity suggests a pathology. Also, unilateral conditions or in-toeing associated pain may be a concern. The most common causes of in-toeing are femoral anteversion, internal tibial

torsion, and metatarsus adductus. Tripping and falling are commonly associated with in-toeing. In-toeing in an infant is most likely due to metatarsus adductus. In children <3, tibial torsion is most common, and in children >3, femoral anteversion is the most likely cause.

Other pathologies such as cerebral palsy, hip dysplasia, and Legg–Calvé–Perthes should be ruled out.

Causes of in-toeing
(Pigeon toes)

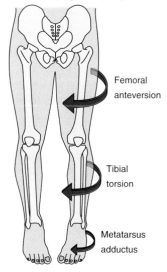

Femoral Anteversion

Femoral anteversion is an inward twisting of the long axis of the femur. An outward twisting of the femur is called femoral retroversion.

Normally, there is 30° of external rotation at birth.

By 8 to 10 years, there is 10° of external rotation (>10° is in-toed).

Patients with in-toeing from femoral anteversion have other distinctive features such as a propensity to sit in the "W" position. They also run with an "eggbeater" or "windmill" type motion, and they have medially pointed "kissing patella."

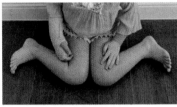

"W" Sitting Position

Hip Rotation

The easiest way is to assess hip range of motion is by using Craig test. The patient lies in the prone position with knees flexed to 90°.

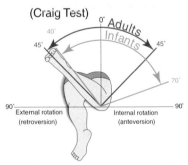

Infants have an average of 40° of external rotation and 70° of internal rotation. By age 8 to 10 years, internal and external rotation are both around 45°.

NOTE: Internal rotation of the hip joint is performed by externally rotating the lower leg.

Internal Tibial Torsion

Internal tibial torsion is an inward twisting of the tibia. An outward twisting of the tibia is called external tibial torsion.

At birth, tibial torsion is 0°.

By 8 to 10 years, there is 15° external rotation.

A test for tibial torsion is the thigh-foot angle.

Thigh-Foot Angle

Patient prone with knees flexed at 90° and the foot dorsiflexed. Measure the angle of a line down the center of the thigh to the heel bisector. Infants average 5° internal rotation by age 8 to 10 years, the adult position of 10° external is achieved.

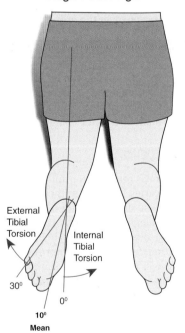

Thigh-Foot Angle

Foot Progression Angle

The angle of the foot relative to an imaginary straight line in the patient's path. Patients who in-toe are assigned a negative value, and patients who out-toe are given a positive value. This value represents the sum total of the rotational profile of the leg. It takes into account femoral torsion, tibial torsion, and foot contour.

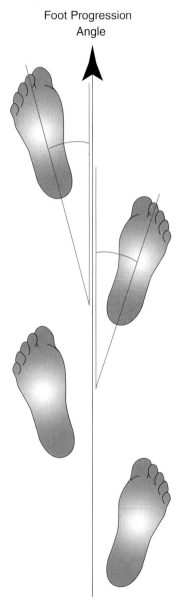

Foot Progression
Angle

Normal:	−5 to +20°
Mild in-toeing:	−5 to −10°
Moderate in-toeing:	−10 to −15°
Severe in-toeing:	> −15°

METATARSUS ADDUCTUS (MTA)

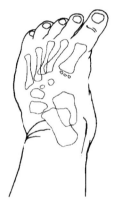

Metatarsus adductus is a single plane (transverse) deformity with adduction of the forefoot at the Lisfranc joints. The rearfoot is normal. Metatarsus adductus is usually idiopathic and rarely associated with neuromuscular disease. Most cases resolve satisfactorily without treatment. Spontaneous improvement should be almost complete at about 3 months. Clinical symptoms include an in-toed gait with frequent tripping and a prominent styloid process. The severity of the adduction progressively decreases from medial to lateral.

Foot is "C" shaped.
Affects 1 in 1,000 live births
Males:females (1:1)
55% bilateral
10% associated with dislocated hip

Differential Diagnosis

Any condition that causes in-toeing. Internal tibial torsion, inter-nal femoral torsion, internal femoral position, femoral anteversion

Cause

Intrauterine position (most cases)
Tight abductor hallucis muscle
Absent or hypoplastic medial cuneiform
Abnormal insertion of anterior tib-ial tendon

Classifications

Type I Mild	Type II Moderate	Type III Severe
Flexible: (Actively cor-rectable) Tickle foot on lateral border and it straightens.	Partial flexibility: (Passively correctable) Does not correct to neutral actively, but does with gentle lat-eral pressure.	Rigid: (fixed) Does not cor-rect to neutral actively or passively.
Tx: none.	Tx: Stretching exercises during diaper changes. Consider casting if not corrected at 4–6 months.	Tx: Casting/bracing.

Heel Bisector (Bleck Classification)

Bisect the heel and extend the line distally to see where it falls on the toes.

Heel Bisector Angle
(Bleck Classification)

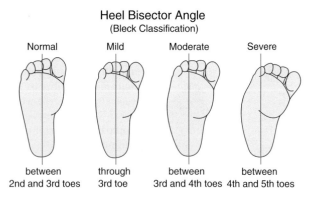

Normal	Mild	Moderate	Severe
between 2nd and 3rd toes	through 3rd toe	between 3rd and 4th toes	between 4th and 5th toes

"V"-Finger Test

The "V"-finger test is a simple imprecise clinical test used to raise suspicion of MTA. By placing the infant's foot between the index and middle finger, metatarsus adductus becomes easier to appreciate.

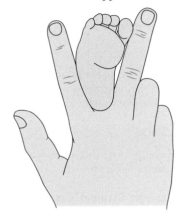

Measuring the Metatarsus Adductus Angle

Classic Method

A line is drawn between the medial-proximal aspect of the 1st metatarsal base and the medial-distal aspect of the talonavicular articulation.

A second line is drawn between the lateral-proximal aspect of the 4th metatarsal base and the lateral-distal aspect of the calcaneocuboid joint.

A third line is drawn between the bisection of these two lines.

Next, the angle is measured between a line drawn perpendicular to this third line and a line drawn down the longitudinal shaft of the 2nd metatarsal.

Metatarsus adductus angle >20° is considered adducted.

MTA angle at birth is 25° to 30°; at 1 year (begin walking), it is around 20°; and by 4 years, it is at the adult normal of around 15°.

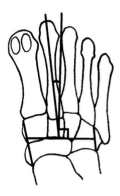

Lepow Technique

Take the perpendicular of a line passing through the lateral base of the 5th and medial base of the 1st metatarsals and compare with the 2nd metatarsal.

Values are comparable to values obtained by the traditional method.

MTA angle at birth is 25° to 30°; at 1 year (begin walking), it is around 20°; and by 4 years, it is at the adult normal of around 15°.

Normal values: 22° to 25° at birth, 15° to 20° in a toddler, and 10° in an adult.

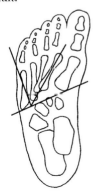

Engel Angle

Bisect the intermediate cuneiform and compare with the 2nd metatarsal. A normal value using this method is 24°.

The angle increases with an adducted foot.

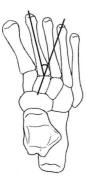

Treatment, Conservative

Conservative (children <3 years old)

Manipulation and serial casting are the standard treatment.

Shoes, orthotics

Splints (Ganley), braces

Treatment, Surgical (Soft Tissue)

Children between 2 and 6 or 8 years of age, soft-tissue procedures are recommended.

Heyman, Herndon, and Strong

Release of all soft-tissue structures at Lisfranc joint, except lateral and plantar lateral ligaments

Initially described using one transverse skin incision, revised to two or three longitudinal incisions

Thompson Procedure

Resection of the abductor hallucis muscle

Release medial head of FHB, if necessary

Lange

Capsulotomy of the 1st metatarsal and the 1st cuneiform joint

Division of the abductor hallucis

Lichtblau

Sectioning of the hyperactive abductor hallucis

Treatment, Surgical (Osseous)

Children 8 years and older—osseous procedures

Berman and Gartland

Laterally based crescentic osteotomies of metatarsal base 1 to 5

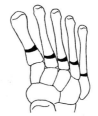

Lepird

Closing wedge osteotomy of the 1st and 5th metatarsal bases

Oblique rotational osteotomies of the three central metatarsals

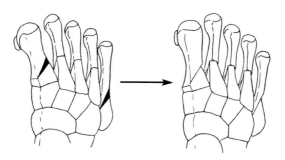

Johnson Osteochondrotomy

Closing abductory base wedge osteotomy of the 1st metatarsal

Resection of osteocartilaginous 2.5 mm wedge from the lesser metatarsals

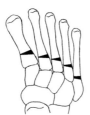

Peabody–Muro

Excision of the base of the central three metatarsals

Osteotomy of the 5th metatarsal

Mobilization of the 1st metatarsal and cuneiform joint

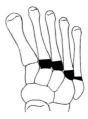

Fowler

Opening wedge osteotomy of the medial cuneiform with insertion of bone graft

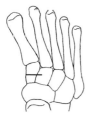

Steytler and Van Der Walt

Oblique osteotomy of all metatarsals

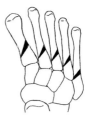

McCormick and Blount

Arthrodesis of the 1st metatarsal and cuneiform joint

Osteotomy of metatarsals 2, 3, and 4

Possible wedge resection of cuboid

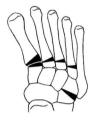

METATARSUS VARUS

Metatarsus varus is metatarsus adductus with a varus component. It tends to be more rigid than simple metatarsus adductus. As a result of the rigid presentation, metatarsus varus often results in a skewfoot due to compensation. Metatarsus varus consists of frontal plane inversion and adduction at the Lisfranc joint. Metatarsus varus is a two-plane deformity, there is no sagittal plane component.

SKEWFOOT (Z FOOT, SERPENTINE FOOT, COMPENSATED METATARSUS ADDUCTUS)

A skewfoot is a foot type with an adducted forefoot, normal midfoot, and a valgus hindfoot. Skewfoot is an acquired deformity resulting from gradual compensation of metatarsus varus. Unlike clubfoot, skewfoot does not involve a sagittal plane deformity. Skewfoot is usually acquired from gradual compensation of a metatarsus varus

that develops with weight-bearing or improper manipulation and casting. Other signs include a fixed hindfoot valgus and severe rigid metatarsus adductus. There is also an increased calcaneocuboid angle.

SKEWFOOT

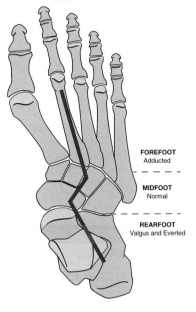

FOREFOOT
Adducted

MIDFOOT
Normal

REARFOOT
Valgus and Everted

Radiographs

Lateral: plantarflexed talus and decreased CIA

AP: abducted forefoot and increased talonavicular coverage angle

Treatment

Infants:

Serial casting in young children, best initiated between 6 and 12 months. Cast the forefoot in the same manner as in a foot with metatarsus adductus but with the ankle in slight plantarflexion and the STJ in slight inversion.

Children:
Symptoms are usually related to toe adducted forefoot. Pain over lateral 5th base and/or medial to the head of the 1st metatarsal. There may also be pain or a callus under the plantarflexed talar head. Rearfoot symptoms mimic signs and symptoms of a flexible flatfoot with a tight Achilles with pain in the sinus tarsi related to the hindfoot valgus and equinus.

OUT-TOEING

Out-toeing is much less common than in-toeing and is caused by the same rotational deformities that cause in-toeing, but in the opposite direction (femoral retroversion, lateral tibial torsion, any foot pathology that causes abduction of the foot).

CLUBFOOT (TALIPES EQUINOVARUS)

Introduction

Clubfoot is a congenital deformity in which the infant's foot is turned inward.
A triplanar deformity involving:
    Ankle equinus
    Hindfoot varus
    Forefoot adduction
1:1,000 live births
Male to female (2:1)

Fifty percent of cases are bilateral.
Occurs in the right foot more than the left
Lowest incident in Asians; highest in Polynesians

Types

Idiopathic	Intrauterine position
Nonidiopathic	Spina bifida, CP, MD, meningitis, postpolio, traumatic, Streeter dz

Evaluation

Sign	Normal	Clubfoot
Kite angle	20°–40°	0°–15°
Meary angle	0°	>0°
Calcaneal inclination angle	20°–25	~17°
Talar head/neck relative to body: Adduction	10°–20°	80°–90°
Plantarflexion	25°–30°	45°–65°

Lateral view of clubfoot: Talus and calcaneus are parallel (Kite angle is 0°).

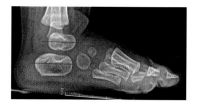

AP view of clubfoot: Note the fore-foot adduction and abnormal Meary angle. Kite angle is close to 0°.

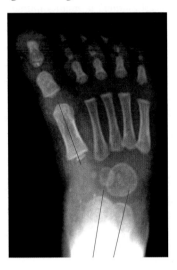

Horizontal Breech

While the talar head and neck are medially deviated, the talar body and trochlear talar surface may be slightly externally rotated within the mortise, leading to an external torsional deformity of the tibia and fibula. The lateral malleolus becomes displaced posteriorly off its articular talar facet, leading to a decrease in the bimalleolar axis. The bimalleolar axis is the angle between the longitudinal bisection of the hindfoot and the malleolar plane. Normal bimalleolar axis values are 75° to 90°; in a clubbed foot, this angle decreases to <75°.

Beatson and Pearson Assessment Method

The talus and calcaneus are longitudinally bisected on a lateral and A/P x-ray. The calcaneus is bisected on the lateral film by using the CIA. The talocalcaneal angle of the A/P view is added to the talocalcaneal angle of the lateral view. If the sum is <40°, the foot is clubbed.

Simon Assessment Method (Simon Rule of 15)

The talus, calcaneus, and 1st metatarsal are longitudinally bisected on an A/P x-ray, with the foot positioned in the maximally corrected position. In a clubfoot, the talo-1st metatarsal angle was >15° and the talocalcaneal angle (Kite ankle) was <15°.

Treatment, Conservative

Serial Casting (Begin As Soon As Possible)

Stretching and manipulation should be performed before cast application.

Apply tincture of benzoin to child's skin to help the undercast stick to the skin.

A cast is applied with 2-inch cast material. (Short or long leg cast may be used; generally in infants, use a long leg to prevent cast from slipping off. Flex knee at 75° to 90°.)

Reduction of the clubfoot deformity should be performed in the following order:

ADDUCTION
VARUS
EQUINUS

> Mnemonic—AVEnue (Adduction, Varus, Equinus)

Ponseti technique serial casting weekly. Percutaneous tendo Achilles tenotomy for *hindfoot stall.* Once corrected abduction foot orthotics worn full time for 12 weeks, then at night and during naps until age 4 years.

Ponseti vs. Kite

Kite method of casting corrected each component one at a time. Ponseti corrects them simultaneously. All the components of a clubfoot are corrected simultaneously, except the equinus. Equinus is corrected last.

Casting should supinate and abduct the foot, not pronate it. In clubfoot, the 1st metatarsal shows excessive plantarflexion, leading to pronation of the forefoot in relation to the hindfoot resulting in a cavus deformity. It is corrected by supinating the forefoot by lifting the head of 1st metatarsal with some abduction, thereby placing the forefoot in proper alignment with the hindfoot.

If there are no signs of improvement after 12 weeks, consider surgical intervention.

Complications of cast treatment:

a. Metatarsus adductus

b. Heel varus

c. Pes planovalgus—overcorrection

d. Rocker-bottom foot, from overzealous correction of the equinus

e. AVN or talar head flattening. Infant connective tissue is stronger than infant bone and cartilage. During casting, tremendous forces are exerted on the navicular and talar head.

f. Navicular subluxation—usually dorsally over talus

Treatment, Surgical

Soft-Tissue Release (Children 3 to 12 Months)

Two most popular incisions

1. Medial hockey stick, with a secondary lateral if necessary

2. Cincinnati incision

Posterior Release

Reflection of the origin of abductor hallucis and plantar fascia

Z-plasty of Achilles tendon

Release of the posterior, medial, and lateral ankle joint

Release of the posterior, medial, and lateral STJ. In doing so, the posterior talofibular and calcaneofibular ligaments are severed.

Medial Release (Talonavicular and Medial STJ Release)

Z-plasty of the posterior tibial tendon

Release of the talonavicular joint. In doing so, the spring ligament and Henry knot are severed.

Release of the entire medial STJ, which will include the superficial deltoid ligament

Lateral Release (Performed Through the STJ in the Single Medial Incision Approach)

Release of the interosseous talocalcaneal ligament

Release of the bifurcate ligament

Release of the lateral STJ

Osseous Procedures (1 to 4 Years)

After the child reaches the age of at least 1 year, bony correction involving a lateral closing wedge may be required to shorten the lateral column and prevent long-term stiffness of the hindfoot.

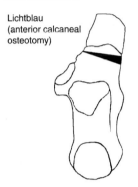

Lichtblau
(anterior calcaneal
osteotomy)

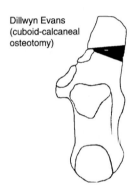

Dillwyn Evans
(cuboid-calcaneal
osteotomy)

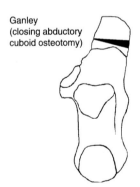

Ganley
(closing abductory
cuboid osteotomy)

CONGENITAL VERTICAL TALUS

■ Also known as congenital convex pes planovalgus, reverse clubfoot, Persian slipper, Rocker-bottom flatfoot

Description

Congenital vertical talus is a condition where there is a fixed dorsal dislocation of the navicular on the talar head and neck and a fixed valgus and equinus contracture of the calcaneus, resulting in a rigid flatfoot deformity. The forefoot is abducted and dorsiflexed at the midtarsal joint. The foot may actually touch the front of the tibia at birth. The talar head is prominent on the medial plantar aspect of foot and may have a callus over it from bearing most of the body weight. *Rigidity is the hallmark* of this deformity. The gastroc-soleus is contracted, and the spring ligament becomes elongated. The majority of cases are bilateral, and the right foot is more commonly affected than the left.

Walking is not delayed because the condition is not painful in childhood; however, gait is awkward, clumsy, and almost peg-like, and shoes may be difficult to wear. Vertical talus often occurs with other congenital deformities, most notably arthrogryposis. Hubscher maneuver will be negative.

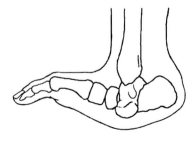

Radiographic Evaluation

Lateral View Vertical Talus

Talus is pointing almost straight down.
Increased Kite angle
Abnormal Meary angle
Navicular (if ossified) will be seen articulating with the dorsal neck of the talus.

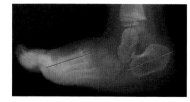

A/P View Vertical Talus

Talocalcaneal angle (Kite angle) is increased, usually >40°, normal is 20° to 40°. Meary angle is abnormal.

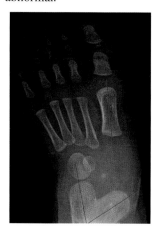

Stress Plantarflexed Lateral View

Vertical talus can sometimes be difficult to distinguish from calcaneovalgus. Definitive diagnosis can be confirmed by taking a stress plantar-flexed lateral radiograph. Calcaneovalgus is a flexible

STRESS PLANTARFLEXED LATERAL VIEW

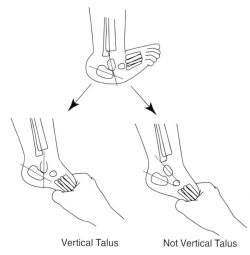

Vertical Talus   Not Vertical Talus

454   Chapter 29 Pediatrics

deformity, and Kite angle and Meary angle will partially or completely correct. With a vertical talus, a stress plantarflexed lateral radiograph will cause the talus to become even more "vertical" because the navicular is dislocated over the top of the talar head and it pushes the talus further into plantarflexion. This test is especially helpful in children under 3, before the navicular has ossified.

Clubfoot Treatment

Closed Reduction

Rarely successful. Manipulation and casting is recommended as a means of stretching the soft tissues for future definitive surgical treatment in an attempt to avoid skin sloughing.

Open Reduction

3 months to 3 years: If closed reduction fails, open reduction should be performed at 3 months of age. Many procedures have been described; they all involve a posterior release and reduction of the talonavicular joint.

3 to 6 years: In addition to open reduction, an extra-articular arthrodesis (Green–Grice type) or arthroereisis may be attempted to maintain reduction and stabilize the STJ.

6 years and up: At this point, it is best to postpone surgery until skeletal maturity (10 to 14 years of age), at which time a triple arthrodesis is performed, which may require removal of the head and neck of the talus to obtain reduction.

FLEXIBLE PES PLANUS (FLATFEET)

Flexible vs. Rigid

Flexible	Rigid
(+) Hubscher maneuver	(−) Hubscher maneuver
(+) Resupination test	(−) Resupination test
Not painful	Painful
Longitudinal arch presents during WB	Causes include coalition, vertical talus

Description

Flexible pes planus deformity is usually asymptomatic. Most infants are flatfooted and develop an arch during the first decade of life. There is a higher incidence in blacks. The foot appears externally rotated in relation to the leg. Weight-bearing axis of the LE is medial to the mid-axis of the foot.

Symptoms

Symptoms are quite varied and are often asymptomatic. When symptoms are present, they may include muscle cramps, especially calf and anterior leg, arch pain, and heel pain.

Radiographic Evaluation

	Normal	Flatfoot
Lateral		
Meary angle	0°	1°–15° mild, >15° severe
CIA	20°–25°	<15°
A/P		
Talocalcaneal angle	<25°	<25°
Talonavicular articulation	<50%	60%–70%

Causes

Compensated FF varus
Compensated FF valgus
RF equinus
Adducted foot
Abducted foot
Neurotrophic feet
Muscle imbalance
Posterior tibial tendon rupture
Ligamentous laxity (Ehlers–Danlos, Marfan, Down, osteogenesis imperfecta)
Calcaneovalgus
Enlarged or accessory navicular

Treatment

Conservative treatment in young children involves manipulation and strapping, whereas in older patients, orthotics are beneficial. Flexible flatfoot with short tendon Achilles is not an indication for orthotics or arch supports because the short tendon Achilles will prevent recreation of the arch and instead cause increased pressure under the talar head. With these, children use a heel cup whose margins have been increased to 25 mm. This keeps the heel in a more vertical position.

Adding a medial flare of about 1/8″ on the rearfoot post will help eliminate some of the excess pronation.

Surgical treatment is based on plane dominance.

Transverse Plane

Evans

Opening osteotomy of the calcaneus 1.5 cm proximal to the calcaneocuboid joint with insertion of a bone graft

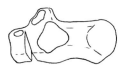

Kidner

Removal of prominent navicular tuberosity or accessory navicular and transplantation of the tibialis posterior tendon into the underside of the navicular bone

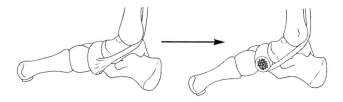

Sagittal Plane

Lowman

Plantarflexory talonavicular wedge arthrodesis performed with a TAL. The tibialis anterior tendon is rerouted under the navicular and sutured into the spring ligament to further support the arch. Next, a slip of the Achilles tendon, which is left attached to the calcaneus, is folded forward along the medial arch as an accessory ligament.

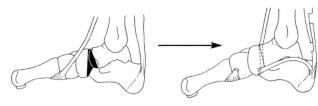

Cotton

Opening dorsal wedge on the 1st cuneiform

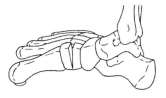

Hoke

Plantarly based wedge arthrodesis of the navicular and the medial and intermediate cuneiforms. Performed with a TAL.

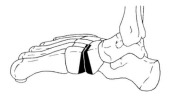

Miller

Naviculo-1st cuneiform–1st metatarsal fusion. Posterior tibial tendon and spring ligament advancement using an osteoperiosteal flap.

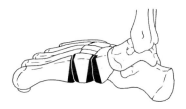

Young (Keyhole Technique)

Reroute the anterior tibial tendon through a keyhole in the navicular without detaching it from its insertion. Posterior tibial advanced under the navicular.

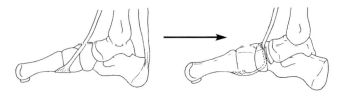

Frontal Plane

Chambers

Raise the posterior facet of the STJ using a bone graft under the sinus tarsi.

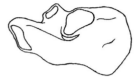

Baker

Osteotomy inferior to the STJ posterior facet with bone graft

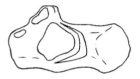

Selakovich

Opening wedge osteotomy of the sustentaculum tali with bone graft, which restricts abnormal STJ motion

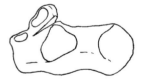

Calcaneal Osteotomies

Gleich

Oblique osteotomy displaced anteriorly. Helps increase the calcaneal inclination angle.

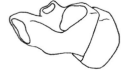

Silver

Lateral opening wedge with graft

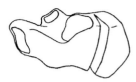

Koutsogiannis

Medial slide calcaneal osteotomy

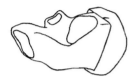

Triple Arthrodesis

Reserved for the second stage salvage procedure

Grice and Green Extra-Articular Subtalar Arthrodesis

A bone graft is inserted laterally in the sinus tarsi between the talus and the calcaneus. This procedure is acceptable for children because it provides excellent stability without interfering with the growth of the tarsal bones.

CAVUS FOOT TYPE (PES CAVUS)

Description

A cavus foot is a foot type with an elevated longitudinal arch. It is primarily a sagittal plane deformity. A cavus foot has less surface area touching the ground, and painful callus may develop under the metatarsal heads. They are also more prone to chronic inversion ankle sprains. Heel, knee, or hip pain may develop secondary to lack of shock absorption from the abnormal architecture of the foot.

Radiologic Evaluation

WB and NWB radiographs should be taken to determine whether the deformity is reducible. A "bullet hole" sinus tarsi seen on lateral radiograph is indicative of a cavus foot.

Signs	Normal	Cavus Foot
CIA	20°–25°	>30°
Angle of Meary	0°	>6°
Angle of Hibbs	135°–140°	>150°

Classification (Based on Apex of Deformity)

Metatarsal cavus	Lisfranc joint
Lesser tarsus cavus	Lesser tarsal bones
Forefoot cavus	Chopart joint
Combination	Apex generalized over lesser tarsals

Causes

Cavus foot is often the first manifestation of many neuromuscular disorders, including spina bifida, Charcot–Marie–Tooth disease, Friedreich ataxia, poliomyelitis, spinal cord tumors, myelomeningocele, CP, infection, syphilis, trauma, and spinal cord lesion.

Treatment, Conservative

Shoe modification and orthotics can alleviate symptoms by increasing the weight-bearing surface of the foot and relieving painful callus under the ball of the foot. Extra depth shoes combined with a metatarsal bar may help alleviate pressure under the ball of the foot. In young patients, passive stretching, manipulation, and casting may be beneficial.

Treatment, Surgical (Soft Tissue)

Soft-tissue procedures may be adequate for flexible deformities.

Plantar Fascial Release

Plantar fasciotomy may relax some of the plantar structures.

Steindler Stripping

Plantar fascia along with the long plantar ligament, abductor hallucis, FDB, and abductor digiti quinti are all stripped from the periosteum of the calcaneus.

Tendon transfers are also effective treatment for flexible deformities:

Jones tenosuspension
Heyman procedure: Transfer of all four extensor tendons to their respective metatarsal heads.
Hibbs procedure
Split tibialis anterior tendon transfer (STATT)
Peroneus longus tendon transfer
Tibialis posterior tendon transfer

Peroneal Anastomosis

In the area of the lateral ankle, the tendon of the peroneus longus is anastomosed to the tendon of the peroneus brevis. This decreases plantarflexion of the 1st metatarsal and increases eversion forces of the foot.

Peroneus Longus and Tibialis Posterior Tendon Transfer to the Calcaneus

Peroneus longus is cut in the area of the cuboid and attached to the lateral boarder of the Achilles tendon, and the tibialis posterior is cut and attached to the medial boarder of the Achilles tendon.

Treatment, Surgical (Osseous)

Cole

Dorsiflexory wedge osteotomy through the naviculocuneiform joint and cuboid bone

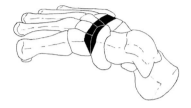

Japas

A V-shaped osteotomy through the entire midfoot. The apex of the "V" is proximal and at the highest point of the cavus, usually in the navicular. The lateral limbs of the "V" extend through the cuboid, and the medial limb of the "V" extends through the cuneiform. No bone is excised; the distal part of the osteotomy is shifted dorsally.

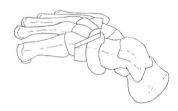

DuVries

Dorsiflexory fusion through the MTJ

Dwyer

Lateral closing wedge or an opening medial wedge

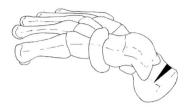

McElvenny–Caldwell Procedure

Dorsiflexory fusion of the 1st metatarsal and medial cuneiform joint. If the deformity is severe, then a naviculocuneiform joint fusion is added.

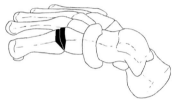

DFWO

Dorsiflexory wedge osteotomy of the 1st metatarsal or all metatarsals

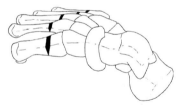

JAHSS

Dorsiflexory wedge osteotomy across the tarsometatarsal joints

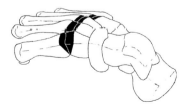

TARSAL COALITIONS

Description

An abnormal bridge between two or more tarsal bones that restrict motion. Incidence is about 1%, and 50% of cases are bilateral. Tarsal coalitions are the most common cause of peroneal spastic flatfoot. The spasm occurs in response to the immobilization of the STJ. A common peroneal block may be required to relax the spastic peroneal muscles and fully evaluate STJ ROM. Coalitions occur more in males than in females. Symptoms, if any, are usually insidious in onset or may follow athletics or minor trauma. Occasionally, anterior and posterior muscles are in spasm, causing a varus deformity. TC and CN coalitions are roughly equal in distribution and account for over 90% of tarsal coalitions. CT scan is the gold standard for diagnosis, but radiographs are very useful.

Conservative treatment for coalitions includes decreasing the motion of the involved joints with shoe modifications or braces, casting, or splints. RICE and NSAIDs.

Cause

Cause is most often congenital due to failure of segmentation of primitive mesenchyme. The condition can be acquired through infection, arthritis, trauma, or iatrogenic.

Coalition Tissue Types

Syndesmosis—fibrous
Synchondrosis—cartilaginous
Synostosis—osseous

Talocalcaneal (TC) Coalitions

Talocalcaneal coalitions account for about 45% of tarsal coalitions, and almost all involve the middle facet. Symptoms usually begin around age 12 to 14 years. Pain is usually located in the sinus tarsi or over the middle facet. There is associated decreased ROM at the STJ and MTJ. Lateral, Harris–Beath, and Isherwood views are the best radiographic views for visualization.

Surgical treatment involves resection of the coalition and interposing soft tissue between bones. Triple arthrodesis may be warranted if previous surgery has failed or joint destruction is severe.

Radiographic signs of a TC coalition on lateral radiograph:

C sign or halo sign: A C-shaped line formed by the medial outline of the talar dome and the inferior outline of the sustentaculum tali. The C sign or halo sign has been shown to be the most sensitive and specific radiographic sign of an STJ coalition.

Absence of the STJ facets: The middle facet may be nonvisualized. There is often joint space narrowing with diminished clarity of the posterior facet even if only the middle facet contains the coalition.

Talar beak sign: Flaring of the superior margin of the talar head

Rounding of the lateral talar process: The lateral process of the talus becomes blunted or flattened.

Shortening of talar neck: Dysmorphic sustentaculum tali. The sustentaculum tali may be ovoid shaped as opposed to its normal brick shape.

Ball-in-socket: Configuration of talus in the ankle mortise takes on a more rounded shape vs. its normal squared off shape. This finding is best viewed on ankle A/P images.

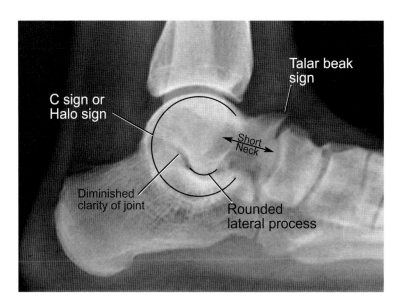

Talar beak sign

C sign or Halo sign

Short Neck

Diminished clarity of joint

Rounded lateral process

Calcaneonavicular (CN) Coalitions

Calcaneonavicular coalitions account for about 45% of tarsal coalitions. CN coalitions are considered extra-articular and, when pain is present, usually begin around 8 to 10 years of age.

Pain is often localized to the area over the coalition. There may be a moderate decrease in ROM at the STJ and MTJ. Medial oblique radiographs may show where the calcaneus and navicular are in close proximity or connected (calcaneonavicular bar). With incomplete fusion, the bone ends are irregular and lack cortical definition. The lateral head of the talus may be hypoplastic. Lateral views show the classic elongated anterior process of the calcaneus, anteater sign.

Surgical treatment involves resection of coalition and placing the EDB muscle belly in void (Cowell procedure).

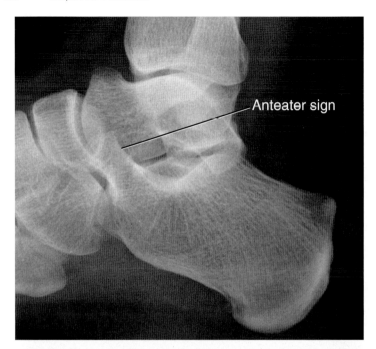

Anteater sign

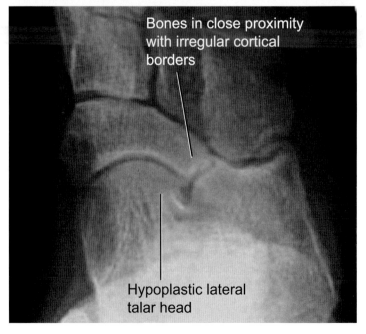

Bones in close proximity with irregular cortical borders

Hypoplastic lateral talar head

Talonavicular (TN) Coalitions

Talonavicular coalitions account for about 2% of tarsal coalitions. They are mostly asymptomatic; when painful, pain begins around 3 to 5 years of age. Chief complaint is usually bump pain from shoe gear rubbing on the medial prominence. Lateral radiographs show the absence of the dorsal portion of the Cyma line. Surgical correction involves resecting the medial prominence.

Calcaneocuboid (CC) Coalitions

Calcaneocuboid coalitions account for about 2% of tarsal coalitions. Radiographically, there is an absence of the CC joint. They are asymptomatic.

POLYDACTYLY

Supernumerary digits
More common in blacks and
    females

Associated with:
    Down syndrome
    Laurence–Moon–Biedl
        syndrome
    Chondroectodermal dysplasia
        trisomies 13 and 18
    Thirty percent have a positive
        family history.

Classification

Preaxial: Involves the hallux (15%)
Central: Involving digits 2, 3, or 4
    (6%)
Postaxial: Involving the 5th digit
    (79%), six subtypes
Postaxial polydactyly can also be
    divided into:
    Type A: Well-formed articulated
        digit
    Type B: Rudimentary often
        without skeletal component

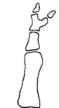

Normal metatarsal
with distal phalangeal
duplication

Normal metatarsal
shaft with wide
head (most common)

Short block
metatarsal

T-shaped
metatarsal

Y-shaped
metatarsal

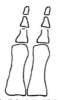

Partial or complete
ray duplication

Treatment

Supernumerary digits are removed for cosmetic reasons and for comfort in shoes.

With all other factors equal, remove the most peripheral digit.

Surgery should be avoided until at least 1 year of age when the full pattern of skeletal involvement becomes clear and when the child can better tolerate anesthesia.

SYNDACTYLY

Webbing between toes

M > F

Traumatic syndactyly may occur, most notably as a result of burns.

Acrosyndactyly—partial joining of digits with proximal opening, usually due to IU environmental factors

Classification

Type I (Most Common)

Zygodactyly

Partial or complete webbing of the 2nd and 3rd toes

Type II

Synpolydactyly

One soft-tissue mass covering the 4th, 5th, and 6th toes

Type III

Associated with metatarsal fusion

Davis and German Classification System

Incomplete—webbing does not extend to distal toes.

Complete—webbing extends to distal toes.

Simple—phalanges not involved

Complicated—phalanges involved

Treatment

If cosmesis is not a concern, no treatment

Desyndactyly procedure (see Chapter 8)

MACRODACTYLY

Local gigantism of one or more toes

Usually unilateral

M > F

Heredity does not play a role in the deformity.

Usually involves toes 1st, 2nd or 3rd

May be associated with neurofibromatosis

Blood vessels and tendons are not affected.

Poor circulation because blood vessels have not enlarged with the digit

Can often affect the metatarsal head as well as the phalanges

Involvement of two or three adjacent digits is more common than single digit involvement.

Classification

Static deformity—growth rate is proportional to other digits (most common).

Progressive deformity—disproportionately fast growth rate until puberty

Treatment

Condition is not painful, and treatment is performed for cosmetic and shoe fitting purposes.

Epiphysiodesis—the soft cartilage of the physis is surgically resected with a scalpel or by multiple drilling; this will stop the bone from lengthening, but the bone will still increase in girth.

Amputation or partial amputation

Plastic reduction/debulking procedures (see Chapter 8)

BRACHYMETATARSIA

Shortened metatarsal

Although the deformity is isolated to the metatarsals, the patient usually perceives the problem to be in the toe itself because the toe is what appears short clinically.

Affected toes are dorsally displaced, often causing problems with shoe gear.

Most commonly affects the 1st or 4th metatarsal

Most commonly B/L and symmetrical

Females to males (25:1)

Becomes evident between ages 4 and 15 years

Plantar callus may develop on adjacent metatarsal heads.

Clinical signs include a floating toe/short toe and a plantar fissure of sulcus where the metatarsal head should be.

Toe is functionless due to a lack of mechanical advantage.

Associated conditions:
Down syndrome
Pseudohypoparathyroidism
Pseudo-pseudohypoparathyroidism
Poliomyelitis
Trauma
Idiopathic
Albright
Turner syndrome

Classification

Type I   Shortening of the 1st metatarsal only

Type II   Shortening of 1st or 2nd of the lesser metatarsals (usually 4th and/or 3rd)

Type III Shortening of the 1st and one or more (but not all) of the lesser metatarsals

Type IV   Shortening of all the metatarsals

Treatment

Palliative treatment includes orthotics and accommodative devices. Surgical treatment consists of reestablishing a normal metatarsal parabola. This can be accomplished by lengthening the short metatarsal via bone graft or callus distraction or shortening long adjacent metatarsals. Surgery correction should be delayed until after skeletal maturity.

Surgical procedure (using a bone graft)
V-Y skin plasty
Z-plasty EDL lengthening; FDL lengthening is not necessary.
Sectioning of the short extensor and interossei
Insert bone graft, up to 1.5 cm, and fixate with K-wire.

Monitor digital circulation for the first 24 hours.

Non–weight-bearing cast for 2.5 to 3 months after surgery

CALCANEOVALGUS

Calcaneovalgus foot is a deformity in infants, which causes the foot to appear pushed up against the front of the leg. It is a flexible deformity caused by an abnormal positioning in the uterus. Characterized by excessive dorsiflexion of the ankle and eversion of the foot. Dorsal surface of the foot may be in contact with the anterior surface of the leg. Must rule out vertical talus. Prognosis is excellent, and the condition usually resolves spontaneously with growth but may require serial casting.

CEREBRAL PALSY

Description

A broad term used to describe several static nonprogressive neuromuscular disorders resulting from brain damage before, during, or immediately after birth

Types of CP include the following:

Spastic CP (most common, 70%)
Athetoid CP (20%)
Ataxic CP (10%)
Rigidity CP
Tremor CP
Atonic CP

Signs and Symptoms

"Scissors gait" due to adductor spasticity
Speech defects, retardation, seizures, visual defects
Ankle equinus

Treatment

PT, OT, splinting, bracing

MUSCULAR DYSTROPHIES

Description

Muscular dystrophy is a group of inherited chronic progressive disorders characterized by progressive weakness and degeneration of the skeletal muscles. Some MDs are seen in infancy or childhood, whereas others may appear in middle age or later.

Symptoms

MD is characterized by progressive weakness, atrophy, loss of DTRs, secondary contractures, and deformity. Proximal muscle weakness involvement is more pronounced than distal. Pseudohypertrophy is an apparent hypertrophy of certain muscles, specifically the calves. The apparent muscle bulk is actually fat deposits. Although these muscles may look overdeveloped, they are actually weaker than normal.

Diagnosis

Diagnosis involves clinical evaluation, EMG, muscle biopsy, and an elevated CPK.

Treatment

There is no cure; treatment is aimed at maintaining ambulation for as long as possible (PT, braces, weight control, surgery to control contractures). Keeping patients active is important; inactivity often leads to worsening of the underlying muscle disease.

Types of Muscular Dystrophies

Age of Onset (Years)	Where Weakness Begins	Pseudohyper-trophy	Contracture	Cardiac Involvement	Progression	Specific Symptoms
Duchenne (sex linked, recessive)						
2–5	Pelvic girdle	80%	Yes	Yes	Rapid: • Wheelchair bound by age 10–12 y • Die around age 20 y, usually from secondary conditions such as resp sepsis or cardiac arrest	• Toe walking • Difficulty climbing stairs • Lordosis • Waddling gait • Gower sign • Decreased IQ • Pulmonary disorders
Becker (sex linked, recessive)						
5–25	Pelvic girdle	90%	Yes (mild)	Yes (mild)	Slow: • Wheelchair bound by age 20–50 y • Die around age 40 y	• A milder form of Duchenne, but no decrease in IQ • Pes cavus (60%) (some have normal life spans)
Emery–Dreifuss (sex linked)						
5–15	Diffuse (maximally in upper arms and peroneals)	None	Yes	Yes (severe)	Slow: • Patients often die of cardiac arrhythmias	• Toe walking • Contracted elbows • Severe cardiac arrhythmias
Facioscapulohumeral (autosomal dominant)						
7–20	Shoulder girdle, face	Uncommon	Rare	Rare	Slow: • Minor disability • Normal life spans	• Foot drop (distal legs weakness) • "Popeye arms" (distal arms spared)
Limb-Girdle (autosomal recessive)						
10–30	Shoulder girdle or pelvic girdle	30%	Yes (late in dz)	Very rare	Variable rate of progression	

Metadductus Angle

Before ossification of the navicular, metatarsus adductus is indistinguishable from forefoot adductus.

Bisection of the 2nd met relative to a line traversing the 1st and 5th metatarsal bases exceeds 25° at birth, 20° at 18 months, and 10° at adulthood.

At 1 year when they begin walking, it is around 20°. By age 4, it is the adult value of 15°.

Using the Engel angle, bisect the 2nd metatarsal and the intermediate cuneiform. Normal is 24°.

Lateral talocalcaneal angle: normal 25° to 45°

When the calcaneus is valgus, it abducts and dorsiflexes. The talus then loses its support and moves medially and plantarward. This caused the lateral Kite angle to increase on lateral view.

When the calcaneus is varus, the calcaneus adducts and plantarflexes. There is more overlap between the talus and the calcaneus, with the calcaneus positioned more medially. This decreases Kite ankle on lateral view. This is seen in cavus foot.

Hindfoot varus: the talocalcaneal angle is decrease and A/P. The long axis of the talus is lateral to the 1st metatarsal and overlaps more with the calcaneus.

The lateral talocalcaneal angle is decreased to <25° in children with hindfoot varus.

Collum tali axis (CTA) should parallel the 1st metatarsal axis. Normal is 0° ± 4°. If it is less, they have pes planus.

Pes planus: talus down in relation to the 1st metatarsal and CIA is decreased to <18°.

Pes cavus: talus is dorsiflexed in relation to the 1st metatarsal and CIA is >30°.

Pes planus: increased Kite angle on AP > 30°, increased Kite on lateral >45°, talus points plantar > 4° in relation to the 1st metatarsal, decreased CIA < 18°. Talonavicular coverage angle is abnormal. Talus points medial to the 1st metatarsal on AP. The navicular is subluxed on the talus > 7°. MPJ and interphalangeal joints are aligned. Cyma line should be a smooth on both lateral and AP. If the Cyma line is broken, it suggests "shortening" of the calcaneus relative to the talus.

Abnormal loading of the medial column leads to collapse of the longitudinal arch and eventually impingement on the lateral column.

Causes of flatfoot: PTTD, Charcot, posttraumatic, RA, neuromuscular disorders, tarsal coalition

Talonavicular coverage angle: Draw lines connecting the articular surfaces of the navicular and talus. Normal is ≤7°.

Calcaneal pitch or inclination angle: Normal is 18° to 20° (range 17° to 32°).

Kite Angle

Usually normal or slightly increased Calcaneocuboid angle

An adducted cuboid could indicate a transverse plane compensation at the midfoot, possible skewfoot deformity.

Pediatric flat foot: Flexible—will have normal arch when NWB and flat when WB.

Skewfoot: An uncommon disorder characterized by severe pronation of the rearfoot and an adductovarus forefoot. Skew foot has characteristics of flatfoot and adductovarus deformity.

Rule out ankle valgus, tibia varum, genu varum, genu valgum, tibial torsion, femoral anteversion, and limb-length discrepancy

Voluntary withdrawal from physical activities

History: clumsiness, frequent falling, difficulty climbing, difficulty arising from the floor (Duchenne muscular dystrophy)

Look for equinus.

Look at heel on toe rise.

Too many toes sign

Differential diagnosis:

Flexible: flexible flatfoot, skewfoot

Rigid: congenital vertical talus, tarsal coalition, peroneal spastic flatfoot without coalition

Flexible flatfeet that are nonpainful are most common.

Radiographically concentrate relationship of the talus and calcaneus

With flatfoot deformity, the talocalcaneal angle increases in size on both AP and lateral. The talus plantarflexes in flatfeet. Talus (midtalar line) should pass through the 1st metatarsal.

Calcaneal inclination angle decreases in flatfoot.

Symptoms may include pain on the medial side of the foot; pain in the sinus tarsi, leg, and knee; and decreased endurance.

Tx: activity modifications and orthotics, stretching exercises for equinus, NSAIDs

R/O other issues: obesity, ligamentous laxity, hypotonia, proximal limb problems

Sx correction can be grouped into three categories: reconstructive procedures, arthrodesis, and arthroereisis.

Recon: Soft-tissue reconstruction of flexible flatfoot is rarely successful. Bony procedures may include lateral column lengthening and/or medial displacement osteotomy of the calcaneus; heel cord lengthening and medial plication are often included.

Arthroereisis: Subtalar joint implants.

Arthrodesis: STJ arthrodesis is typically performed as the primary procedure. Triple may be used later as a salvage procedure.

Clinically

The infant will have a high arch, and the big toe has a wide separation from the 2nd toe and deviates inward.

Metatarsus adductus often resolves spontaneously without treatment. There are also stretching and passive manipulation exercises that can be performed by the parents during diaper change. Casting is also an option. Special shoes.

Serial casting

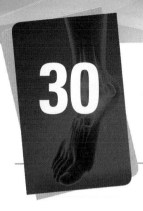

30 ANKLE EQUINUS

EQUINUS

Definitions

1. A limitation of passive ankle joint dorsiflexion to <90°
2. At least 10° of dorsiflexion past 90° is required for normal gait.

Anatomy

Gastrocnemius muscle originates on the femur and crosses three joints (knee, ankle, STJ).

Soleus muscle originates on the tibia/fibula and crosses two joints (ankle, STJ).

Plantaris muscle originates on the femur and crosses three joints (knee, ankle, STJ). Plantaris runs between the gastrocnemius and soleus muscles and inserts on the medial aspect of the posterior calcaneus. This muscle is absent 7% of time.

The triceps surae muscle is referred to the two heads of the gastrocnemius muscle and the soleus muscle.

Silfverskiold Test

■ Tests for gastrocnemius equinus

Passive dorsiflexion is measured with the knee extended and again with the knee flexed. If the amount of dorsiflexion increases with knee flexion, there is an equinus due to a tight gastrocnemius, because the gastrocnemius crosses the knee joint and the soleus does not.

Types/Causes of Ankle Equinus

Muscular

Spastic equinus
    CP (hyperreflexia, Babinski, clonus)

Duchenne (post muscle contractions, weak/atrophic
muscles, absent reflexes)
Congenital equinus
Birth history, childhood diseases
Note: Toe walking for the first 3
to 6 months of ambulation is
a normal variant.
Acquired
Improper casting with the foot
plantarflexed
Repetitive use of high-heel
shoes
Iatrogenic
Pseudoequinus
Pseudoequinus is not a true ankle
equinus. The deformity is in the
foot, not in the ankle. It is caused
by a cavus foot that causes the
midfoot and/or forefoot to be
plantarflexed more than normal.
On weight bearing, the ankle
must compensate for this deformity by dorsiflexing. If the forefoot deformity is severe enough,
the patient will present with a
functional equinus.

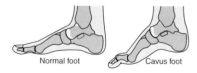

Normal foot   Cavus foot

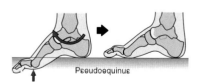

Pseudoequinus

Osseous

Talotibial exostosis
Clinically, there is a hard and
abrupt end ROM upon
dorsiflexion.
Stress lateral x-ray may aid
diagnosis.
Pseudoequinus
Apparent equinus due to cavus
foot type

Symptoms

Toe walking/early heel off/short
stride length
Plantar fasciitis/arch pain
Calf cramping/fatigue
Retrocalcaneal tendinitis
(possible calcifications in
Achilles tendon)
Calcaneal apophysitis (young
patients)
Secondary signs
Lumbar lordosis
Hip flexion
Genu recurvatum
Digital contractures
Knee flexion
Abducted angle of gait

GAIT AND PHYSICAL EXAMINATION

Biomechanics: Look for STJ ROM,
ankle joint ROM, rigid vs. flexible
deformity.

Equinus		
Uncompensated	**Partially Compensated**	**Fully Compensated**
Hypertrophic calves	Early heel off	Forefoot supinatus
STJ supinated	STJ pronation	STJ pronation
Walking plantarflexed	Mild HAV	Heel valgus, HAV deformity
Smaller steppage gait		*most pathologic*
RF inverted		

Treatment

Conservative
   Stretching, braces, heel lifts
Surgical

GASTROCNEMIUS RECESSION

These procedures do not lengthen the soleus muscle and are used strictly for a gastrocnemius equinus. Indicated for patients with a positive Silfverskiold test.

Vulpius and Stoffel

Inverted V-shaped cut through the gastrocnemius aponeurosis

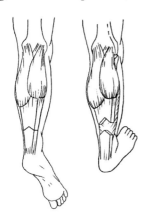

Strayer

Transverse cut through the gastrocnemius aponeurosis

Suture proximal flap to soleus

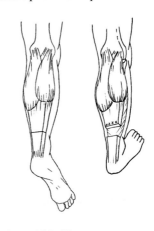

Fulp and McGlamry

Tongue in groove (tongue portion proximal)

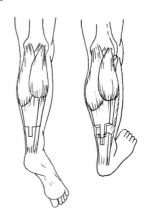

Baker

Tongue in groove (tongue portion
   distal)

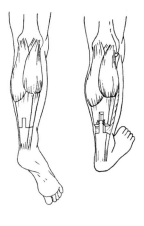

Silfverskiold

Release origin of gastrocnemius
   from femoral condyles
Reinsertion to proximal tibia

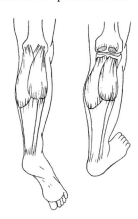

MURPHY PROCEDURE

Indicated in a spastic equinus.
By advancing the insertion of the
Achilles anteriorly on the calcaneus, the muscles lose some mechanical advantage and decrease
the equinus.

Transfer Achilles insertion to
dorsum of calcaneus just posterior
to posterior facet of STJ. This weakens the triceps surae at the ankle
joint by 50% but weakens toe-off
ability by only 15%. A modification
of this procedure is to reroute the
Achilles tendon deep (anterior) to
toe FHL tendon.

Several fixation techniques have
been described.

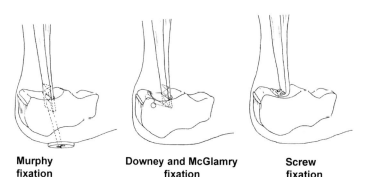

Murphy
fixation

Downey and McGlamry
fixation

Screw
fixation

TENDO ACHILLES LENGTHENING

Performed on the conjoined tendon of the gastrocnemius and soleus muscle. Indicated for patients with a negative Silfverskiold test.

Z-Plasty (Sagittal Plane)

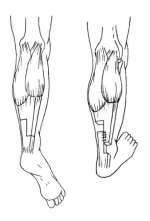

Z-Plasty (Frontal Plane)

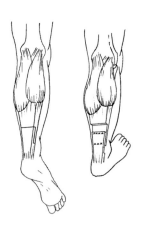

Hauser

Section posterior 2/3 proximally and medial 2/3 distally

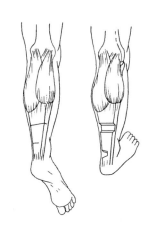

White

Section anterior 2/3 distally and medial 2/3 proximally

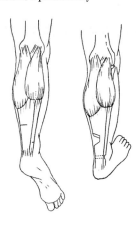

Hoke

Triple hemisection with first and last cut medially and second cut laterally

These incisions are made through skin stab incisions.

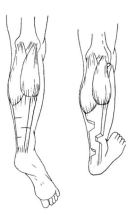

Conrad and Frost

Sectioning the medial 3/4 at the distal end and lateral 3/4 proximally

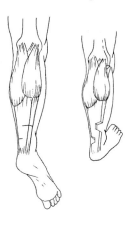

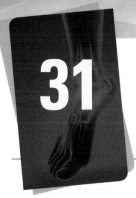

31 TRIPLE ARTHRODESIS, ARTHROEREISIS, AND ANKLE ARTHROSCOPY

TRIPLE ARTHRODESIS

Fusion of three joints in the foot:

Talonavicular joint
Talocalcaneal joint
Calcaneocuboid joint

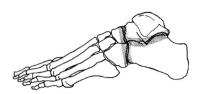

Fixation varies but is often with 6.5- or 7.0-mm cannulated screws for the STJ and two staples at 90° for the CC and TN joints. Hindfoot should be positioned in slight valgus position, about 5°. The body can compensate for valgus. Varus foot should be avoided at all cost; these patients end up with pain and callus formation under the lateral midfoot and forefoot. The TN fusion requires the longest time for revascularization. As a result of a triple arthrodesis, there is extra stress on the ankle joint. For this reason, the ankle joint should be free of DJD pre-op. Sliding the calcaneus posteriorly on the talus will raise the arch, and sliding the calcaneus anteriorly on the talus will lower the arch.

Indications

Pes cavus
Residual clubfoot
Neuromuscular dz
Calcaneal fx
Tarsal arthritis
Tarsal coalition
Collapsing pes valgo planus
Ruptured posterior tibial tendon

Incisions

Lateral incision (Ollier incision): Extends from the tip of the lateral malleolus to the base of the 4th metatarsal, providing access to STJ and CC joint

Medial incision: Extends from medial gutter of the ankle joint to the 1st metatarsal base, providing access to TN joint and TC fixation.

Order of Joint Resection and Fixation

1. Resect MTJ (CC then TN); this allows access to the STJ.
2. Resect STJ.
3. Temporarily fixate STJ.
4. Temporarily fixate MTJ (TN then CC).
5. Fixate STJ.
6. Fixate MTJ.

Post-op

Apply Jones compression dressing immediately post-op for 2 to 3 days; casting is generally avoided because of swell.

Change dressing at 48 hours.

At 2 to 3 days, pull drain and apply a BK NWB cast.

At 3 weeks, apply D/C cast and remove sutures.

Apply removable BK NWB cast for an additional 4 weeks.

Progressive WB and PT for an additional 3 months

Return to work 6 months.

Complications

Pseudoarthrosis, nonunion, malunion, inadequate correction, continued instability, gait disturbances, adjacent joint degeneration

SUBTALAR ARTHROEREISIS IMPLANTS

Subtalar joint arthroereisis implants are designed to limit subtalar joint pronation by blocking the anterior–inferior displacement of the talus. Although they are commonly referred to as subtalar joint implants, they are not inserted into the joint. They are inserted into the sinus tarsi between the posterior and middle facets of the STJ. The goal of STJ arthroereisis implants is to limit pronation and reduce heel valgus by blocking contact of the lateral talar process against the calcaneal sinus tarsi floor. They are sometimes described as an "implantable orthotic." All subtalar implants are considered both "direct impact" and "axis-altering" implants. They are considered direct impact implants because the implants physically block the motion of the talus. This decreased motion alters the spatial orientation of the STJ axis during gait, making them "axis altering" too.

Classifications

Intraosseous

Intraosseous implants have a stem that is fit into a hole drilled into the floor of the sinus tarsi and requires some bone resection. These intraosseous implants are falling out of favor and slowly being discontinued.

Extraosseous

Extraosseous implants are simply screwed into the sinus tarsi with no

bone resection required. Extraosseous subtalar arthroereisis implants
are further divided into type I and
type II.

Type I

Type I implants are inserted into the
sinus portion of the sinus tarsi.

Type II

Type II implants have a narrower
distal (medial) portion to the
implant, allowing them to fit
into both the sinus and the
deeper canalis portion of the
sinus tarsi.

Indications

Flexible pes planus
PTTD

Complications

Device migration (backing out)
Lateral foot and ankle soft-tissue
strain
Synovitis/arthrosis/cyst formation
Overcorrection/undercorrection
Sinus tarsi pain
Talar neck fracture

Contraindications

Angular deformity of knee
Torsional leg deformities
Metatarsus adductus
Valgus ankle

INTRAOSSEOUS TYPE

Lundeen Subtalar Implant (LSI)

Polyethylene
Intraosseous
Sgarlato labs

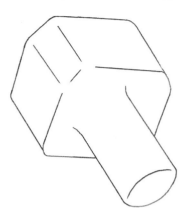

STA-Peg Subtalar Implant

Polyethylene
Wright Medical

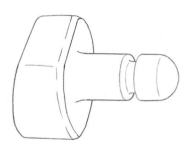

**Future Angled Subtalar Implant
(ASI)**

Angled intraosseous subtalar implant
Polyethylene
Wright Medical

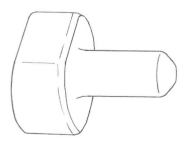

EXTRAOSSEOUS TYPE I
BioArch

Cannulated

Conical tapered design

Blunt thread design for limited bone impingement and irritation

Horizontal slots designed to allow fibrous in-growth to hold the device in place

Smooth proximal surface designed to minimize arthrosis and sinus tarsitis

Wright Medical

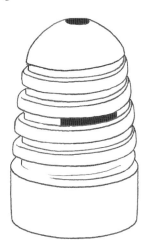

Horizon Subtalar Implant

Titanium

Cannulated

Smooth proximal surface slightly tapered from medial to lateral. Designed to minimize arthrosis and sinus tarsitis.

A hybrid design is also available, which comes with a polyethylene sleeve over the lateral portion, offering a softer more forgiving interface.

BioPro

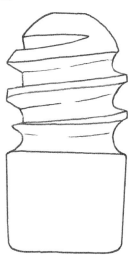

BMA

Titanium

Cannulated

Soft threaded device

Slotted design allows for some shock absorption while also allowing fibrous in-growth to hold the device in place.

Bioabsorbable version called the Bio-Block also available, made of PLLA

Integra LifeSciences

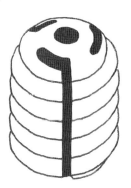

Conical Subtalar Implant (CSI)

Titanium
Cannulated
Progressively softened threads
Apertures allow soft-tissue
    in-growth.
Wright Medical

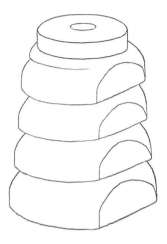

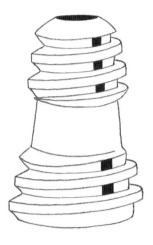

TruArch Subtalar Implant System

Titanium
Cannulated

GaitWay Sinus Tarsi Implant

Titanium
Cannulated
Flat sides are designed to improve
    load-bearing distribution that
    may decrease incident of reactive
    synovitis.
Undercut threads designed to resist
    extrusion forces
This product has been
    discontinued.
Wright Medical

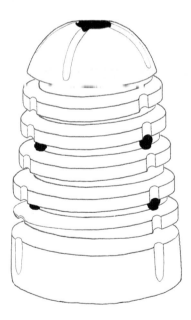

Conical Subtalar Spacer System (CSTS)

Titanium
Cannulated
Center nonthreaded portion is grit blasted to improve soft-tissue encapsulation.
OrthoPro

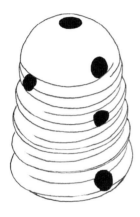

Talar-Fit

Titanium, cone shaped
Cannulated
Blunt threads for reduced bone irritation
OsteoMed

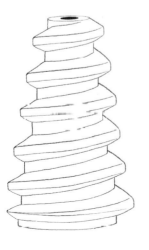

SubFix

Titanium, cone shaped
Cannulated
Fine medial threads allow immediate soft-tissue fixation.
Lateral portion is smooth to limit trauma to the periosteum of the lateral process of the talus and calcaneus.
Stryker

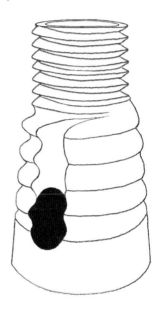

Twist

Titanium
Blunt, inverted threads. Inverted meaning the threads become thicker as they extend out from the body of the implant.
Trestle structure—there are holes from top to bottom through the threads, where they meet the body of the implant. Designed for soft-tissue in-growth.

Trilliant surgical

Wright medical

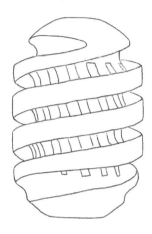

Talus of Vilex (TOV)

Titanium, cone shaped
Cannulated
Fully threaded
Vilex

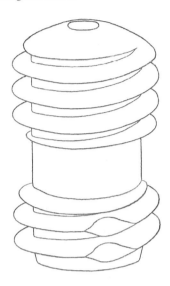

ProStop

Titanium, cone shaped
Cannulated
Soft threads
Concave head allows easy pin and
    screwdriver placement.
Bioabsorbable version called the
    ProStop Plus also available,
    made of PLLA
Arthrex

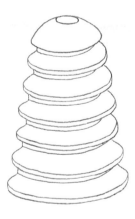

Subtalar Spacer System (STS)

Titanium
Cannulated
Nonthreaded middle por-
    tion to allow soft-tissue
    encapsulation

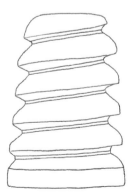

EXTRAOSSEOUS TYPE II
HyProCure

Titanium
Cannulated
GraMedica

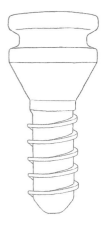

Talex

Titanium
Cannulated
Vilex

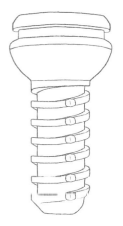

Disco Subtalar Implant System

Titanium
Cannulated

Trestle design intended for tissue
    integration
Deep distal anchor thread for
    canalis
Trilliant Surgical

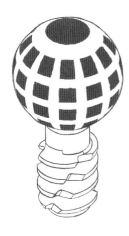

PitStop

Peek
Cannulated
The implant has two tantalum
    markers inside to help guide po-
    sitioning radiographically.
This implant is pushed in vs. being
    screwed in as with most other
    STJ implants.
In2Bone

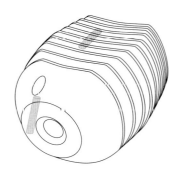

ANKLE ARTHROSCOPY

Terminology

Cannula

Rigid hollow tube used to establish and maintain portal for both the scope and instruments

Trocar

Sharp pyramidal tipped solid rod placed in the cannula and used to pierce the soft tissue and capsule. After the portal has been established, the trochar is removed, leaving the cannula in place.

Obturator

Same as a trochar but with a blunt tip. Less destructive when bone contact is made. Used to penetrate the joint when placing the cannula in an already established portal.

Scope

With ankle arthroscopy, usually, a 4.0-mm scope is used with a 30° viewing radius.

Instruments

Sweeping

Side-to-side and up-and-down movement of the scope to view anatomic areas

Pistoning

Moving the scope in for magnification and moving the scope out for better orientation

Triangulation

Triangulation refers to bringing the scope and another instrument together, through two different portals at a specific site in the joint.

Irrigation

Normal saline or Ringer solution may be used, but Ringer is preferred because it is less damaging to chondrocyte metabolism. Ingress refers to where the irrigation fluid enters the joint, and egress refers to where the irrigation leaves the joint.

Common Portals

Anteromedial Portal

The anteromedial portal is made medial to the anterior tibialis tendon and lateral to saphenous vein and saphenous nerve. This is classically the first portal created.

Anterolateral Portal

The anterolateral portal is made just lateral to the peroneus tertius tendon. Care should be taken to avoid the superficial peroneal nerve branches (medial and intermediate dorsal cutaneous nerves). Transillumination can assist with the placement of this portal. Transillumination is a technique where the arthroscope is inserted through the medial portal and directed laterally to transilluminate the soft tissues. This technique is useful for proper portal placement and avoiding critical structures.

Posterior–Lateral Portal

The posterior–lateral portal is created 1.0 to 1.5 cm lateral to the Achilles tendon at the level of the distal tip of the lateral malleolus. The sural nerve, lesser saphenous vein, and peroneal tendons should all be lateral to the portal.

Less Common Portals

Anterior–Central Portal

This portal is made just lateral to the EHL tendon and medial to the EDL tendon. Avoid the anterior tibial artery, the deep peroneal nerve.

Posterior–Medial Portal

Medial to the Achilles, lateral to the tarsal canal. This is a high-risk portal due to the proximity to the neurovascular structures.

Posterior–Central Portal

Also called the trans-Achilles, portal is created directly through the posterior aspect of the Achilles tendon at the level of the ankle. While this portal involves splitting the Achilles tendon, it is farther from any local nerves as compared with the other portals.

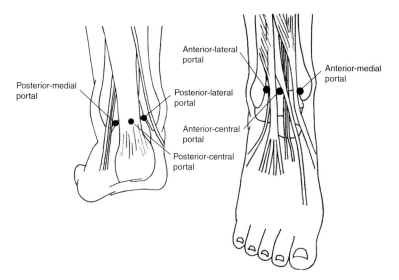

Gutters

Medial Gutter

The medial gutter is the space between the medial articular surface of the talus and the tibia.

Lateral Gutter

The lateral gutter is the space between the lateral articular surface of the talus and the fibula.

Anterior Gutter

The most anterior portion of the ankle joint

Posterior Gutter

The most posterior portion of the ankle joint

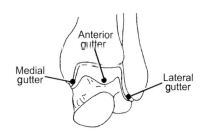

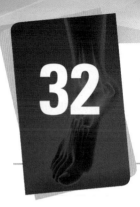

32 TRAUMA

OPEN FRACTURE

An open fracture, also called a compound fracture, is a fracture resulting in the bone penetrating through the skin. These injuries are considered contaminated, but if they are left without treatment for 6 to 8 hours, they are considered infected. Open fractures are considered a medical or surgical emergency, and patients should be admitted for antibiotics, closed reduction/open reduction internal fixation (ORIF), and/or debridement.

Ottawa Rules

The Ottawa rules were developed as a way to decrease unnecessary diagnostic imaging.

1. Rules state ankle x-rays are only required if there is any pain in the malleolar zone and any of the following findings:
    a. Bone tenderness at the distal 6 cm of the posterior edge of the tibia or tip of the medial malleolus (A)
    b. OR, bone tenderness at the distal 6 cm of the posterior edge of the fibula or tip of the lateral malleolus (B)
    c. OR, inability to bear weight immediately after injury and in ED
2. Rules state that foot x-rays are only required if there is any pain in the midfoot zone and any of the following findings:
    a. Bone tenderness at the base of the 5th metatarsal (C)
    b. OR, bone tenderness at the navicular bone (D)
    c. OR, inability to bear weight immediately after injury and in ED

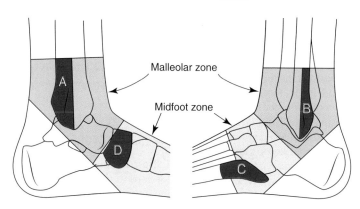

Malleolar zone

Midfoot zone

Gustilo and Anderson (Classification System for Open Fractures)

Type I

Open fx, clean, <u>wound < 1 cm</u>, simple transverse or oblique fracture

Type II

Open fx, <u>wound ≥ 1 cm but < 10 cm</u>, simple transverse or oblique fracture

All type III fractures have a wound > 10 cm and subclass by

the amount of soft-tissue damage. They are usually caused by high-energy trauma such as a gunshot or farming accident with extensive soft-tissue damage with comminution.

Type IIIA

Open fx, >10 cm, adequate soft-tissue coverage

Type IIIB

Open fx, >10 cm, periosteal stripping, inadequate soft-tissue coverage, requires free or rotational flaps

Type IIIC

Open fx, >10 cm, arterial injury requiring repair

Treatment

Begin ABX ASAP.
Tetanus prophylaxis
Debridement/irrigation/
   culture/C&S
When possible, skin defects overlying the open fractures should be closed at the time if initial debridement. If a skin grafting or soft-tissue transfers are required (Gustilo type IIIB), it is recommended that coverage be completed within severe days of injury.
Stabilize fracture.
Appropriate wound coverage

Antibiotic Therapy

Begin ASAP, within 3 hours of injury.

Type I:	cephalosporin
Type II:	cephalosporin or cephalosporin + aminoglycoside (if contaminated)
Type III:	cephalosporin + aminoglycoside

Skin flora (Gram-positive organisms) are the most likely infectious agent in open fractures, so a first-generation cephalosporin is a good choice. Cefazolin 1 to 2 g IV followed by 1 g IVPB q8h until cultures are available.

If penicillin allergic, use clindamycin 900 mg IV q8h.

For type III (*and contaminated type II*), add an aminoglycoside to cover Gram negatives. Tobramycin 5.1 mg/kg IV q24h.

If there is any chance of fecal or Clostridial contamination, such as farming accidents, penicillin should be added to cover anaerobes. Penicillin G 2 to 4 million units IV q4h.

Duration of prophylaxis (controversial): 24 hours. In cases of severe contamination, antibiotics may be continued for as long as 72 hours.

Open fracture >8 hours old should automatically be considered a type III and presumed infected.

For type III fractures, stop ABX 72 hours after injury or within 24 hours of soft-tissue coverage.

Study shows changing to vanc + cefepime to cover MRSA and *Enterococcus*

STRESS FRACTURE

A stress fracture is a fracture that develops due to cyclical loading on a bone. These forces are seen in people with overuse and repetitive activities, such as runners and athletes. Ninety-five percent of stress fractures occur in the lower extremity, most notably the neck of the 2nd metatarsal. They may take 14 to 21 days to present radiographically after a bony callus has developed. If x-rays are inconclusive, a three-phase technetium bone scan may be positive as early as 2 to 8 days after the onset of symptoms. MRI may show early signs within 1 to 2 weeks, and exposes patient to less radiation.

GREENSTICK FRACTURE

A greenstick fracture is an incomplete fracture in which the cortex on only one side of the bone is cracked. They are more commonly seen in children due to their soft bones.

FRACTURE CLASSIFICATIONS

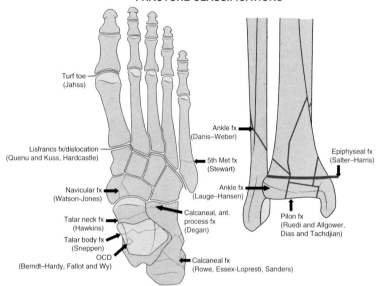

TURF TOE

Turf toe is a sprain or tear of the plantar structures of the 1st MPJ caused by forced hyperextension of the big toe. Turf toe results in plantar capsular and ligamentous injury. Turf toe is a type of plantar plate tear of the 1st metatarsophalangeal joint.

Grade I: The ligaments and joint capsule are stretched, localized pain and swelling.

Grade II: The ligaments and capsule are partially torn. Pain with weight bearing, mild-to-moderate edema, and bruising.

Grade III: The ligaments and joint capsule are completely torn. Severe tenderness, swelling, and bruising. Pain on ROM. Sesamoids may be retracted on radiograph or fractured, positive Lachman test. May require surgical repair.

Note: Another injury called **sand toe** is a sprain of the 1st MPJ caused by hyperflexion of the hallux. Tends to occur when barefooted in sand.

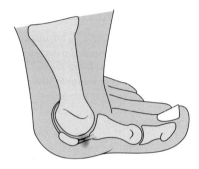

GREAT TOE DISLOCATION

Great toe dislocation occurs with axial loading on a dorsiflexed hallux. This drives the metatarsal head through the plantar capsule. A dislocation differs from a Turf toe in that there is an actual dislocation of bone.

JAHSS Classification of Great Toe Dislocation

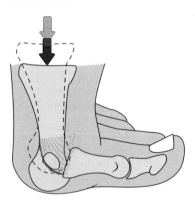

Type I

Dorsal dislocation of the proximal phalanx, in which the metatarsal head punctures through the plantar capsule

The intersesamoidal ligament remains intact, and there are no fractures.

The deformity is tight and unable to be closed reduced due to the intact intersesamoidal ligament, requires ORIF.

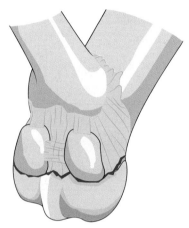

Type IIA

Dorsal dislocation of the proximal phalanx, in which the metatarsal head punctures through the plantar capsule

The intersesamoidal ligament is ruptured, and the sesamoids no longer remain opposed to one another. The deformity is loose and easier to close reduce.

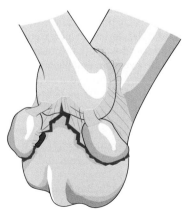

Type IIB

Dorsal dislocation of the proximal phalanx, in which the metatarsal head punctures through the plantar capsule

The intersesamoidal ligament remains intact, and there is a transverse avulsion fracture of one of the sesamoids. The deformity is close reducible.

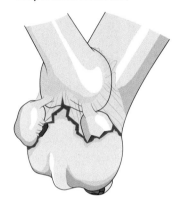

Treatment

ORIF type I and close reduction types IIA and IIB

RICE

Strapping/splinting

Protective padding (i.e., dancer's pad)

Shoes with a firm sole or add a carbon fiber plate to prevent dorsiflexion of MPJs

MPJ SEQUENTIAL RELEASE FOR A HAMMERTOE

1. Release of extensor expansion
2. Tenotomy/lengthening of extensor digitorum longus/extensor digitorum brevis
3. Transverse MPJ capsulotomy
4. Release of collateral ligaments
5. Plantar plate release—metatarsal (McGlamry) scoop

SEQUENTIAL RELEASE FOR AN OVERLAPPING 5TH TOE

1. Z-plasty or V-Y skin plasty
2. Z-tendon lengthening (for severe cases, transfer tendon to metatarsal head)
3. Release of extensor hood
4. Capsulotomy (dorsally and medially)
5. Plantar plate release (McGlamry elevator)
6. Plantar skin wedge excision

SESAMOID FRACTURE

A fractured sesamoid must be distinguished from a bipartite sesamoid, which has an incidence of 20%. The easiest way to make the distinction is to compare current radiographs with previous films, if available. When earlier films are not available, comparing the contralateral foot can be useful. Fractured sesamoids may show irregular jagged edges of separation with interrupted peripheral cortices, longitudinal or oblique division lines, or a bone callus formation.

Treatment

Conservative treatment includes splinting, dancer's pad, post-op shoe, and non–weight bearing (NWB).

Surgical treatment usually involves removal of the sesamoid.

Complications of Sesamoid Excision	
Tibial sesamoid removal	Hallux valgus
Fibular sesamoid removal	Hallux varus

(*continued*)

Complications of Sesamoid Excision

Tibial and fibular sesamoid removal	Hallux malleus (hammering)[a]

[a]If both sesamoids are removed, consider performing an IPJ fusion and Jones tenosuspension to prevent hammering at the IPJ.

Sesamoid Fracture vs. a Bipartite Sesamoid

Note: *These general signs can also be used to distinguish between a posterior process fracture of the talus from an os trigonum.*

Sign	Fracture	Bipartite
Radiographic appearance		
Larger than the other sesamoid	No	Yes
Bilateral	No	Often (25% are bilateral)
Edges	Sharp/irregular/less distinct	Smooth/clear/distinct
Changes on serial x-rays	Yes (due to evolving callus formation)	No
MRI or CT to conclusively diagnose	Yes	Yes

ANKLE SPRAINS

Ankle sprains occur when the ligaments of the ankle are stretched or torn. There are three main types of ankle sprains:

Inversion sprains
Eversion sprains
High ankle sprains (syndesmotic injury)

Ankle Sprain Classification

Grade I—stretching of the ligaments
Grade II—partial tear of the ligaments
Grade III—complete tear of the ligaments

Inversion Ankle Sprains (Most Common)

Most ankle sprains are inversion sprains, where the foot inverts and the lateral ligaments are damaged. The position of the foot at the time of an inversion sprain determines which ligaments are damaged. When the foot is plantarflexed at the time of injury, the anterior talofibular (ATF) ligament is damaged. This accounts for 95% of ankle sprains. When the foot is dorsiflexed at the time of injury, the calcaneofibular ligament (CFL) is most likely damaged. With a CFL sprain, the peroneal tendon sheath may also be damaged because it overlies this structure.

CLINICAL TESTS

Anterior Drawer Test—Test for Damage to the ATF

Brace the lower leg and attempt to anteriorly translate the foot on the leg. This tests the integrity of the ATF. Compare with the other leg, test is positive with excessive gapping or pain.

NOTE: There is also a radiographic version of this test.

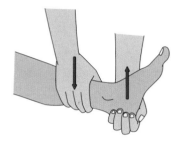

Talar Tilt Test—Tests for Damage to the CFL

Stabilize the leg and invert the foot. Perform the test with the foot at 90°. This tests the integrity of the CFL. Pain is positive for a possible ligamentous injury. The test can also be performed with the foot in plantarflexion to test for the ATF.

Note: There is also a radiographic version of the talar tilt test.

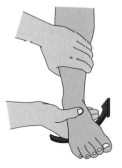

Radiographic Testing

Arthrograms

Arthrograms are useful only in acute ruptures while the ligaments are still damaged; after 5 to 7 days, fibrosis may seal off injury and arthrograms will be of no use. Dye is injected into the ankle joint and should remain in the ankle joint on x-ray. Some individuals have a normal connection between the ankle joint and the peroneal tendon sheath, which should not be misdiagnosed as a rupture. The integrity of the articular cartilage should also be inspected with an arthrogram. The dark bands of the articular cartilage should be apparent with the radiopaque dye between them forming the "Oreo cookie sign." If the articular cartilage is damaged, the dye will extend into the subchondral bone.

Radiographs

Anterior drawer view is useful in diagnosing ATF ligament ruptures. A positive test is a ≥6 mm between the posterior lip of the tibia and the nearest part of the talar dome, or >3 mm difference compared to the contralateral side. An ankle block may be required for this test due to pain.

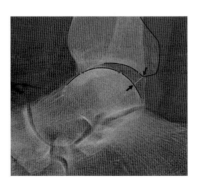

Talar tilt test/inversion stress test is used to diagnose a calcaneofibular ligament rupture. With the foot at 90°, stabilize the distal tibia and invert the foot. An ankle block may be required for this test due to pain. Measure the angle between a line drawn across the tibial plafond and across the talar dome. A measurement >5° is indicative of a CFL tear or rupture.

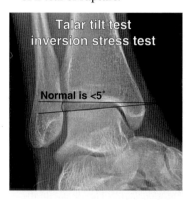

Treatment

Nonsurgical treatment is aimed at decreasing inflammation, splinting, and supporting the damaged tissues to prevent reinjury.

Surgical treatment involves procedures that reinforce and stabilize the damaged and elongated ligaments. This often involves tendon transfers.

Surgical Treatment for Inversion Sprains

Broström Procedure
Consists of reconstruction of torn or elongated lateral ankle ligaments and retinaculum by imbrication (overlapping) and suturing in a "pants-over-vest" manner

Other Surgical Treatment for Inversion Sprains

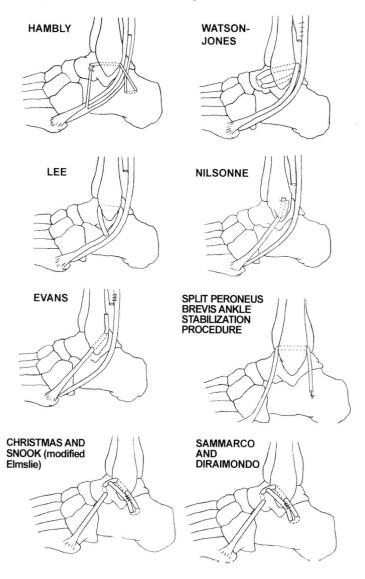

HAMBLY

WATSON-JONES

LEE

NILSONNE

EVANS

SPLIT PERONEUS BREVIS ANKLE STABILIZATION PROCEDURE

CHRISTMAS AND SNOOK (modified Elmslie)

SAMMARCO AND DIRAIMONDO

SUPPAN
(use plantaris)

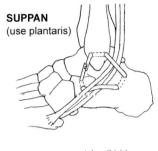

LARSEN

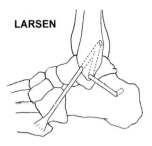

MERCADO

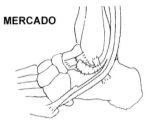

SEEBURGER

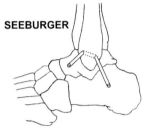

WHINFIELD

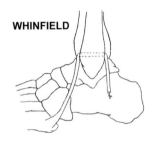

KELIKIAN
(use plantaris)

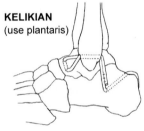

ELMSLIE

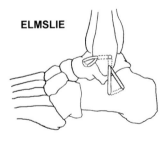

Eversion Ankle Sprains

Eversion sprains are rare for two reasons. First, the deltoid ligament on the medial side of the ankle is very strong. Second, the fibula prevents the foot from everting; hence, when they do occur, they may be associated with a fibular fracture.

Clinical tests:

"Eversion" talar tilt test—tests the integrity of the Deltoid ligament

Stabilize the leg and evert the foot. Pain over the medial ankle is positive for a possible deltoid ligament injury.

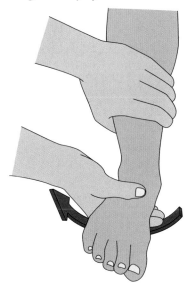

Radiologic Evaluation of the Deltoid ligament

Medial Clear Space

Used to predict a deltoid ligament injury. Evaluated on either the ankle mortise or ankle A/P radiograph. Medial clear space is the distance between the lateral border of the medial malleolus and the medial border of the talus. This measurement should be <4 to 5 mm and should also be equal to the dorsal clear space (distance between the tibial plafond and the talus). Widening of the medial joint space >4 to 5 mm indicates lateral talar translation that occurs with a deltoid ligament injury.

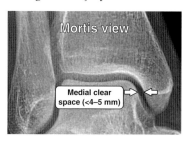

Mortis view

Medial clear space (<4–5 mm)

Surgical Treatment for Eversion Sprains

Schoolfied Procedure

The deltoid ligament is detached from the tibia, the foot is maximally inverted, and the ligament is reattached superiorly to the detachment site. The deltoid ligament is effectively advanced.

DuVries Procedure

A large cruciate form incision is made in the deltoid ligament and then sutured back together. The theory behind the procedure is that the resultant scar tissue will effectively reinforce and stabilize the medial ankle.

Wittberger and Mallory Procedure

The tibialis posterior (TP) tendon is split longitudinally down to its insertion. Half the tendon is detached proximally and passed inferiorly to superiorly through a drill hole in the distal tibia and sutured back on itself with the foot forcibly inverted.

HIGH ANKLE SPRAINS (DISTAL TIBIOFIBULAR SYNDESMOTIC INJURY)

A distal tibiofibular syndesmotic injury is also called a high ankle sprain and accounts for 10% of all ankle sprains. The distal tibiofibular syndesmosis is a fibrous joint connecting the bones just above the ankle joint. The mechanism of injury is external rotation of the foot on the leg. Commonly occurring in sports where the foot is planted on the ground and the knee is hit from the lateral side. This causes the "square" talar dome to rotate in the mortise, forcing the tibia and fibula apart from one another and rupturing the syndesmosis.

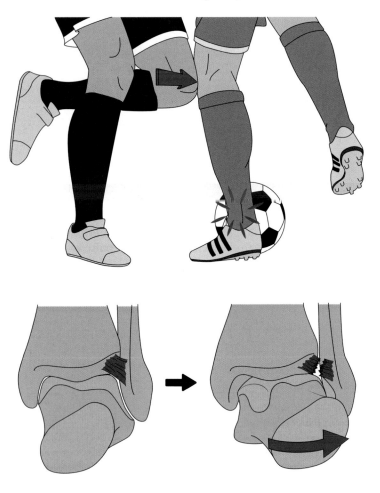

Tibiofibular Syndesmosis Anatomy

Composed of the following four ligaments, listed from anterior to posterior:

Anterior inferior tibiofibular ligament (AITFL)

Tibiofibular interosseous ligament
Inferior transverse tibiofibular ligament
Posterior inferior tibiofibular ligament (PITFL; strongest)

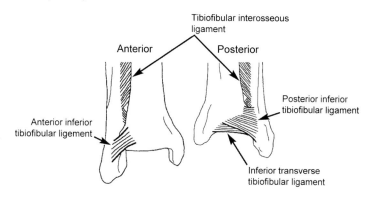

The talar dome is wider anteriorly than posteriorly, and the syndesmosis shows elasticity of 1 to 2 mm when the foot moves from plantarflexion to dorsiflexion. Extreme dorsiflexion can also cause separation of the distal tibiofibular articulation and injure the ligamentous structures.

Clinical Tests

Dorsiflexion may elicit pain as the wider anterior portion of the talus is rotated into the mortise and separates the bones. There may also be palpable tenderness between the distal tibia and the fibula.

External Rotation Test

Also called **Kleiger test**. With the foot at 90° or slightly dorsiflexed and the leg stabilized, externally rotate the foot. This test recreates the mechanism of injury and will elicit pain at the site of the syndesmosis. This is the most reliable test for diagnosing a syndesmotic injury.

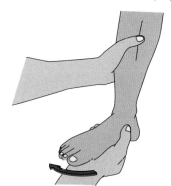

Distal Compression Test

Medial lateral compression at the level of the malleoli elicits pain due to compression of the ligaments

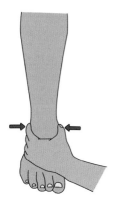

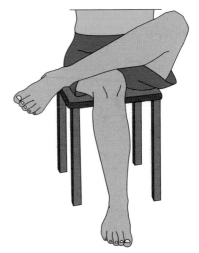

Squeeze Test

Also called the **Hopkins test** or proximal compression test. Medial lateral compression at the midcalf level elicits pain due to a slight distraction that results distally at the syndesmosis. There is also the **"crossed-leg test,"** which mimics the mechanism of the squeeze test. In this test, the patient crosses the bad leg over the good leg, and the pressure from the knee on the mid-calf mimics the squeeze test.

Diagnosis, Radiographic

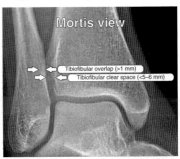

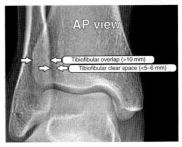

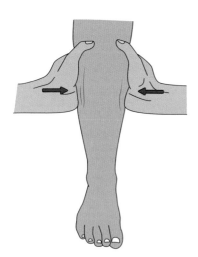

Tibiofibular Overlap

Measure the tibiofibular overlap at a point 1 cm above the plafond. The amount of overlap should be >10 mm on the A/P radiograph and >1 mm on the mortise view.

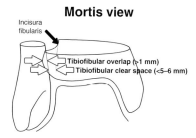

Mortis view

Incisura fibularis

Tibiofibular overlap (>1 mm)
Tibiofibular clear space (<5–6 mm)

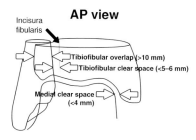

AP view

Incisura fibularis

Tibiofibular overlap (>10 mm)
Tibiofibular clear space (<5–6 mm)

Medial clear space (<4 mm)

Tibiofibular Clear Space
Take the width between the medial aspect of the fibula and the lateral border of the posterior tibia (fibular notch or incisura fibularis) 1 cm proximal to the plafond.

This distance should be <5 to 6 mm on both the A/P and mortis view (easier to see landmarks on the mortise view). A value >5 to 6 mm indicates a syndesmotic injury.

Treatment

Surgical treatment may include fixation with a fully threaded 4.5-mm cortical transsyndesmotic screw through four cortices. Fixation should be placed with the ankle fully dorsiflexed to allow the widest part of the talus to be accommodated. Transsyndesmotic fixation is placed from posterolateral to anteromedial between 2 and 4 cm from the ankle joint. Screws are removed at 3 to 4 months. Screws

left in tend to fail due to the normal motion between the tib and the fib. Screws may be placed through only three cortices of the fibula and lateral tibia. The theory being that this will allow some toggle motion, preventing the screw from breaking. Bioresorbable screws are also available. There are also suture button devices available, such as the TightRope by Arthrex.

The actual ligaments of the syndesmosis may require primary repair, and a plantaris graft can be utilized to reinforce the structures. Syndesmotic fusion and ankle fusion are also options for patients with continued pain and instability.

ANKLE FRACTURES

1. **Bosworth fracture**: Lateral malleolar fracture with posterior displacement of proximal fibula
2. **Cedell fracture**: Fracture of the posterior medial process of the talus
3. **Cotton fracture**: Trimalleolar fracture
4. **Dupuytren fracture**: Pott fracture (bimalleolar fracture)
   Foster: Entire posterior process
5. **Maisonneuve fracture**: Proximal 1/3 fibular fracture (fibular neck), associated with syndesmotic injury. Often involves medial malleolar fracture or rupture of the deltoid ligaments
6. **Pott fracture**: Bimalleolar fracture
7. **Shepard fracture**: Fracture of posterior lateral talar process
8. **Tillaux–Chaput fracture**: Avulsion fracture of anterior inferior lateral tibia

9. **Wagstaffe fracture:** Avulsion fracture of anterior inferior medial fibula

10. **Volkmann fracture:** Avulsion fracture of the posterior malleolus

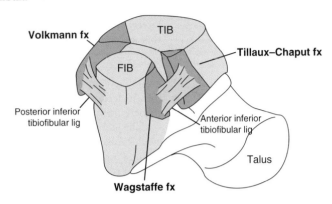

11. **Butterfly fragment (fracture):** A triangular fragment of bone produced in long bone fractures. Mechanism of injury is bending, causing compression on one side of the bone and tension on the other side. Seen in Lauge–Hansen PAB stage 3.

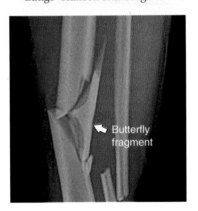

Ankle Fracture Classifications

Classification (Danis–Weber)

This is based on the location of the fibular fracture with respect to the syndesmosis. The more proximal the fibular fracture, the increase the risk of syndesmotic disruption and ankle instability

Type A
Infrasyndesmotic fibular fracture
(below the level of the syndesmosis)
Cause: Supination and adduction (internal rotation and adduction injury)
Transverse avulsion fracture
Syndesmosis intact
Stable

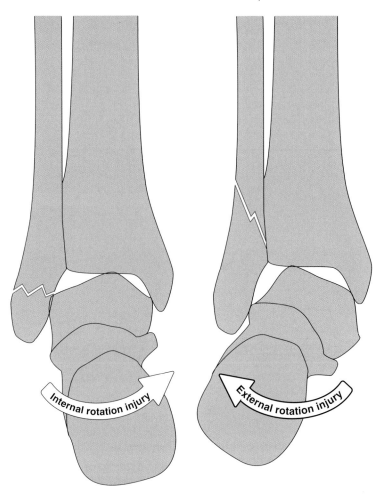

Type B

Transsyndesmotic fibular fracture *(at the level of the syndesmosis)*

Cause: Supination and external rotation

OR

Pronation and abduction

(external rotation injury)

Oblique fracture

Syndesmosis intact or partially torn

Variable stability

Type C

Suprasyndesmotic fibular fracture *(above the level of the syndesmosis)*

Cause: Pronation with external rotation

(abduction injury)

Syndesmosis disrupted

Unstable and requires ORIF

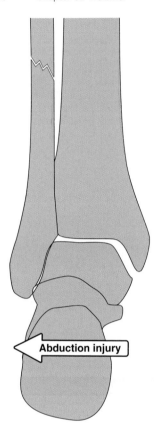

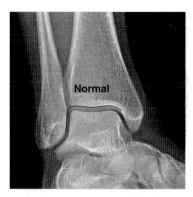

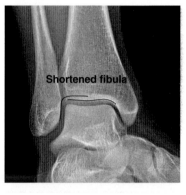

Talocrural angle: The angle should be ~83° plus or minus 4°. The contralateral side should be within 2° to 3° of the injured side.

Three intraoperative techniques to help assure the fibula is brought out to length during fracture repair:

Shenton line: The subchondral bone should form a continuous curved line between the fibula and the tibia around the talus. With a short fibula, Shenton line is broken.

Note: *Do not confuse this Shenton line with the Shenton line that is used to evaluate infants for hip dislocations.*

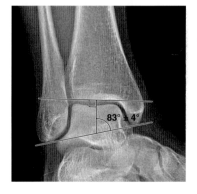

Dime test/Ball sign: On an AP ankle view, there should be an unbroken curve between the lateral talus and the peroneal groove of the **fibula**. With a malreduced fibula, the fibula will be shortened and the dime sign is absent.

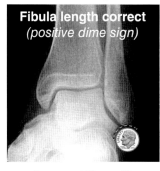

Fibula length correct
(positive dime sign)

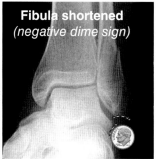

Fibula shortened
(negative dime sign)

Volkmann fracture, Wagstaffe fracture, and Tillaux–Chaput fracture are all avulsion fractures of the distal tibiofibular syndesmosis.

Classification (Lauge–Hansen)

NOTE: Regarding the Lauge–Hansen classification:

1. Injuries cannot skip steps, if a radiograph reveals a stage 3 injury, then they have the injuries of stages 1 and 2.

2. Classifications may not always reflect clinical reality.

Supination-Adduction (Aka: SAD or SA) 10% to 20% of Malleolar Fractures

Stage 1: Rupture of lateral ankle ligament or transverse lateral malleolus fracture

Stage 2: Vertical medial malleolar fracture

Supination-Adduction (SAD)

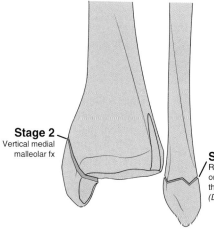

Stage 2
Vertical medial malleolar fx

Stage 1
Rupture of lateral ankle lig's or transverse fib fx below the syndesmosis
(Danis–Weber Type A)

Supination-External Rotation (Aka: SER or SE, Supination-Eversion)

40% to 75% of malleolar fractures—most common

Stage 1: Rupture of anterior inferior tibiofibular ligament with or without an associated avulsion fracture of its tibial or fibular attachments (Tillaux–Chaput fracture or Wagstaffe fracture)

Stage 2: Oblique spiral fracture of the fibula beginning at the level of the syndesmosis anteriorly and progressing proximally and posteriorly (posterior spike); SER stage 2 is the most common fracture.

Stage 3: Posterior inferior tibiofibular ligament rupture or a posterior malleolar fracture (Volkmann fracture)

Stage 4: Transverse fracture of medial malleolus or rupture of the deltoid ligament

Supination-External Rotation (SER)

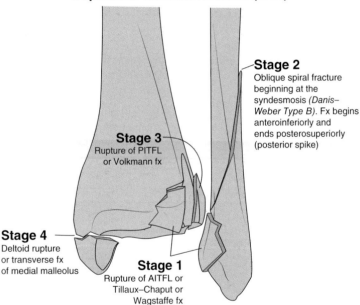

Stage 2
Oblique spiral fracture beginning at the syndesmosis *(Danis–Weber Type B)*. Fx begins anteroinferiorly and ends posterosuperiorly (posterior spike)

Stage 3
Rupture of PITFL or Volkmann fx

Stage 4
Deltoid rupture or transverse fx of medial malleolus

Stage 1
Rupture of AITFL or Tillaux–Chaput or Wagstaffe fx

Pronation-Abduction (a.k.a.: PAB or PA) 5% to 20% of Malleolar Fractures

Stage 1: Transverse fracture of medial malleolus or rupture of the deltoid ligament

Stage 2: Rupture of the anterior inferior and posterior inferior tibiofibular ligaments or an avulsion fracture of its tibial or fibular attachments (Tillaux–Chaput fracture, Wagstaffe fracture, or Volkmann fracture). Interosseous ligament remains intact.

Pronation-Abduction (PAB)

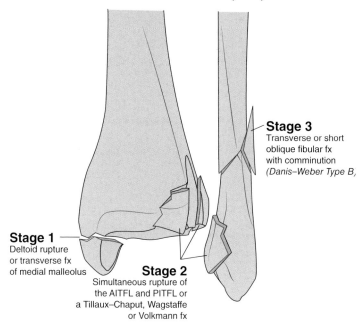

Stage 3
Transverse or short oblique fibular fx with comminution
(Danis–Weber Type B,

Stage 1
Deltoid rupture or transverse fx of medial malleolus

Stage 2
Simultaneous rupture of the AITFL and PITFL or a Tillaux–Chaput, Wagstaffe or Volkmann fx

Stage 3: Transverse or short oblique fracture of the fibula at or above the level of syndesmosis, often with comminution or a butterfly fragment

Pronation-External Rotation (aka: PER, PE, Pronation-Eversion)

5% to 20% of malleolar fractures—Worst Kind

Stage 1: Transverse fracture of medial malleolus or rupture of the deltoid ligament

Stage 2: Rupture of the anterior syndesmosis and rupture of the interosseous ligament or Tillaux–Chaput fragment or Wagstaffe fragment

Stage 3: Interosseous membrane tear with a spiral fracture of the fibula above the level of the syndesmosis; can be as high as the fibular neck (Maisonneuve fracture)

Stage 4: Posterior talofibular ligament rupture or fracture of the post malleolus (large fragment) ANKLE DIASTASIS

Pronation-External Rotation (PER)

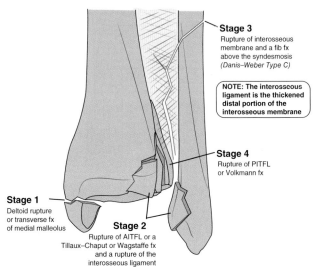

Stage 3
Rupture of interosseous membrane and a fib fx above the syndesmosis *(Danis–Weber Type C)*

NOTE: The interosseous ligament is the thickened distal portion of the interosseous membrane

Stage 4
Rupture of PITFL or Volkmann fx

Stage 1
Deltoid rupture or transverse fx of medial malleolus

Stage 2
Rupture of AITFL or a Tillaux–Chaput or Wagstaffe fx and a rupture of the interosseous ligament

Danis–Weber/Lauge–Hansen Classification Crossover

Weber A	Lauge–Hansen SAD (supination-adduction)
Weber B	Lauge–Hansen SER (supination-external rotation) PAB (pronation-abduction)
Weber C	Lauge–Hansen PER (pronation-external rotation)

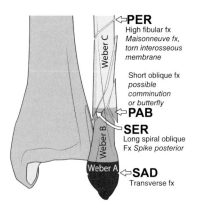

PER
High fibular fx *Maisonneuve fx, torn interosseous membrane*

PAB
Short oblique fx *possible comminution or butterfly*

SER
Long spiral oblique Fx *Spike posterior*

SAD
Transverse fx

Weber C *Weber B* *Weber A*

EPIPHYSEAL PLATE FRACTURES

Classification (Salter–Harris)

Associated with 35% of all skeletal injuries in children

Type I (6%) Fracture Through Growth Plate

No shortening

Type I

Type II (75% Most Common)

Through growth plate and traveling above into the metaphysis

Extra-articular

Minimal shortening, with no functional limitations after healing

Results in a Thurston–Holland fragment, which is a portion of the metaphysis remaining with the epiphysis in the physeal fracture

Type II

Type III (8%)

Through the growth plate and traveling below into the epiphysis
Intra-articular
Tillaux–Chaput type fracture that can cause shortening

Type III

Type IV (10%)

Oblique fracture through the epiphysis and metaphysis/diaphysis
Intra-articular

Type IV

Type V (1%)

Crush injury of the growth plate
Growth plate disturbance that can cause shortening and is associated with poor prognosis

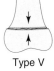
Type V

Type VI

Type VI

Type VII

Type VII

I	**S**ame
II	**A**bove
III	**L**ower
IV	**T**hrough
V	**R**eally bad

CALCANEAL FRACTURES

Calcaneal fractures account for 1% to 2% of all fractures and typically occur as a result of axial loading, such as a fall from a height or an MVA. The mechanism of injury is by way of the lateral process of the talus being driven down into the neutral triangle. Twenty percent of calcaneal fractures are associated with a spinal fracture between T12 and L2, with L1 being the most common. Lumbar radiographs are, therefore, recommended in all fall/calcaneal injury patients presenting with back pain. Surgical repair should be performed within 5 hours of injury before acute swelling begins. If this window is missed, surgery should be delayed until swelling subsides, usually around 7 to 10 days, but before the 3-week mark when consolidation of the fracture begins. The goal of ORIF is to reestablish height and length to the calcaneus and realign the articular cartilage. These patients should be monitored for compartment syndrome.

Clinical Signs

Mondor sign is a clinical indicator for a calcaneal fracture. Patients present with ecchymosis extending from the malleoli to the sole of the foot.

Radiographic Signs

Lateral View

Böhler angle is useful in evaluating calcaneal fractures. On a lateral x-ray, a line is drawn from the highest point of the anterior process to the highest point of the posterior articular surface and a line drawn between the same point on the posterior facet and the most superior point of the tuberosity. Normal values range between 20° and 40°; average is around 30° to 35°. Measurements <20° are seen in calcaneal fractures. Surgeons should strive to correct Böhler angle during ORIF for optimal outcome.

Gissane (critical) angle is useful in evaluating calcaneal fractures. On a lateral x-ray, a line is drawn along the posterior facet and a second line at the point of the sinus tarsi through the highest point of the anterior process. Normal is 120° to 145°; a fractured calcaneus will cause this angle to increase. Surgeons should strive to correct Gissane angle during ORIF for optimal outcome.

HARRIS–BEATH VIEW: Ski jump view used to view the posterior and middle STJ facets, varus/valgus angulation of tuberosity, increased heel width, and loss of height.

BRODEN VIEW: Special calcaneal views to show the congruency of the subtalar joint. Often taken intraoperatively to monitor calcaneal fracture reduction.

CT Scan

Semicoronal Plane

(Perpendicular to the posterior facet) Visualizes: articular surface of the posterior facet, the sustentaculum tali, shape of the heel, and position of the peroneal and FHL.

Note: This is the plane used when determining the Sander Classification.

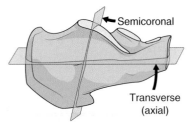

Best CT planes for a calcaneal fracture

Semicoronal

Transverse (axial)

Transverse (Axial) Plane

Visualizes: calcaneocuboid joint, the anterior inferior aspect of the posterior facet, and the sustentaculum tali

Fracture Lines

Primary Fracture Line

The primary fracture line extends obliquely through the calcaneus from anterolateral to posteromedial. The anteromedial fragment consists of the anterior process, the sustentaculum tali, and a portion of the posterior facet. The posterolateral segment contains the tuberosity, the lateral wall, and variable portion of the posterior facet. The primary fracture line is a vertical fracture oriented from superior to inferior at the Gissane angle and is the result of the lateral process of the talus being driven down into the calcaneus.

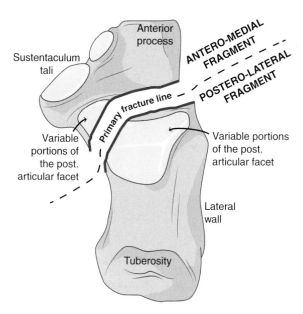

Secondary fracture lines are determined by the direction of force. They can extend into the calcaneocuboid joint separating the anterior process into anteromedial and anterolateral fragments, or it can extend medially separating the sustentacular fragment from the anteromedial fragment.

Fragments

a. *Constant fragment* (a.k.a. superomedial fragment, sustentacular fragment). Because of its strong ligamentous and tendon support, this fragment remains constant as far as its location relative to the talus. This is the fragment to which all other fragments are fixated.

b. *Anteromedial fragment*

c. *Anterolateral fragment*

d. *Lateral articular fragment (thalamic fragment)* is found with a joint depression type of injury where a fragment consisting of the lateral portion of the posterior facet develops.

e. *Lateral wall fragment* develops as a result of a hydraulic tangential burst that occurs when the posterior facet is driven down into the body of the calcaneus.

f. *Tuberosity (tuber) fragment* is typically displaced varus and laterally.

CALCANEAL FRACTURE CLASSIFICATIONS

Rowe Classification

Primarily used to describe extra-articular fractures. While Rowe types IV and V are intra-articular, most clinicians use Essex-Lopresti when describing intra-articular fractures.

NOTE: For the purposes of describing calcaneal fractures, any fracture not involving the STJ posterior facet is considered extra-articular.

Type IA

Medial calcaneal tuberosity fracture
MOI axial loading with the heel in valgus

Type IB

Sustentaculum tali fracture
MOI axial loading with inversion

Type IC

Anterior process fracture
Most common type I fx
MOI inversion and plantarflexion
Usually caused by avulsion of bifur-cate ligament

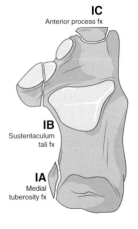

IC
Anterior process fx

IB
Sustentaculum tali fx

IA
Medial tuberosity fx

Type IIA

Post beak fx (Achilles not involved)
MOI direct trauma

Type IIB

Post beak avulsion fx (Achilles involved)
Medical emergency due to potential for overlying soft-tissue necrosis
MOI Achilles contracture on a fixed foot

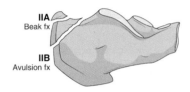

IIA
Beak fx

IIB
Avulsion fx

Type IIIA

Simple extra-articular body fx
MOI fall from a height with heel varus or valgus

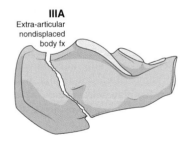

IIIA
Extra-articular nondisplaced body fx

Type IIIB

Comminuted/displaced extra-articular body fx
MOI fall from a height with heel varus or valgus

IIIB

Extra-articular
displaced
body fx

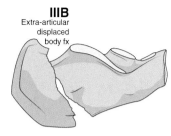

Type IV

Intra-articular body fx involving
the STJ without depression
MOI fall

IV

Intra-articular
nondisplaced
body fx

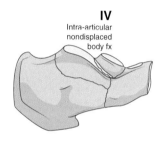

Type V

Intra-articular body fx with depression (comminution)
MOI fall

V

Intra-articular
displaced
body fx

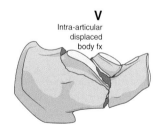

Classification (Essex-Lopresti)

(Intra-articular calcaneal fractures)

Type A (Tongue Fracture)

Occurs when talus is driven straight
down into the neutral triangle

Primary fracture is from Gissane
angle down to inferior surface of
the calcaneus.

Secondary fracture extending from
primary fracture out the posterior aspect of calcaneus

Medical emergency due to potential for overlying soft-tissue
necrosis

Type A

Tongue fx

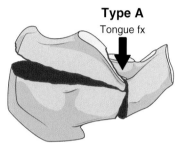

Type B (Joint Depression)

The vector of force is more
anteroposterior.

Primary fracture same as type A

Secondary fracture around posterior facet with possible comminution involving the STJ

Worse prognosis

Type B

Joint depression

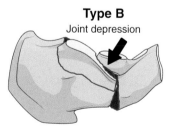

Essex-Lopresti Maneuver

The Essex-Lopresti maneuver is a
percutaneous fracture reduction
technique for a type A fracture. A
Schanz or Steinmann pin (sometimes called a Gissane spike)
is inserted posteriorly into the

tongue fragment just lateral to the Achilles. The pin is used as a lever to reduce the fracture and restore congruency to the posterior facet.

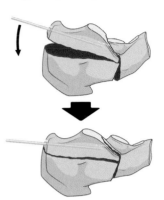

Essex-Lopresti maneuver

Sanders CT Classification

Based on CT coronal and axial sections

The posterior facet is divided into three sections: A, B, and C at the widest point of the posterior facet at the level of the sustentaculum tali.

Fractures are classified according to the number and location of intra-articular fragments.

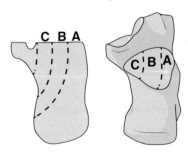

Type I

Any articular fractures with <2 mm displacement, regardless of number of fractures

Type II

One fracture through posterior facet (creating two fragments)

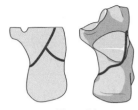

Type 2A

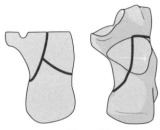

Type 2B

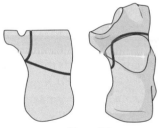

Type 2C

Type III

Two fracture through posterior facet (creating three fragments)

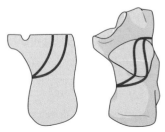

Type 3AB

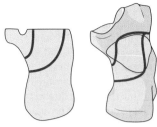

Type 3AC

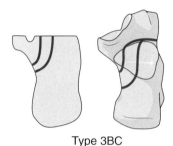

Type 3BC

Type IV

Fractures with three or more articular fractures that are displaced and severely comminuted

Calcaneal Fracture Repair

Fracture repairs are usually delayed 1 to 3 weeks until swelling and fracture blisters have subsided. Look for return of skin lines (wrinkles) and epithelialization of fracture blisters. The most common approach is the lateral extensile incision, which consists of a 90° incision placed over the lateral aspect of the calcaneus. This incision is full thickness to bone, and the flap is lifted subperiosteally. While the lateral extensile incision protects the peroneal tendons, sural nerve, and the extensor retinaculum, it was specifically developed as a way of preserving the lateral calcaneal artery, which supplies blood to the flap.

Goals of surgical correction:

Restore the height
Restore length
Decrease any widening
Correct angulation of the tuberosity fragment (fractures result in varus)
Restore articular congruency

Order of reduction (can vary):

1. Temporarily remove or fold back the lateral wall fragment to gain exposure to the other bone fragments.

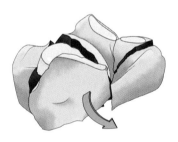

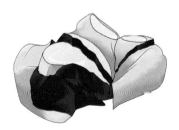

2. The first step is to create an intact anterior process. If present, the anterolateral and anteromedial fragments are reduced and temporarily fixated to the constant fragment.

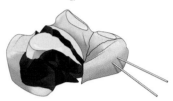

3. Next, insert a Schanz pin or Steinmann pin into the posterior tubercle. The pin is inserted laterally and bicortically. Calcaneal fractures cause the tuber to become varus and laterally displaced. To reduce the tuberosity fragment, use the Schanz pin as a "joystick" to reduce the primary fracture line. Manipulate the fragment posteriorly, inferiorly, valgus, and then medially in that order. Temporarily fixate the tuberosity to the constant fragment with pins.

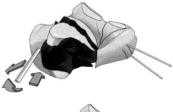

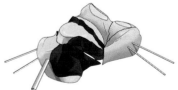

4. Next, reduce the articular fragment (thalamic fragment). Use an elevator to lift up the posterior facet and restore the subchondral bone plate. K-wires are driven transversely through this fragment into the sustentacular fragment. Subchondral lag screws are inserted at this time from lateral to medial to compress the articular fragments.

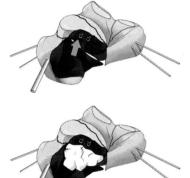

After fixating the articular fragment, a bone void often results beneath the fragment in the area of the neutral triangle. This area can be filled with bone graft. The use of bone graft is subjective and somewhat controversial.

5. Lastly, the lateral wall is put back in place. Permanent fixation is then applied. Temporary K-wires fixation is then removed.

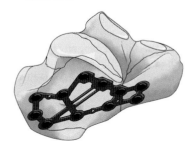

OSTEOCHONDRITIS DISSECANS (OCD LESIONS)

Necrosis of bone beneath an area of cartilage. In the foot, it usually refers to a lesion in the talar dome.

Talar Dome OCD Lesions

Mechanism of Injury	Location of Injury
Dorsiflexion-inversion	Anterior-lateral
Plantarflexion-inversion	Medial-posterior

mnemonic-DIAL-A-PIMP

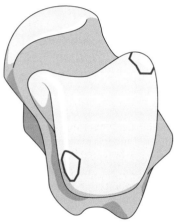

Classification (Berndt–Harty)

Type I

Small area of subchondral bone compression with the overlying cartilage intact

Type II

Partial detached osteochondral fragment

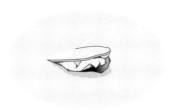

Type III

Completely detached fragment remaining in crater

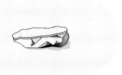

Type IV

Displaced osteochondral fragment

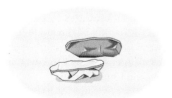

TALAR FRACTURES

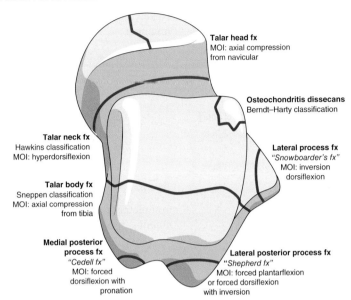

Talar head fx
MOI: axial compression
from navicular

Osteochondritis dissecans
Berndt–Harty classification

Talar neck fx
Hawkins classification
MOI: hyperdorsiflexion

Lateral process fx
"Snowboarder's fx"
MOI: inversion
dorsiflexion

Talar body fx
Sneppen classification
MOI: axial compression
from tibia

**Medial posterior
process fx**
"Cedell fx"
MOI: forced
dorsiflexion with
pronation

Lateral posterior process fx
"Shepherd fx"
MOI: forced plantarflexion
or forced dorsiflexion
with inversion

TALAR NECK FRACTURES "AVIATOR'S ASTRAGALUS"

Mechanism of injury: forced hyperdorsiflexion resulting in impingement of the talar neck on the distal anterior tibia. However, it has been found in laboratories to be caused by axial loading of the ankle in the neutral position while compressing the calcaneus against the overlying talus and tibia.

Best x-ray view for talar neck: **Canale view.** Foot in maximum equinus, 15° pronated, x-ray 15° cephalad from vertical.

Complications: AVN radiographic evidence takes about 8 weeks to show. In all, 20% to 30% of talar neck fractures have an associated medial malleolar fracture, especially in type III.

Fixation is accomplished either from anterior to posterior or from posterior to anterior with two 3.5-mm cortical screws. Because the talar surface is 60%, articular cartilage fixation should be performed with headless screws or the heads should be countersunk to prevent interference with joint movement.

Hawkins sign: A radiolucent subchondral band in the talar dome that develops 6 to 8 weeks after a talar AVN. This is a good prognostic sign, indicative of bone resorption and revascularization.

Normal Joint	Hawkins Sign	AVN
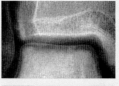	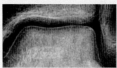	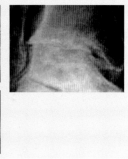
Congruent joint space, normal-appearing bone	Radiolucent subchondral band	Sclerotic bone Flattening of articular surface Narrowing joint space

Treatment for AVN

With a Hawkins type III fracture, the medial malleolus is often fractured as the talar body squeezes out the back of the ankle between the medial malleolus and the Achilles tendon. During surgical relocation, a medial malleolar osteotomy may be required to relocate the talar body. Avoid cutting the deltoid ligaments to preserve as much remaining blood supply to the talus as possible.

Talar neck fractures that result in AVN require a talectomy with either a Blair fusion or a tibio-calcaneus fusion

With talar neck fractures, the head is usually spared from AVN. A Blair fusion involves a sliding tibial graft that is fixated to the remaining viable talar head and neck.

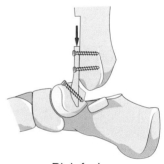

Blair fusion

If there is insufficient talar head for a Blair fusion, a tibio-calcaneus fusion may be indicated. This results in significant shortening of the limb.

Classification (Hawkins)

Useful for predicting long-term outcome and development of AVN

Type	Description	AVN Occurrence
Hawkins I	Nondisplaced neck fx	0%–13%
Hawkins II	Displaced neck fx with STJ dislocation	20%–50%
Hawkins III	Displaced neck fx with STJ and ankle joint dislocation	80%–100%
Hawkins IV	Displaced neck fx with STJ, ankle joint, and talonavicular joint dislocation	80%–100% Possible disruption of blood supply to head

Type I: Nondisplaced talar neck fracture

Disrupts only blood vessels entering the body via the dorsal talar neck and intraosseous vessels crossing the neck, 0% to 13% chance of AVN. Type I is the only type that can be treated nonoperatively with casting and non–weight bearing.

TYPE I

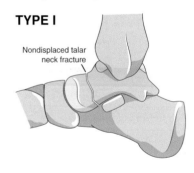

Nondisplaced talar neck fracture

Disrupts only the vessels entering the dorsal and lateral aspects of the neck of the talus

Type II: Displaced Talar Neck Fracture With Subluxed or Dislocated STJ

Disrupts dorsal neck arterial branches plus branches entering inferiorly from the sinus tarsi and tarsal canal, medial blood supply often spared, 20% to 50% chance of AVN

Disrupts the blood supply from the dorsal and lateral aspects of the talar neck and from the vascular sling in the sinus tarsi and tarsal canal

TYPE II

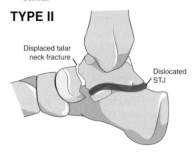

Displaced talar neck fracture

Dislocated STJ

Type III: Displaced Talar Neck Fracture With Dislocation of the STJ and Ankle Joint

The talar body dislocated posteriorly and medially.

All three major blood supplies are disrupted, 20% to 100% chance of AVN.

Disrupts blood supply of the entire talar body

TYPE III

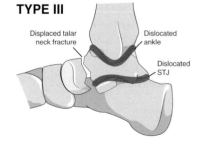

Displaced talar neck fracture

Dislocated ankle

Dislocated STJ

Type IV: Displaced Talar Neck Fracture With Dislocation of the STJ, Ankle Joint, and the Talonavicular Joint

The talar body dislocated posteriorly and medially.

All three major blood supplies are disrupted, 70% to 100% chance of AVN. Plus blood supply to the talar head is affected.

TYPE IV

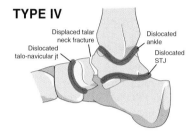

Displaced talar neck fracture
Dislocated talo-navicular jt
Dislocated ankle
Dislocated STJ

TALAR BODY FRACTURES

Talar body fractures are intra-articular injuries. Talar body fractures occur from axial compression of the talus between the tibial plafond and the calcaneus. They usually occur as a result of a fall from a height or an MVA. While less common, the prognosis of a talar body fracture is much worse than a talar neck fracture. Comminuted fractures of the talar body have poor long-term results and are often best treated with a talectomy and calcaneotibial fusion. As an alternative, to maintain height of the ankle, a Blair fusion may be preferred. A *Blair fusion* involves a sliding graft from the anterior surface of the tibia into the remnant head and neck of the talus.

Sneppen Classification

Five types based on anatomic location

Type 1: Transchondral and osteochondral dome fractures (includes OCD)

Type 2: Coronal, sagittal, or horizontal shear fractures (whole-body fractures)

Type 3: Posterior tubercle fractures (Shepherd fracture)

Type 4: Lateral process fracture

Type 5: Crush fractures

TALAR LATERAL PROCESS FRACTURE "SNOWBOARDER'S FRACTURE"

Mechanism of injury: Inversion and dorsiflexion

MOI: Axial-loaded dorsiflexed foot becomes externally rotated and/or everted.

Best views are ankle AP or ankle mortise. Often missed on lateral views due to overlapping bone. Having said that, look for the "V sign" on lateral films. The lateral process normally makes a distinct "V" shape. A disruption of this is a positive V sign and suggests a lateral process fracture.

Treatment: For nondisplaced lateral process fractures, non–weight-bearing cast 6 weeks. If displaced > 2 mm or fragment over 1 cm, treatment is ORIF.

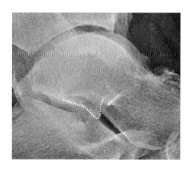

TALAR POSTERIOR PROCESS FRACTURE

Lateral Tubercle: Stieda Process, Shepherd Fx

Involves the lateral tubercle of the posterior process. The lateral tubercle serves as the attachment of the posterior talofibular ligament.

This type of fracture must be differentiated from an os trigonum. A test for this type of fracture is to plantarflex the foot and dorsiflex hallux. This maneuver will elicit pain at the fracture site due to the FHL, which courses between the medial and lateral posterior talar processes.

Another test is the nutcracker sign. The nutcracker sign is pain with forced plantarflexion of the ankle. The posterior process of the talus can be fractured in two ways. Forced plantarflexion, which leads to impingement between the posterior malleoli and the calcaneal tuber. These fractures also occur from excessive dorsiflexion, which leads to avulsion-type fracture due to the posterior talofibular ligament.

Excessive plantarflexion, which leads to impingement against the PT plafond

OR

Excessive dorsiflexion, especially with inversion, which leads to an avulsion-type fracture due to the posterior talofibular ligament

Medial Tubercle: Cedell Fracture

An avulsion fracture from the medial tubercle of the talus caused from forced dorsiflexion and pronation.

The fracture is a result of an avulsion fracture from the posterior talotibial ligament (one of the ligaments making up the deltoid).

A test for this type of fracture is to plantarflex the foot and dorsiflex hallux. This maneuver will elicit pain at the fracture site due to the FHL, which courses between the medial and lateral posterior talar processes.

FIFTH METATARSAL FRACTURES

Zone I (93% of Fractures)

Avulsion fractures (pseudo-Jones fracture)

Occurs PROXIMAL to the 4th and 5th metatarsal articulation

MOI plantarflexion and inversion

Avulsion fracture due to either the peroneus brevis tendon or the lateral plantar aponeurosis

Low risk for nonunion

Tx: WB in ortho shoe 4 to 6 weeks

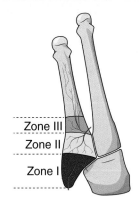

Zone II (4% of Fractures)

Jones fractures

Occurs at the metaphyseal–diaphyseal (occurs at the level of the 4th and 5th metatarsal articulation)

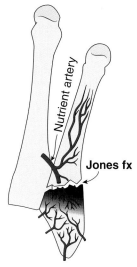

Nutrient artery

Jones fx

MOI plantarflexion and adduction
High risk of nonunion due to their
location at a vascular watershed
area
Tx: non–weight bearing for 6 to
8 weeks, 20% to 50% become
nonunions

Zone III (3% of Fractures)

Stress fractures
Proximal shaft (DISTAL to the
4th and 5th metatarsals
articulation)
Tx: non–weight bearing for 6 to
8 weeks, 20% to 50% become
nonunions
MOI: repetitive use, athletes

TIBIAL PLAFOND FRACTURE (PILON FRACTURE)

A pilon fracture is a distal tibial
metaphyseal fracture involving the
weight-bearing articular surface of
the ankle joint. Plafond fractures
tend to result in a varus deformity
due to the extra lateral stability of
the fibula. Fibula is also fractured in
80% of pilon fractures.

Pilon fractures are grossly divided into two groups based on
mechanism of injury: axial and
rotational.

Type	Mechanism	Examples	Prognosis	Soft-Tissue Damage
Axial	High energy	Fall from height, MVA	Worse	Likely
Rotational	Rotational	Skiing	Better	Less likely

There is usually an anterolateral fragment that subluxes or dislocates from the joint and remains
attached to the fibula.

If the injury occurs with the
ankle plantarflexed, the fragment
is posteriorly. If the ankle is dorsiflexed, the fragment is anteriorly.
If the foot is neutral, there are two
fractures front and back.

Classification Systems
Rüedi and Allgöwer

Type I
Distal tibial fracture
without displacement

Type II
Distal tibial fracture
with significant
displacement

Type III
Distal tibial fracture
with significant
displacement and
comminution

AO/OTA classification (Arbeitgemeinschaft für Osteosynthesefragen/Orthopedic Trauma Association)

Three categories (A, B, or C) based on the degree of articular involvement

These three categories are further divided (1, 2, and 3) based on the amount of comminution.

AO/OTA CLASSIFICATION

Type A (Extra-Articular) *Type A's are bending/twisting injuries*

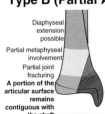

Diaphyseal extension possible

Metaphyseal fracture

Joint intact
No articular fractures

A1
Metaphyseal simple

A2
Metaphyseal wedge

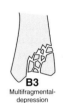

A3
Metaphyseal complex

Type B (Partial Articular) *Type B's tend to be shearing injuries*

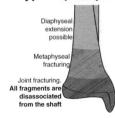

Diaphyseal extension possible

Partial metaphyseal involvement
Partial joint fracturing
A portion of the articular surface remains contiguous with the shaft

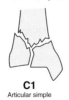

B1
Pure split

B2
Split-depression

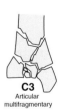

B3
Multifragmental-depression

Type C (Complete Articular) *Type C's are from axial load*

Diaphyseal extension possible

Metaphyseal fracturing

Joint fracturing.
All fragments are disassociated from the shaft

C1
Articular simple

C2
Metaphyseal multifragmentary

C3
Articular multifragmentary

General

Immediate ORIF is not recommended because the soft tissue is usually bad. Initial treatment is usually closed reduction and splinting. Followed by staged ORIF. First stage: apply x-fix (A-frame), then get CT scan.

When internal fixation is used, it is better to use minimally invasive fixation.

Soft-tissue condition should improve before definitive Sx. 1 to 3 weeks.

Superficial peroneal nerve

With a pilon fx and tibial shaft fracture, fixate the articular surface, and IM rod.

Most approaches are some form of anterior approach. Swing the Chaput fragment laterally on a AITFL hinge to access deeper fragments. Fixate the postero-lateral fragment (Volkmann) to the fibula. This fragment is usually relatively constant due to the PITFL. Fixate the medial malleolar fragment to the pos-terolateral fragment (this may require another incision). Then fixate any central impacted frag-ments (die-punch fragments). Then close down the anterolat-eral fragment. Then secure the articular segment with screws or a small plate. Then fixate the articular block the diaphysis.

For the medial malleolar fragment, it may require an additional incision or at least some per-cutaneous incisions for screw placement. May require bone graft if there is a metaphyseal void.

With the foot dorsiflexed, the frag-ment is anterior but also worth noting, the anterior fragment is anterior impaction.

Fracture Pattern

Fracture patterns depend on the degree of trauma and position of the ankle during impact.

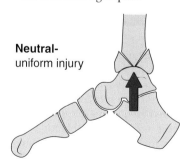

Neutral-
uniform injury

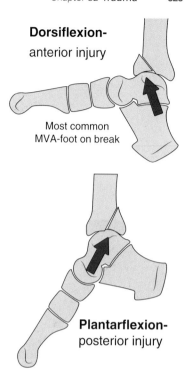

Dorsiflexion-
anterior injury

Most common
MVA-foot on break

Plantarflexion-
posterior injury

Consistent Fragments of a Pilon Fracture

The three classic articular compo-nents of a tibial pilon fracture are the anterolateral (Tillaux–Chaput) fragment, the posterolateral (Volk-mann) fragment, and the medial (malleolar) fragment. They present in a "Y" shaped configuration. Of-ten times with some central com-minution in the middle. A fibular avulsion fracture (Wagstaffe) may also be present.

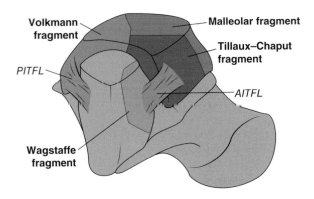

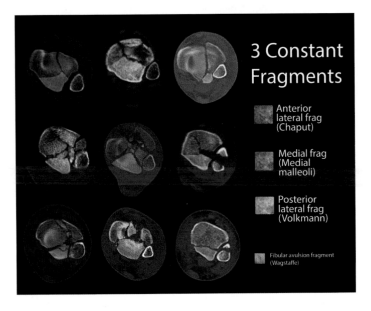

Incisional Approach

Incisional approach to a pilon fracture is largely determined by the location and orientation of the fracture pattern. An anterior approach is most common due to the degree of exposure, and it provides better visualization of the articular surface of the talar plafond. There are two main anterior approaches and two posterior approaches in addition to a medial approach directly over the medial malleoli. More than one of these incisions is often required for adequate reduction. The most common combination is a posteromedial approach combined with an anterolateral approach. While somewhat controversial, it is generally recommended to leave a 7-cm bridge between incisions.

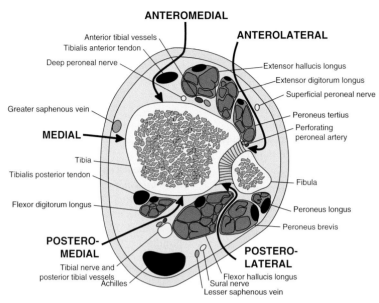

Pilon Fracture Incisional Approaches

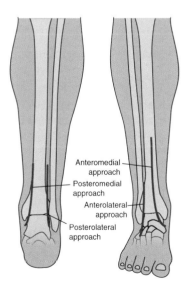

Anteromedial approach
Posteromedial approach
Anterolateral approach
Posterolateral approach

Anteromedial approach: Incision is along the medial border of the anterior tibialis tendon about 1 cm lateral to the tibial crest and ends with a hockey stick turn under the medial malleolus. Soft-tissue structures are retracted laterally to allow exposure and the anterior distal tibia. Avoid violating the anterior tibial tendon sheath to decrease the chances of soft-tissue necrosis.

Advantages:	Excellent exposure to tibia shaft and articular surface. Good visualization of medial malleolus
Disadvantages:	Poor visualization of Chaput fragment
	High-risk area for wound breakdown due to the thin soft-tissue envelope over the shin bone

Anterolateral approach (Böhler incision): This incision is centered at the ankle joint, extends between the tibia and the fibula, and is directly in line with the 4th ray.

Advantages: Medial malleolus cannot be accessed through this approach.

Improved soft-tissue coverage compared to anteromedial approach

Useful when there is a large lateral (Tillaux–Chaput) fragment

Disadvantages: Superficial peroneal nerve is directly in the path of this incision.

Limited access proximally due to crossing muscles. Usually does not extend >7 cm above the ankle.

Medial approach: Directly over the medial malleolus

Advantages: Limited vital soft-tissue structures other than saphenous vein and nerve

Disadvantages: This incision must extend far proximally enough to allow displacement of the medial fragment (malleolus) in order to access to the ankle joint.

Posteromedial approach: Uncommon approach. Incision is made just posterior to palpated boarder of the tibia, and dissection is between the FDL and neurovascular bundle.

Advantages: Good for a severely displaced posteromedial fragments, which are challenging to reduce from the front

Disadvantages: Poor visualization of articular surface

Posterolateral approach: Uncommon approach. Incision between the Achilles tendon and the lateral malleolus. Between the peroneus brevis and FHL.

Advantages: Provides good visualization of a Volkmann fragment

Disadvantages: Poor visualization of articular surface

Repair Axial Injuries-Staged Treatment

There is usually significant soft-tissue injury with pilon fractures. The soft-tissue envelop around the ankle is thin to begin with, and 30% of Pilon fractures are open fractures. Tissue necrosis is common, especially anteromedially where the soft tissue is especially thin. For this reason, pilon fracture treatment has evolved into a two-stage approach to avoid violating the soft-tissue envelop immediately after injury. Stage I involves acute application of a spanning fixator with optional plating of the fibula. Stage II is performed about 2 to 4 weeks later with definitive fixation with ORIF and/or MIPO after the soft tissues have recovered.

MIPO (Minimally Invasive Plate Osteosynthesis)
MIPO is minimally invasive ORIF where smaller incisions are made and plates are slid up along the bone just above the periosteum. Plates are fixated with percutaneous screws through stab incisions.

Stage I

Performing surgery while there is acute swelling makes it much more difficult to align bone fragments and increases the risk of infection and soft-tissue damage. Acute injuries are initially treated with application of a spanning fixator. A spanning fixator is an external fixator that spans the ankle joint. It provides traction to help realign the bone fragments (ligamentotaxis) and hold the length of the extremity until the soft tissue has a chance to recover. If the pilon fracture is open, I&D should be performed at this time as well.

Spanning fixators are usually in a Delta frame or A-frame configuration with two medial-based threaded bicortical pins in the tibia and one centrally threaded transfixation pin in the calcaneus. The calcaneal pin is inserted medial to lateral. Some surgeons opt to stabilize the foot with a second pin in the foot, usually through the cuneiforms. When applying the fixator, keep the pins and bars away from areas of future incisions and plate placement.

Definitive ORIF of the fibula is often performed initially along with the spanning fixator. Fibula plating adds stability to the fixator and re-established proper length of the lateral column.

Order a CT Scan

Once the injury is stabilized with the spanning fixator, a CT is performed. It is important to order the CT AFTER the spanning fixator is applied. Application of the fixator will change the orientation of fragments, making an earlier CT less useful. CT scans are essential for planning incisional approach and hardware construct. The most distal axial cuts of the tibial plafond are particularly useful for this purpose.

Stage II

Stage II involves definitive fixation that can occur at 2 to 4 weeks after the soft tissues have recovered. Indication of soft-tissue recover includes the return of skin wrinkle lines and epithelialization of fracture blisters.

Repairing the Articular Block

With the fibula having been previously fixated out to length in stage I, the lateral column becomes the starting point for repair. The anterolateral (Chaput) and posterolateral (Volkmann) fragments are usually in their anatomically correct position due to the AITFL and PITFL, respectively. Anterior access to the tibial plafond is essential in the majority of high energy pilon fractures, which makes the posterolateral fragment the most logical fragment to use as the constant fragment. The posterolateral fragment in a pilon fracture is similar to the sustentaculum fragment in a calcaneus fracture in this regard.

Establishing the posterolateral fragment as the constant fragment can be achieved in different ways.

1. Surgical reconstruction of the fibula may result in reduction of the posterolateral fragment through ligamentotaxis.
2. The posterolateral fragment may be accessed through the anterior approach and can be reduced to the shaft.
3. Finally, a posterolateral approach may allow for a direct reduction of this fragment and can convert a C-type pilon fracture into a B-type fracture.

Definitive correction begins with establishing an intact articular plafond. Each fragment is separately lagged to the stable fragment. Reconstructing the articular block from an anterior approach begins by folding back the anterolateral (Tillaux–Chaput) fragment. The anterolateral fragment is "booked" open on an AITFL hinge. Temporarily remove any other fragments to allow access into the fracture and reduction of central impaction.

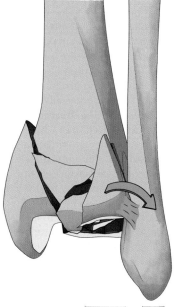

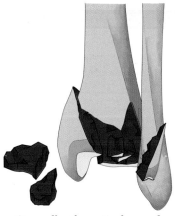

Generally, the articular surface is reconstructed from lateral to medial and from posterior to anterior, starting with the posterolateral fragment. The posterolateral fragment or Volkmann fragment is somewhat constant due to its attachment to the fibula.

Once exposure to the fracture is achieved, all hematoma and small fragments are cleared from the field. Fracture fragments are mobilized. The medial fragment containing the medial malleolus is temporarily fixed to the posterolateral fragment.

reduce with ligamentotaxis. These small osteochondral fragments are repositioned back into place like a jigsaw puzzle and can be fixated with flush-cut pins or buried wires.

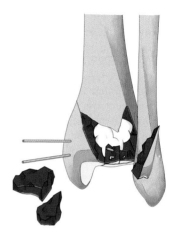

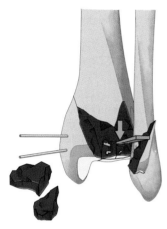

Bone graft is then packed into the metaphyseal void left after reducing the impacted articular fragments.

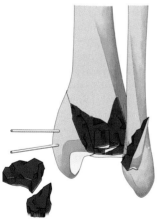

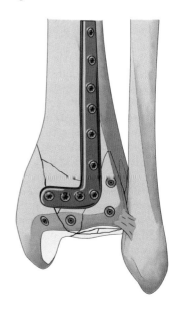

Next, an osteotome or elevator is used to disimpact the centrally compressed articular fragments. These fragments are purely articular and have no soft-tissue attachments. These fragments are called die-punch fragments, and they do not

Sequential reduction is completed by "closing the book," folding back the anterolateral fragment. Cannulated lag screws and small plates can be used to fixate the articular block.

Finally, a buttress plate is used to connect the articular block to the diaphysis (shaft). These plates should be applied using percutaneous techniques (MIPO) when possible. Through the incision used to reconstruct the articular block, an epiperiosteal tunnel is created proximally along the medial tibial shaft. Placement of plate will vary based on fracture pattern. A cloverleaf plate is then slid through the tunnel and fixated percutaneously with screws.

Distal Articular Block

There are many precontoured plates available for pilon injuries. Plates can be applied anteriorly, medially, or posteriorly depending on the injury. Generally, injuries that present with a primary valgus deformity require an anterolateral buttress, whereas primary varus deformities require a medial buttress. Anterior crush injuries should be plated with an anterior pilon plate, while a posterior crush injury would do better with a posterior plate. A combination of several plates may be the best option for other injuries. In other situations, an IM nail is preferred.

The spanning fixator usually comes off at the time of definitive fixation as the bars and pins get in the way of fixation.

LISFRANC FX/DISLOCATION

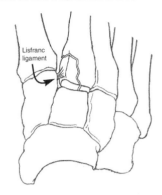

A Lisfranc injury is an injury to the midfoot that can involve broken bones or damaged ligaments. They can be subtle injuries that are often misdiagnosed as simple sprains but are severe injuries that can require months to heal and may require surgery. Most injuries occur from forced dorsiflexion. The Lisfranc ligament is the strongest interosseous tarsometatarsal ligament, and the integrity of the Lisfranc joint depends on this ligament. Its disruption can result in the lateral displacement of the rest of the tarsometatarsal joints. There is no interosseous ligament between the 1st and 2nd metatarsals.

Lisfranc Ligament

Also called the medial interosseous tarsometatarsal ligament. It attaches the medial cuneiform to the 2nd metatarsal. This ligament plus the recessed 2nd metatarsal are responsible for most of the stability at the Lisfranc joint. It is the strongest interosseous tarsometatarsal ligament. The Lisfranc ligament is responsible for the avulsion-type fracture of the base of the medial aspect of the 2nd metatarsal.

Diagnosis

Patient presents with a history of trauma, although it may be relatively minor. There may be swelling and bruising on the top and bottom of the arch. A dorsal or plantar deviation of the 2nd metatarsal base from the medial cuneiform may be palpated. Lisfranc injuries may be subtle, and a CT scan may be required for proper diagnosis.

Radiographic Evaluation

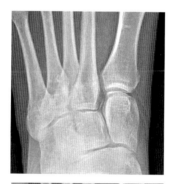

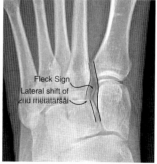

Fleck Sign
Lateral shift of
2nd metatarsal

Subtle dislocations can be difficult to diagnose. Weight-bearing films and/or abductory radiographs will accentuate the fracture dislocation deformity. On AP, the lateral border of the 1st metatarsal base should be aligned with the lateral border of the medial cuneiform and the medial 2nd metatarsal base should be in line with the medial border of the intermediate cuneiform. Also, look for a fleck sign. A *fleck sign* is a small subtle bone fragment seen between the medial cuneiform and the 2nd metatarsal base as a result of an avulsion of the Lisfranc ligament.

Treatment

Open or closed anatomic reduction with percutaneous pinning as close to the time of injury as possible is the treatment of choice. Casting unstable joints without fixation or making primary arthrodesis is rarely effective. The 2nd metatarsal is reduced first followed by the 1st and then 3rd through 5th. Inadequate reduction results in long-term arthrosis. The long-term sequela of this injury, when not adequately reduced, is arthrosis at which time arthrodesis is indicated.

Classification (Hardcastle)

Type A—Total Incongruity

Disruption of the entire Lisfranc joint complex in a sagittal or transverse plane, usually lateral but can be medial. This is the most common type.

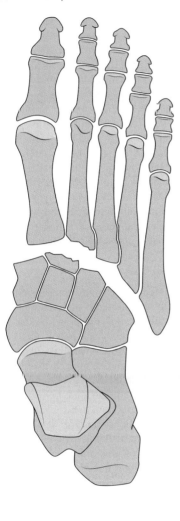

Type A

Entire Lisfranc joint in the sagittal or transverse plane. Usually lateral, but can be medial. This is the most common type.

Type B—Partial Incongruity

Partial incongruity involving the 1st ray medial dislocation only

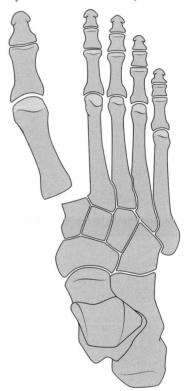

Type C—Divergent

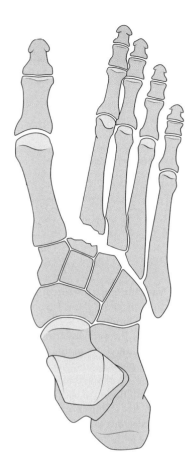

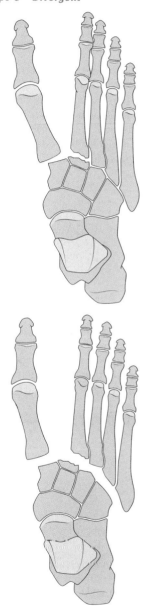

Type B1 (Partial Incongruity)

Type B2 (Partial or Complete Incongruity)

Involving 1st ray medially

Involving lateral displacement of lesser rays

Type C1 (Partial Displacement)

Type C2 (Total Displacement)

NAVICULAR FRACTURES

Central third of the navicular is avascular due to the extensive articular surfaces on the bone.

1. **Cortical Avulsion Fracture**: It is usually caused by excessive plantarflexion or eversion of the midfoot and results in an avulsion of the dorsal lip of the navicular. If it is a small fragment and painful, it can be removed.

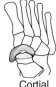

Cortial
Avulsion Fracture

2. **Tuberosity Fracture**: This is caused by forced eversion, resulting in an avulsion fracture from the posterior tibial tendon. There may be associated CC impaction.
Tx: ORIF if displaced

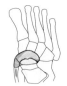

Tuberosity Fracture

3. **Navicular Body Fracture**: High-energy trauma with axial loading. ORIF if displaced. Anteromedial incision along the medial aspect of the tibialis

anterior. A second anterolateral incision may also be necessary. Severe intra-articular fractures may require arthrodesis to adjacent bones.

Sangeorzan Navicular Body Fracture Classification

Sangeorzan Navicular
Body Fx Classification

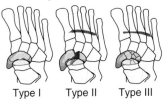

Type I   Type II   Type III

Type I: Primary fracture line is in the transverse plane. No angulation of forefoot.

Type II: Primary fracture line is dorsolateral to plantar medial with medial displacement of major dorsomedial fragment and adduction of the forefoot.

Type III: Comminuted fracture of navicular body in the sagittal plane with forefoot laterally displaced; possible CC impaction

4. **Stress Fracture**: It occurs in the sagittal plane in the relatively avascular middle third of the navicular. It often presents as an incomplete fracture without displacement.

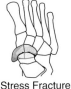

Stress Fracture

ACHILLES TENDON RUPTURE

Description

The Achilles tendon inserts on the middle 1/3 of the posterior aspect of the calcaneal tuberosity. Rupture of the Achilles tendon usually occurs in the area of poorest blood supply, 2 to 6 cm proximal to the calcaneal insertion. Patients usually remember the precipitating traumatic incident and may hear a pop at the time of rupture. Symptoms include pain, swelling, and weakness. There may be excessive dorsiflexion of the ankle when compared with the opposite foot. Active plantarflexion of the foot is still sometimes possible with a full rupture due to the posterior and lateral muscle groups.

The Achilles tendon consists of the gastrocnemius, soleus, and plantaris muscle tendons. The Achilles tendon has an internal rotation as one follows the tendon distally. This results in the gastrocnemius inserting laterally on the posterior aspect of the calcaneus, while the soleus inserts medially and the plantaris far medially and anterior. This anterior position of the plantaris means the calcaneus is a shorter lever arm for this tendon, and often after a complete rupture, the plantaris fibers will be the only tendon still intact. The plantaris muscle is absent in about 7% of the population.

Diagnosis

Thompson test: When the calf muscle is squeezed, the foot should plantarflex. If the foot does not plantarflex, this is a positive test and indicative of a rupture.

Kager triangle: On lateral radiograph, there should not be anything in the triangle. With an ATR, there is an increased soft-tissue density in the triangle because the flaps of the tendon fall into the triangle. The apex of the triangle may be blunted from the retracted tendon.

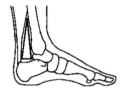

Toyger angle: A line drawn down the posterior aspect of the Achilles tendon should produce a straight line (180°); with an ATR, this angle decreases.

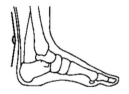

Palpable dell: There may be a palpable dell on palpation of the Achilles tendon.

Treatment

Conservative Treatment

Preferred treatment for older, sedentary patients. Begin with an NWB gravity below knee equinus cast and gradually bring foot up to neutral position by successive casting every 2 weeks.

Surgical Treatment

Preferred treatment for young, athletic patients. The ruptured tendon is reapproximated and sutured. After the tendon is repaired, the foot must be casted in equinus and worked up to neutral.

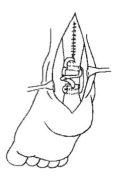

Bosworth

A 20-cm strip of the gastrocnemius aponeurosis is freed proximally, flapped distally, and woven through the proximal and distal tendon stumps to bridge the Achilles tendon.

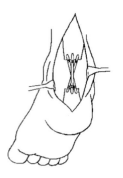

Bugg and Boyd

Three 1-cm fascia lata strips from ipsilateral thigh join the ruptured tendon defect and are sutured in tube-like manner around the Achilles tendon.

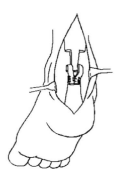

Lindholm

Two outer strips of the gastrocnemius aponeurosis are flapped distally to reinforce the tendon repair.

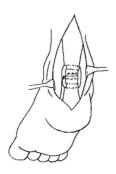

Repair Using Peroneus Brevis Tendon

Peroneus brevis is detached from its insertion and placed through a drill hole in the posterior calcaneus.

PERONEAL SUBLUXATION/ DISLOCATION

Skiing is the most common sports-related injury. The patient usually complains of a "snapping" sensation during and thereafter the traumatic incident. Spontaneous relocation is common but usually results in chronically dislocating peroneal tendon. During dislocation, there may be a "snapping" sensation. An avulsed cortical fleck fracture may be seen lying parallel to the lateral malleolus on a mortise view.

Normal anatomy

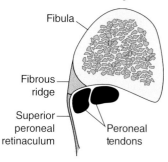

Classification (Eckert and Davis)

Grade I	Grade II	Grade III
(Most common) The retinaculum separates from the fibrocartilaginous ridge.	Involves the fibrocartilaginous ridge along with the retinaculum detaching from the fibula	(Least common) Involves an avulsion fracture of the fibula

Treatment

DuVries—Sliding Osteotomy of the Distal Fibula

Kelly—Distal Fibular Osteotomy With Rotation and Posterior Displacement Creating a Posterior Lip

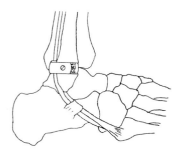

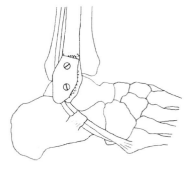

*Jones—Strip of Achilles Tendon
Used to Recreate the Superior
Peroneal Retinaculum*

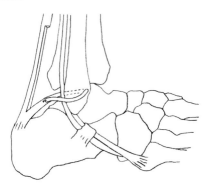

*Zoellner and Clancy—Groove
Deepening Procedure*

Groove deepening procedure (Zoellner and Clancy)

Dislocated or
dislocatable
peroneals

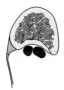

TIBIALIS POSTERIOR TENDON RUPTURE

Usually occurs at the zone of decreased vascularity, which is behind the medial malleolus. TP tendon rupture results in the collapse of the longitudinal arch. Patient may notice a progressive unilateral flattening of their arch, loss of forceful plantarflexion, and inversion. A clinical test for a TP rupture is to have the patient stand on their tiptoes. The heel should invert; if not, the TP may be ruptured.

Treatment

Surgical treatment involves primary end-to-end repair. The TP tendon can be reinforced by cutting the flexor digitorum longus (FDL) tendon and suturing it to the TP tendon. The distal end of the FDL can then be sutured to the FHL tendon to maintain active plantarflexion of digits 2 through 5.

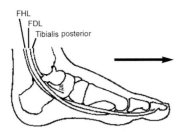 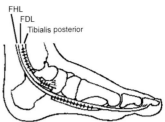

TIBIALIS ANTERIOR TENDON RUPTURE

Rupture of the tibialis anterior tendon is rare, but when it occurs, active dorsiflexion and inversion are decreased. Foot drop and steppage gait may be present. Tibialis anterior tendon rupture usually occurs 1 to 2 cm from tendon insertion. Surgical repair is often necessary in young active patients.

HYPOTHERMIA

Presentation at Various Temperatures

98.6°F	37°C	Average body temperature
95°F	35°C–35.5°C	Patient unaware of one-third of events around them
93.2°F	34°C	Extreme judgment errors, amnesia to current events
91.8°F	33.2°C	Frequent cardiac dysrhythmias-A fib
87.8°F	31°C	Loss of shivering
82.4°F	28°C	Pupils dilated
80.6°F	27°C	Flaccid body
78.8°F	26°C	Loss of consciousness
77.7°F	25°C–24°C	Loss of DTRs and vasoconstriction
68°F	20°C	Loss of pupil reflex to light
64.4°F	18°C	Flat EEG
51.9°F	10.5°C	Lowest cardiac activity
48.2°F	9°C	Lowest survival temperature recorded

Treatment

Hypothermia can be dangerous to treat due to:

Cardiac irritability

Afterdrop—paradoxical drop of core temperature occurring during rewarming

Methods of Rewarming

Passive	Warm environment, insulation (blankets)
Active external	Bodily contact, hot water bottle, electric blanket, immersion, radiant warmer
Active core	Warm IV, warm GI lavage, inhalation of heated humidified oxygen, peritoneal lavage

Electrocardiogram and electroencephalogram are not valid tools for determining death during hypothermia, and all available techniques of advanced life support should be continued until the patient is rewarmed to 35°C. "They're not dead until they're warm and dead."

FROSTBITE

Injury of the tissue due to freezing. Cellular damage occurs as a result of direct injury (jagged ice crystals) and ischemia. If there is any possibility of refreezing, the frostbitten area should not be thawed; refreezing increases tissue necrosis.

Classification

First degree: Superficial freezing without blistering. Pallor and waxy skin is occasionally present along with anesthesia, surrounding redness, and swelling.
Second degree: Superficial freezing with clear blistering
Third degree: Deep freezing with death of skin, hemorrhagic blisters, and subcutaneous involvement
Fourth degree: Full-thickness freezing, resulting in loss of function/body part

Symptoms

Firm/hard and cool to the touch
Affected area appears waxy white or blotchy blue gray.

Treatment

Symptoms of pain, burning, and pruritus may not be apparent until the body part is thawed. Analgesics are usually required during thawing. Profound edema, hemorrhagic blisters, necrosis, and gangrene may occur. Superficial frostbite (frostnip) can be rewarmed by applying constant warmth with gentle pressure from a warm hand (without rubbing) or by placing the affected body part against another part of the body that is warm. Full-thickness frostbite is best treated by rapid thawing at temperatures slightly above body temperature. Immerse body part in warm water 40°C to 42°C (104°F to 107.6°F) until it has returned to normal temperature (~30 minutes).

Keep affected area elevated at room temperature uncovered or with a loose sterile dressing. Amputation or debridement should not be performed until a line of demarcation between viable and dead tissue is established; this may take 3 to 5 weeks. Massage, application of ice water, or extreme heat is contraindicated.

CHILBLAINS (PERNIO)

A recurrent localized inflammation of small blood vessels resulting from cold. It is seen more commonly in cold climates with high humidity. Lesions are usually painful, pruritic, and burning. Lesions are edematous, erythematous, or violaceous and may blister and ulcerate. Treatment includes protecting area from trauma and secondary infection.

TRENCH FOOT (IMMERSION FOOT)

Caused by prolonged immersion in cool or cold water. The affected limb becomes swollen and appears waxy and mottled. Symptoms initially include numbness and tingling, and tissue death can occur. Treatment includes elevating the extremity and gently rewarming the limb, resulting in hyperemia followed by erythema, intense burning, and tingling. Blistering, swelling, erythema, ecchymosis, and ulceration may occur. A posthypothermic phase occurs at 2 to 6 weeks, resulting in cyanosis to the limb.

BURNS

Intact blisters should be left alone. Circumferential burns of the extremities may restrict blood flow, causing increased tissue pressure with resultant ischemia. In these cases, escharotomy is indicated. Dressings are applied to encourage healing and prevent infection; topical medications for this purpose include silver nitrate solution, silver sulfadiazine, and sodium mafenide.

Burn Size

Rule of Nines

Used to estimate the percentage of body burned in adults

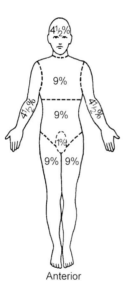

Anterior

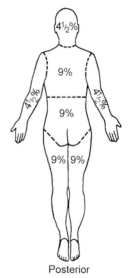

Posterior

Rule of Palm

Scattered burns can be estimated by comparing size of the patient's hand, which constitutes about 1.25% of the body surface. When one entire foot is burned, it is approximately equivalent to 3.5% of the body.

Burn Depth

Thickness	Degree	Depth	Appearance	Texture	Pinprick Sensation	Healing
Partial-thickness burns	First degree (involves only the epidermis)	Superficial epidermis	Erythematous painful	Normal to dry	Yes	3–5 d without scar
	Second degree (involves the dermis but does not penetrate the dermis)	Superficial partial—thickness epidermis, partial dermis	Edematous Erythematous blistered	Edematous Will blanch with pressure	Yes	10–21 d with minimal scar
		Deep partial thickness Entire epidermis and most of dermis	Pink or white	Thick Without blanching	Possibly	25–60 d dense scar Will usually require skin graft after excision of nonviable skin
Full-thickness burns	Third degree (damage extends through dermis)	Full thickness to the level of subcutaneous tissue layer	White, black, or brown Without blanching	Leathery	No	No spontaneous healing (usually requires skin graft) Dense scar

Treatment

Damage continues to progress from the burn site even after the source has been eliminated. Cooling the area with cold water (25°C or 77°F) can shorten this period of burn progression. Extremely cold water or ice is contraindicated. Blisters should be left intact and covered with sterile gauze impregnated with petroleum (i.e., Adaptic) or antiseptic petroleum (i.e., Xeroform). Circumferential wounds of the leg may have an eschar that constricts and impedes circulation; escharotomy and, possibly, fasciotomy may be necessary. Effective topicals for burns are silver nitrate solution, silver sulfadiazine, and mafenide acetate. Skin grafts may also be required. Months or years later, contractures and scarring may need to be released to maintain a plantigrade foot. Xenografts or allografts may be effective in extensive burns to impede dermal ischemia and provide protection of wound surface. Tetanus prophylaxis should also be considered.

DOG BITES

Responsible for 80% of bite wounds, 5% become infected
Most common organism:
  Pasteurella multocida

CAT BITES

Responsible for 10% of bite wounds
Most common organism:
  P. multocida
Thirty percent become infected because feline teeth are sharp and narrow (puncture wounds). Wounds caused by cat claws are considered equivalent to bites with regard to infection because cats are constantly grooming themselves and have saliva on their claws.
P. multocida is responsible for the majority of infections. *Pasteurella* infections advance rapidly (within 24 hours). This can be an important diagnostic tool because most other pathogens take >24 hours to manifest.

Cat-Scratch Disease (Fever)

Infectious organism is *Bartonella henselae.*
Symptoms: Tender raised papule at the site of inoculation followed by local lymphadenopathy, low-grade fever, and malaise

HUMAN BITES

Responsible for 3% of bite wounds
Thirty percent become infected.
Most common organism: *Streptococcus viridans*

Bite Categories

Occlusional injuries are actual bites of another person or self.
Clenched fist injuries (CFIs) occur when one person strikes another in the mouth with a clenched fist. Despite their innocuous appearance, they can result in serious infections because once the long extensor tendons over the knuckles retract, they carry bacteria deep into the tendon sheath. Human bites are also capable of transmitting infectious disease such as hepatitis B or HIV.

Treatment for Human/Animal Bites

Wound Management

Aerobic/anaerobic cultures, Gram stain

X-ray (check for fractures, OM-baseline)

Irrigate copiously

Suturing the wound is controversial; facial wounds are usually sutured for cosmetic reasons.

Antibiotic Prophylaxis

Recommended for all human bites, most cat bites, but only in high-risk dog bites. A high-risk dog bite includes bites on the hand and bites extending into a joint or to bone.

Penicillin is the drug of choice.

Amoxicillin/clavulanic acid (Augmentin) 250 to 500 mg PO tid will cover most bite pathogens.

Vaccinations

The need for tetanus and rabies prophylaxis should be evaluated. Bites by household pets do not usually require vaccination as long as the pet is healthy and available for observation for 10 days. For other animal bites, consider contacting the local health department and consult about the prevalence of rabies in the species of animal involved.

Puncture Wounds

Puncture wounds resulting in cellulitis are usually caused by *Staphylococcus aureus.*

Puncture wounds resulting in osteomyelitis are usually caused by *Pseudomonas aeruginosa.*

COMPARTMENT SYNDROME

Compartment syndrome results from an increase in the hydrostatic pressure of one of the osteofascial compartments of the leg or foot. This increase in compartment pressure results in decreased perfusion to the compartment, resulting in ischemia, infarction, and subsequent contractures (Volkmann contractures). The sequelae of an untreated compartment syndrome can result in lifelong disabilities, including chronic pain, neuropathy, claw toes, cavus foot, and chronic ulcers. Compartment syndrome is considered one of the few orthopedic medical emergencies, and it must be diagnosed and treated in a timely manner to prevent lifelong disabilities.

Compartment syndrome is more common in the leg than the foot. Tibial fractures are the most common cause of compartment syndrome in the lower extremity, and the anterior compartment of the leg is the most common compartment affected. The deep posterior compartment being the second most common.

Compartment syndrome can cause kidney damage secondary to myoglobinuria. Myoglobinuria results from the protein myoglobin being released during skeletal muscle necrosis (rhabdomyolysis). The iron byproducts of myoglobin can cause tubular obstruction and acute kidney injury. Myoglobinuria can present after 4 hours, and kidney function should be monitored.

Causes

Trauma (most notably crush injuries), surgery, burns, exercise, and tight cast

Diagnosis

Compartment syndrome requires rapid diagnosis and treatment to avoid irreversible nerve and muscle damage. Signs and symptoms can be vague and unreliable, especially in the foot.

Blood Tests

CK levels should be monitor to assess the degree of rhabdomyolysis.

Creatinine levels and urine protein level should be monitored to assess kidney function.

Signs/Symptoms

Six P's

Pain: Pain is the most reliable and earliest symptom. Pain from compartment syndrome is agonizing and poorly localized and does not response to pain medication. Pain presents out of proportion to the injury and is severely exacerbated with passive stretching of muscles. This would involve bending of the toes for foot compartment syndrome and flexing and extending the ankle for a leg compartment syndrome.

Paresthesia: Numbness, pins and needles. This is also a relatively early sign. There will be loss of 2 points discrimination and vibratory sensation.

Pallor: A poor prognostic indicator and a late finding. Foot may become pale due to loss of blood flow.

Paralysis: Late finding; at this point, the nerves have been damaged to a point where the patient cannot move their toes. Often permanent.

Poikilothermia: Late finding. Inability of the limb to thermoregulate. The foot may feel cold from ischemia.

Pulselessness: Late finding, indicates that compartmental pressure has risen enough to surpass systolic blood pressure and occlude a major artery.

The six P's are unreliable and most are signs of an established compartment syndrome. If all six P's are present, your window of opportunity has passed, and it is probably too late for a fasciotomy. The most important symptom for early diagnosis of an impending compartment syndrome is *pain disproportionate to that expected for the injury with increase in pain on passive muscle stretching.*

Timeline for Tissue Damage

Window of Opportunity for a Fasciotomy Is Within 8 Hours of the Compartment Pressure Being ≥30 mm Hg

Within the first 3 to 4 hours of compartment syndrome, muscular changes are still reversible. After 6 hours, there is clear muscle damage, and recovery is questionable depending on additional insults. After 8 hours of established compartment syndrome, irreversible changes have occurred to the muscles and nerves.

Muscle and Nerve Damage From Compartment Syndrome

Time	Muscle	Nerves
4 hours	Reversible	Neuropraxia (reversible)
6 hours	Variable	Variable
8 hours	Irreversible	Axonotmesis (irreversible)

Compartment Pressures

Absolute pressure theory: Compartment pressure $\geq$30 mm Hg is positive for a compartment syndrome.

Pressure gradient theory (DP): If the diastolic blood pressure minus the compartment pressure is <30 mm Hg, it is positive for compartment syndrome.

Regardless of which theory you subscribe to, it is prudent to be aware of the diastolic pressure because a higher diastolic pressure means you can maintain continued perfusion at a higher compartment pressure.

Normal resting compartment pressure	0 to 12 mm Hg
Compartment pressure during exercise	20 to 30 mm Hg

(within 5 to 10 minutes after exercise, it returns to normal)

Measuring Compartment Pressures

Compartment pressures are measured with a handheld manometer. Various types exist (Wick catheter, Stryker Stic, Slit catheter). Each compartment needs to be measured and remeasured at regular intervals. Anesthesia may be required. Open fractures do not preclude the possibility of a compartment syndrome. Pressure within each compartment is not uniform, and pressure is highest around the injury (fracture). When measuring compartment pressure, you should be within 5 cm of the injury (fracture) for an accurate reading. It is not good enough to simply be in the compartment. In the foot, the calcaneal compartment typically has the highest pressures and should always be measured. In calcaneal fractures, it is usually the calcaneal compartment that develops into a compartment syndrome. It is thought that it develops from rupture of the medial calcaneal artery.

Locations for Insertion Needle to Measure Foot Compartment Pressure

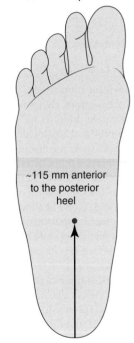

Superficial and deep central compartments

~115 mm anterior to the posterior heel

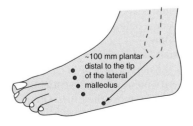

~100 mm plantar distal to the tip of the lateral malleolus

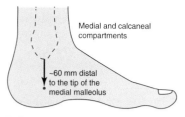

Medial and calcaneal compartments

~60 mm distal to the tip of the medial malleolus

EXERTIONAL COMPARTMENT SYNDROME

A form of compartment syndrome that develops from activity involving repetitive motion, such as swimming, tennis, or running. Pain or cramping when exercising is the most common symptom. Symptoms usually dissipated within 30 minutes after exercising.

Diagnosis of the condition requires putting the patient on a treadmill until symptoms develop and then taking compartment pressures.

Treatment included modification of activity, splinting, and elective fasciotomies. In contrast to acute compartment syndrome, minimally invasive surgical techniques may be attempted and only the affected compartment needs to be released.

Treatment

For a developing compartment syndrome, initial treatment should include removing any dressings or cast and keeping the foot at heart level, but not elevated above heart level. Elevating the extremity above heart level will further decrease the arterial pressure, increasing ischemia.

Compartment syndrome is a medical emergency, and once established, an emergency and immediate fasciotomy is indicated. The only effective way to decompress an acute compartment syndrome is by surgical fasciotomy. Open

fasciotomy should be performed as soon as possible to prevent necrosis and contractures. Long incisions are made into the foot and/or leg and left open to depressurize the compartments. Regardless of which compartment is involved, all four compartments should be decompressed if the condition is in the leg, and all nine if it is in the foot. No tourniquet is used during the procedure, and incisions are left open.

Patients are returned to the OR in about 2 to 5 days to debride necrotic tissue. Depending on the appearance of the site, loose closure of the incisions may be performed. Once perfusion has been reestablished and all necrotic tissue has been debrided, delayed primary closure or skin grafts may be applied.

If you miss your window of opportunity and do not perform a fasciotomy within 8 hours, it is probably best not to perform one at all. By this point, the damage has been done. Performing a fasciotomy would only expose the patient to the risk of infection.

Four Leg Compartments

Compartment	Content
Anterior	Tibialis anterior muscle Extensor hallucis longus Extensor digitorum longus
Lateral	Peroneus longus muscle Peroneus brevis muscle
Superficial posterior	Gastrocnemius muscle Soleus muscle
Deep posterior	Tibialis posterior muscle Flexor hallucis longus muscle Flexor digitorum longus muscle

In the leg, a fasciotomy is typically performed using two incisions.

Fasciotomy for compartment syndrome of the leg

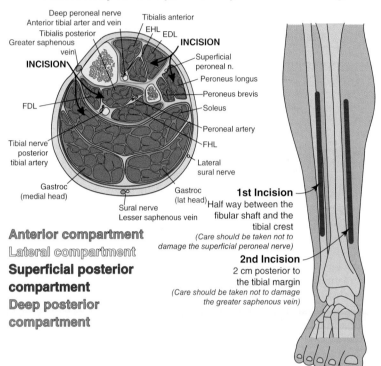

Deep peroneal nerve
Anterior tibial arter and vein
Tibialis posterior
Greater saphenous vein
INCISION
FDL
Tibial nerve
posterior tibial artery
Gastroc (medial head)

Tibialis anterior
EHL EDL
INCISION
Superficial peroneal n.
Peroneus longus
Peroneus brevis
Soleus
Peroneal artery
FHL
Lateral sural nerve
Gastroc (lat head)
Sural nerve
Lesser saphenous vein

Anterior compartment
Lateral compartment
Superficial posterior compartment
Deep posterior compartment

1st Incision
Half way between the fibular shaft and the tibial crest
(Care should be taken not to damage the superficial peroneal nerve)

2nd Incision
2 cm posterior to the tibial margin
(Care should be taken not to damage the greater saphenous vein)

Fasciotomy for Compartment Syndrome of the Foot

The most common approach involves two dorsal incisions and one medial.

Nine Foot Compartments

Compartment	Content
Medial	Flexor hallucis brevis Abductor hallucis
Lateral	Abductor digiti quinti Flexor digiti minimi
Superficial	Flexor digitorum brevis Lumbricals, FDL tendons
Interosseous (×4)	Dorsal and plantar interosseous muscles
Adductor (deep)	Adductor muscle
Calcaneal	Quadratus plantae Lateral plantar nerve

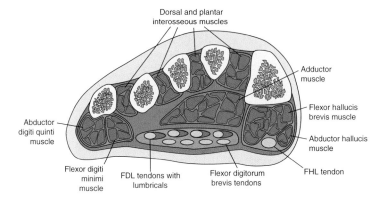

Dorsal and plantar
interosseous muscles

Adductor
muscle

Flexor hallucis
brevis muscle

Abductor
digiti quinti
muscle

Abductor hallucis
muscle

Flexor digiti
minimi
muscle

FDL tendons with
lumbricals

Flexor digitorum
brevis tendons

FHL tendon

Dorsal Incisions

Consists of two incisions, one incision is placed just medial to the 2nd metatarsal and one just lateral to the 4th metatarsal. This allows access to all the interosseous compartments and the adductor compartment with an adequate tissue bridge. The medial, lateral, and superficial compartments can theoretically be accessed through the dorsal incisions, but they are more easily accessed through a separate incision over the medial side of the foot.

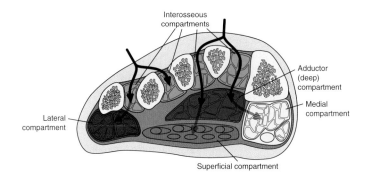

Interosseous
compartments

Adductor
(deep)
compartment

Medial
compartment

Lateral
compartment

Superficial compartment

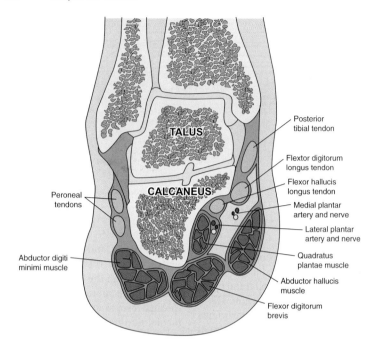

Peroneal tendons

Abductor digiti minimi muscle

TALUS

CALCANEUS

Posterior tibial tendon

Flexor digitorum longus tendon

Flexor hallucis longus tendon

Medial plantar artery and nerve

Lateral plantar artery and nerve

Quadratus plantae muscle

Abductor hallucis muscle

Flexor digitorum brevis

Medial Incision

The medial incision begins about 4 cm from the posterior aspect of the heel and 3 cm above the plantar surface. The incision is about 6 cm long and parallels the plantar surface. The fascia of the abductor hallucis muscle (medial compartment) is visible and should be split longitudinally. The muscle belly is then stripped from the fascia and retracted superiorly. This exposes the calcaneal compartment, which is decompressed. The superficial compartment is also visible lateral to the abductor hallucis muscle. The fascia of the flexor digitorum brevis (superficial compartment) is incised, and the muscle is retracted plantarly, exposing the lateral compartment.

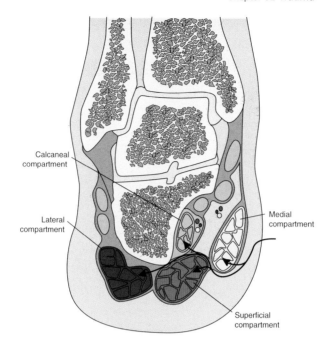

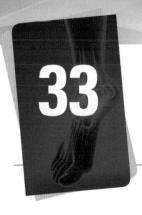

33 EMERGENCY MEDICINE

INSULIN SHOCK

Insulin shock is an acute condition from excessive insulin in the blood, resulting in low blood glucose levels (<50 mg per dL), convulsions, weakness, and coma.

Causes

Overdose of insulin

Skipped meal in an insulin-dependent diabetic

Strenuous exercise in an insulin-dependent diabetic

Symptoms

Tachycardia

Hunger

Increased irritability (nervousness)

Sweating and clammy (fainting)

Mental confusion and bizarre behavior

Seizures

Mild hypothermia

Coma

Treatment

If conscious, give fruit juice (orange juice).

If unconscious, IV 50% dextrose (50 mL at 10 mL per min). Most patients regain consciousness in 5 to 10 minutes.

DIABETIC KETOACIDOSIS

Diabetic ketoacidosis (DKA) results from excessive ketones in the blood as a result of the body's inability to manage insulin. Diabetics either lack the ability to make insulin (type 1) or their body lacks the ability to response to insulin (type 2). As a result, blood glucose levels rise. With the cells unable to use the glucose in the blood, the body begins to metabolize fat cells (which does not require insulin) for energy, a process called ketosis. Metabolizing fat cells for energy produces ketones as a byproduct. In diabetics, ketones can reach toxic levels and the body's pH begins to drop.

Symptoms

Altered mental status: From the brain being starved of energy
Weakness: From being starved of energy
Polyphagia (hunger): Because the cells are starving, they send signals to the brain that they are hungry.
Polyuria (excessive urination): This is the body's attempt to eliminate excess glucose and ketones in the blood. May result in orthostatic hypotension with tachycardia and poor skin turgor due to dehydration.
Electrolyte imbalance: Polyuria also causes a depletion of potassium (K^+) and other electrolytes.
Polydipsia (excessive thirst): As a result of the polyuria
Kussmaul breathing: Deep rapid respiratory pattern. This is the body's attempt to eliminate CO_2 that helps increase pH. The breath has a classic "acetone or fruity" smell consistent with ketones.

Causes

Failure to take adequate amounts of insulin

First manifestation of an undiagnosed diabetic
Conditions that increase the patient's requirements for insulin (infection, trauma)

Diagnosis

Test blood sugar, urine test to test for ketones in urine.

Treatment

Insulin, IV fluids, in severe cases, give bicarbonate to correct pH.

SYNCOPE

Temporary inadequate supply of blood to the brain from a vasovagal response (fainting)

Causes

Fear/anxiety
Pain
Hot airless room

Symptoms

Prodrome (Before Fainting)

Lightheaded, yawning
Nausea
Patient complains of feeling hot.
Dimming of vision
Skin is cool, clammy, pale, and diaphoretic.
Tachycardia

Unconsciousness

Slow weak pulse (bradycardia replaces tachycardia)
Abnormal movements may be noted during unconsciousness.

Treatment

Lay patient flat.

Loosen neckwear.

Inhalation of aromatic spirits of
ammonia

On recovery, rest the patient and
administer sips of water.

Syncope may reoccur, especially
if the patient stands up within
30 minutes after the attack.

MALIGNANT HYPERTHERMIA

Malignant hyperthermia is a rare
but potentially life-threatening
condition that can occur as a result
of exposure to certain anesthetic
agents during general anesthesia.
The muscle relaxant involved is
usually succinylcholine, and the
inhalational anesthetic is most often halothane, although isoflurane,
sevoflurane, or desflurane may be
responsible. Malignant hyperthermia is an autosomal dominant inherited trait, which affects about 1
per 20,000 people. When patients
with this trait are exposed to anesthetic agents, the calcium stored
in their muscles is released, causing the muscles to fasciculate and
contract. This rapid acceleration
of muscle metabolism causes very
high fever, muscle breakdown, and
increased acidosis. Without prompt
diagnosis and treatment, the condition can be fatal.

Symptoms

Dramatic rise in body temperature

Rigid or painful muscles, especially
the jaw

Fasciculations

Profuse sweating

Tachycardia, tachypnea, unstable
BP, arrhythmias, acidosis, shock

Cyanosis (mottled skin, dark blood
at op-site)

Treatment

Surgery and anesthesia are discontinued as soon as malignant
hyperthermia is suspected.

IV dantrolene given 2.5 mg per kg
rapid IV bolus. Dantrolene is a
muscle relaxant that stops the
dangerous increase in muscle
metabolism.

Patients must be cooled with IV
iced saline (not Ringer) and surface cooling with ice.

Oral dantrolene 1 to 3 days after
episode

LOCAL ANESTHETIC TOXICITY

Cause

Exceeding toxic dose levels

Accidental intravascular injection

Symptoms

Primarily involves the central
nervous system and, at higher
plasma concentrations, the cardiovascular system

CNS Stimulation

Restlessness, agitation, confusion,
dizziness, perioral paresthesias,
tinnitus, and tremors of the face
and distal extremities; tonic–
clonic (grand mal) convulsions
may follow.

CV Toxicity

CV stimulation (HTN, tachycardia)
usually begins after signs of CNS
toxicity develop and is more a
result of hypoxia than a direct
action of the anesthetic. Further

increase in blood concentration leads to CV depression, bradycardia, hypotension, and heart block, which may lead to cardiac arrest.

Treatment

Maintain airway
   O_2
Twitching/convulsions
   Valium 5 to 10 mg IV/IM
Cardiac depression
   Atropine 0.4 mg IV
   Epinephrine or metaraminol
      2 mg IV/IM

ACUTE ASTHMATIC ATTACK

Characterized by a variable and intermittent degree of lower airway obstruction caused by a narrowing of bronchioles due to smooth muscle hyperactivity and edema of the mucosa

Symptoms

Breathlessness with expiratory wheezing
Cyanosis

Cause

Allergies (grass, pollen, animal hair)
Drugs
Emotional stress

Treatment

Reassurance, rest, O_2
At-risk patients may carry an aerosol inhaler containing a bronchodilator (salbutamol, terbutaline).
Epinephrine (same dosage/concentration as in anaphylaxis)
   SC every 20 minutes up to three doses. If no relief, aminophylline (theophylline) IV 5 to 6 mg per kg over 20 minutes.

ANAPHYLAXIS

Anaphylaxis is a life-threatening allergic response to a substance the body views as foreign (antigen). The reaction is a direct result of the release of chemicals (e.g., histamines and leukotrienes) from mast cells and basophils. Anaphylaxis occurs only after a patient has been previously exposed to the antigen. It requires sensitization to the antigen through immunoglobulin E (IgE) antibodies.

Causes—Can Be Just About Anything

Narcotic analgesics
Local anesthesia (esters greater than amides)
Drugs (PCN, sulfonamides, ASA)
Foods (nuts, strawberries, shellfish, eggs)
Bee stings

Symptoms

Symptoms typically begin within 1 to 15 minutes following exposure to the triggering agent.
Patient feels uneasy and becomes agitated and flushed. Local urticarial and pruritus may develop. Angioedema occurs, which is similar to urticaria but over a larger area, involving the SC as well as the dermis and often occurring in the eyelids, lips, or tongue. Dyspnea/apnea due to laryngeal edema and bronchospasm (responsible for most fatalities).

Treatment

Inject 0.3 to 0.5 mL (0.3 to 0.5 cc) 1:1,000 epinephrine IM or SC. Epinephrine can also be given IV, but use caution due to possible arrhythmias. If anaphylaxis is due to a reaction on an extremity (i.e., bee sting, vaccination, or other injection), apply tourniquet and inject another 0.25 mL epinephrine 1:1,000 SC at site. PO/IM/IV antihistamines are also recommended.

ANAPHYLACTOID REACTION

Similar to anaphylaxis, but can occur after the first exposure. It does not require sensitization or the presence of IgE antibodies. These reactions have a dose-related toxic idiosyncratic mechanism rather than an immunologically mediated one. Substances that can initiate an anaphylactoid reaction such contrast dye, NSAIDs, and ASA cause a direct breakdown of the mast cells and basophil cells.

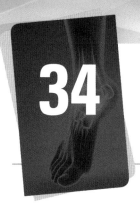

34 PODIATRIC ABBREVIATIONS

ā	before
AAA	autolyzed antigen-extracted allogeneic
AAO	alert, awake, and oriented
AACPM	American Association of Colleges of Podiatric Medicine
AAWM	American Academy of Wound Management
AAT	activity as tolerated
Ab	antibodies
ABC	absolute blood count
	absolute basophil count
	aneurysmal bone cyst
	airway, breathing, circulation
ABPOPPM	American Board of Podiatric Orthopedics and Primary Podiatric Medicine
Abd	abdomen
	abductor
ABE	acute bacterial endocarditis
ABG	arterial blood gas
ABI	ankle brachial index
ABPO	American Board of Podiatric Orthopedics
ABPS	American Board of Podiatric Surgery
ABR	absolute bed rest
ABS	Accu-Chek blood sugar at bedside
ABSSSI	acute bacterial skin and skin structure infections
ABX	antibiotics
AC	before meals
ACD	allergic contact dermatitis
ACE	angiotensin-converting enzyme
ACFAOM	American College of Foot and Ankle Orthopedics and Medicine
ACFAS	American College of Foot and Ankle Surgeons
ACh	acetylcholine
ACL	anterior cruciate ligament
ACLS	advanced cardiac life support
ACU	ambulatory care unit

AD	admitting diagnosis
	Alzheimer disease
	antidepressant
	atopic dermatitis
ADA	American Diabetic Association
ADD	adduction
	attention deficit disorder
	average daily dose
ADM	admission
ADR	adverse drug reaction
AFB	acid-fast bacilli
AF	afebrile
AFL	atrial flutter
AFO	ankle fixation orthotic
	ankle–foot orthosis
AFP	α-fetoprotein
AHCPR	Agency for Health Care Policy and Research
AITFL	anterior inferior tibiofibular ligament
AIIS	anterior inferior iliac spine
AK	above knee
AKA	above knee amputation
	alcoholic ketoacidosis
a.k.a.	also known as
A-line	arterial catheter
ALL	allergies
ALP	alkaline phosphatase
ALS	acute lateral sclerosis
	advanced life support
ALT	alanine transaminase (SGPT)
ALZ	Alzheimer disease
AM	morning
AMA	against medical advice
	American Medical Association
AMB	ambulate
AMI	acute myocardial infarction
ANA	antinuclear antibody
AO	Arbeitgemeinschaft für Osteosynthesefragen (translated: Association for the Study of Internal fixation)
AOA	All Orthopedic Appliances
AODM	adult-onset diabetes mellitus
AP	anterior-posterior (x-ray)
A&P	assessment and plan
APAP	N-acetyl-para-aminophenol (acetaminophen)
APMSA	American Podiatric Medical Students Association
APMSB	American Podiatric Medical Specialties Board
APGAR	appearance (color), pulse, grimace (reflex irritability), activity (muscle tone), and respiration
aPTT	activated partial thromboplastin time
ARC	AIDS-related complex
	American Red Cross

ARDS	adult respiratory distress syndrome
ARIF	arthroscopic reduction and internal fixation
ART	Achilles reflex test
ASA	acetylsalicylic acid (aspirin)
ASIF	Association for the Study of Internal Fixation
ASIS	anterior superior iliac spine
ASO	arteriosclerosis obliterans
AST	aspartate transaminase (a.k.a. serum glutamic oxaloacetic transaminase [SGOT])
ATF	anterior talofibular (ligament)
ATL	Achilles tendon lengthening
ATR	Achilles tendon rupture
	Achilles tendon repair
AVB	atrioventricular block
AVD	aortic valve disease
AVN	avascular necrosis
AVSS	afebrile, vital signs stable
AZT	azidothymidine (zidovudine)
B	black
b/4	before
B9	benign
Bab	Babinski
BAND	band neutrophil
BaS	barium swallow
BB	β-blocker
	blood bank
	blue bloater
	both bones
	breast biopsy
BBB	blood–brain barrier
	bundle branch block
B/C	because
BCC	basal cell carcinoma
BCP	birth control pills
	blood cell profile
BD	birth date
	birth defect
	brain dead
	UK abbreviation for twice a day
BG	basal ganglion
	blood glucose
	bone graft
BGL	blood glucose level
bid	twice a day ("bis in die")
BIL	bilateral
BK	below knee
BKA	below knee amputation
BKWP	below knee walking plaster (cast)
B/L	bilateral

BLE	both lower extremities
BLS	basic life support
BM	black male
	bowel movement
BMK	birthmark
BMP	basic metabolic panel
BP	bathroom privileges
	blood pressure
	birth place
BPM	beats per minute
BPN	bacitracin, polymyxin B, and neomycin sulfate
BPR	blood per rectum
BR	bathroom
	bedrest
BRB	bright red blood
BRP	bathroom privileges
BS	barium swallow
	bedside
	blood sugar
	bowel sounds
	breath sounds
BT	bleeding time
BUN	blood urea nitrogen
	bunion
Bx	biopsy
BZD	benzodiazepine
c̄	with ("cum")
CI-CV	controlled substance (schedules I–V)
CA	cancer
	Candida albicans
CABG	coronary artery bypass graft
CABP	community-acquired bacterial pneumonia
CAD	coronary artery disease
CAL	callus
	calories
CANC	canceled
CASPR	Central Application Service for Podiatric Residencies
CAT	computed axial tomography
CBC	complete blood count
CBR	complete bedrest
CC	chief complaint
	creatinine clearance
C&C	cold and clammy
	chip and clip
CCI	correct coding initiative
CCU	coronary care unit
	critical care unit
CCV	cell conductivity volume
CDC	Centers for Disease Control and Prevention

CDH	congenital dislocation of the hip
CDS	controlled dangerous substances
CEA	carcinoembryonic antigen
CF	cystic fibrosis
	calcaneofibular (ligament)
CFI	clenched fist injury
C&H	curette and hyfrecation
CHEM 6	lab test for (glu, BUN, K, Na, Cl, and CO_2)
CHEM 7	lab test for (glu, BUN, creatinine, K, Na, Cl, and CO_2)
CHEM 12	lab test for (glu, BUN, uric acid, Ca, P, total protein, albumin, chol, total bilirubin, alkaline phosphatase, SGOT, and LDH)
CHEM 18	CHEM 12 + CHEM 6
CHEM 23	CHEM 12 + (Na, K, CO_2, Cl, direct bilirubin, indirect bilirubin, triglyceride, SGPT, R fraction, BUN/creatinine ratio)
CHF	congestive heart failure
CHI	closed head injury
chol	Cholesterol
CIA	calcaneal insufficiency avulsion
	calcaneal inclination angle
CIG	cigarettes
Circ	circulation
CK	creatine kinase
CKC	closed kinetic chain
CKD	chronic kidney disease
CLIA	Clinical Laboratory Improvement Act
CLI	critical limb ischemia
CLTI	chronic limb-threatening ischemia
CMI	cell-mediated immunity
CMT	Charcot–Marie tooth
CMV	cytomegalovirus
CN	cranial nerve
C/O	complained of
COCCIO	coccidioidomycosis
COMP	complications
	compound
	compress
conc	concentration
COPD	chronic obstructive pulmonary disease
COTH	Council on Teaching Hospitals
COX-1	cyclooxygenase isoenzyme 1
COX-2	cyclooxygenase isoenzyme 2
CP	cerebral palsy
	chest pain
	chronic pain
CPK	creatine phosphokinase
CPK-1	creatine phosphokinase MM fraction
CPK-2	creatine phosphokinase MB fraction
CPM	continuous passive motion
CPMA	California Podiatric Medical Association
CPME	Council of Podiatric Medical Education

CPMM	constant passive motion machine
CPPD	calcium pyrophosphate dehydrate (pseudo gout)
CREST	calcinosis, Raynaud disease, esophageal dysmotility, sclerodactyly, and telangiectasia
CRIF	closed reduction and internal fixation
crit.	hematocrit
CRP	C-reactive protein
CRNA	Certified Registered Nurse Anesthetist
CROW	Charcot restraint orthotic walker
CRTX	cast removed take x-ray
CS	cervical spine
	cesarean section
	cigarette smoker
CSF	cerebrospinal fluid
cSSSI	complicated skin and skin structure infection
C&S	culture and sensitivity
C/S	culture and sensitivity
CT	computed tomography
	Coombs test
CTD	connective tissue disease
CVA	cerebrovascular accident
CVD	cardiovascular disease
CWS	Certified Wound Specialist
CXR	chest x-ray
D	dextrose
DASA	distal articular set angle
DC	discharge
	dihydrocodeine
d/c	discontinue
DC'd	discontinued
DCMO	distal chevron metatarsal osteotomy
DCP	dynamic compression plate
DD	differential diagnosis
	dry dressing
DDI	dressing dry and intact
DDx	differential diagnosis
DEA#	Drug Enforcement Administration number
DF	dorsiflexion
DFU	diabetic foot ulcer
DFWO	dorsiflexory wedge osteotomy
DHEA	dehydroepiandrosterone
DI	diabetes insipidus
D&I	debridement and irrigation dry and intact
DIC	disseminated intravascular coagulation
DIPJ	distal interphalangeal joint
DISH	diffuse idiopathic skeletal hyperostosis
DJD	degenerative joint disease
DKA	diabetic ketoacidosis
dL	deciliter (100 mL)
DLE	discoid lupus erythematosus

D₅LR	dextrose 5% in lactated Ringer
DM	diabetes mellitus
DMAA	distal metatarsal articular angle (a.k.a. PASA)
DMD	Duchenne muscular dystrophy
DMERC	Durable Medical Equipment Regional Carrier
DMSO	dimethyl sulfoxide
D5NS	dextrose 5% in 0.9% sodium chloride
D5½NS	dextrose 5% in 0.45% sodium chloride
DNR	do not resuscitate
DO	doctor of osteopathy
	doctor's orders
DOA	date of admission
DOACs	dead on arrival
	direct oral anticoagulants
DOB	date of birth
DOC	drug of choice
DOI	date of injury
DP	dorsal-plantar (x-ray)
	diastolic pressure
	discharge planning
	dorsalis pedis
DPM	doctor of podiatric medicine
DPP	dorsalis pedis pulse
DPT	diphtheria, pertussis, and tetanus
DS	discharge summary
	double strength
DSD	discharge summary dictated
	dry sterile dressing
DTaP	diphtheria and tetanus toxoids with acellular pertussis vaccine
DTP	diphtheria, tetanus toxoids, and pertussis vaccine
DTM	dermatophyte test medium
DTR	deep tendon reflex
DTwP	diphtheria and tetanus toxoids with whole-cell pertussis vaccine
DVT	deep venous thrombosis
D₅W	5% dextrose in water
Dx	diagnosis
dz	disease
EBL	estimated blood loss
EBV	Epstein–Barr virus
ECCE	extracapsular cataract extraction
ECG	electrocardiogram
ECT	European Compression Technique
EDB	extensor digitorum brevis
EDCP	eccentric dynamic compression plate
EDG	electrodynography
EDIN	endoscopic decompression of intermetatarsal neuroma
EDL	extensor digitorum longus
EDQ	extensor digiti quinti
EDS	Ehlers–Danlos syndrome
EDTA	ethylenediaminetetraacetic acid (anticoagulant in blood specimens)

EEE	edema, erythema, and exudate
EEG	electroencephalogram
EENT	eyes, ears, nose, and throat
EES	erythromycin
EFB	elevate foot of bed
e.g.,	exempli gratia (for example)
EHB	extensor hallucis brevis
EHL	extensor hallucis longus
EKG	electrocardiogram
ELISA	enzyme-linked immunosorbent assay
EMG	electromyogram
EMS	emergency medical services
EMT	emergency medical technician
ENG	electroneurogram
ENT	ears, nose, and throat
EOM	extraocular muscles
EOMI	extraocular muscles intact
EPF	endoscopic plantar fasciotomy
epi	epinephrine
EPO	Exclusive Provider Organization
ER	emergency room
ES	extra strength
ESBL	extended spectrum β-lactamase
ESR	erythrocyte sedimentation rate
ESWT	extracorporeal shock wave therapy
ET	enterostomal therapy
EtOH	alcohol
FACFAS	Fellow of American College of Foot and Ankle Surgery
FACFAOM	Fellow American College of Foot and Ankle Orthopedics and Medicine
FB	fasting blood (sugar)
	foreign body
FBS	fasting blood sugar
FDB	flexor digitorum brevis
FDI	flexible digital implant
FDL	flexor digitorum longus
FDM	flexor digiti minimi
FF	forefoot
FFD	focal film distance
FFF	flexible forefoot
FFF-STA	flexible forefoot with short tendo-Achilles
FFP	fresh-frozen plasma
FH	family history
FHB	flexor hallucis brevis
FHL	flexor hallucis longus
FOB	foot of bed
FROM	full range of motion
FS	fingerstick
	full strength
FSH	follicle-stimulating hormone

FT	filling time
	foot
F/U	follow-up
FUO	fever of undetermined origin
fx	fracture
FYI	for your information
GA	general anesthesia
	general appearance
Ga	gallium
GAG	glycosaminoglycan
GB	gallbladder
GBS	Guillain–Barré syndrome
GC	gonococci (gonorrhea)
GDM	gestational diabetes mellitus
GFR	glomerular filtration rate
GG	γ-globulin
GH	growth hormone
GHb	glycosylated hemoglobin
GI	gastrointestinal
GS	general surgery
	Gram stain
GTT	glucose tolerance test
GU	genitourinary
HAI	hospital-acquired infection
HAV	hepatitis A virus
	hallux abducto valgus
Hb	hemoglobin
HbA$_{1c}$	glycosylated hemoglobin
HBcAb	hepatitis B core antibody
HBcAg	hepatitis B core antigen
HBIG	hepatitis B immune globulin
HBO	hyperbaric oxygen
HBsAg	hepatitis B surface antigen
HBV	hepatitis B vaccine
	hepatitis B virus
HCA	health care associated
	Hospital Corporation of America
hCG	human chorionic gonadotropin
Hct	hematocrit
HCTZ	hydrochlorothiazide (a thiazide diuretic)
HD	heloma durum
HDCV	human diploid cell rabies vaccine
HDL	high-density lipoprotein
HEENT	head, eyes, ears, nose, and throat
Hg	hemoglobin
Hgb	hemoglobin
HHS	Health and Human Services
HIV	human immunodeficiency virus
HL	hallux limitus
HLA	human leukocyte antigen

	human lymphocyte antigen
HM	heloma molle
HMO	Health Maintenance Organization
HMP	Health Maintenance Plan
H/O	history of
H_2O_2	hydrogen peroxide
HOPI	history of present illness
H&P	history and physical
HPI	history of present illness
HR	hallux rigidus
	heart rate
HS	bedtime ("hora somni")
	half strength
	heel spur
HSV	herpes simplex virus
HT	hammertoe
	heart
	height
HTN	hypertension
HV	hallux valgus
Hx	history
I	impression
	intact
IBS	irritable bowel syndrome
IC	between meals
ICCU	intensive coronary care unit
ICS	intercostal space
ICU	intensive care unit
ID	identification
	infectious dz
I&D	incision and drainage
IDDM	insulin-dependent diabetes mellitus
i.e.,	id est (that is)
Ig	immunoglobulin
IGTN	ingrown toenail
IM	intermetatarsal intermuscular
IMA	intermetatarsal angle
IMN	intermetatarsal neuroma
INAD	in no apparent distress
INF	infarction
	infection
	inferior
	infusion
INR	international normalized ratio (for anticoagulant monitoring)
INT	internal
INV	inversion
IO	intraoperative
I&O	ins and outs
IOL	intraocular lens

IP	in plaster
	interphalangeal
IPD	inflammatory pelvic dz
IPJ	interphalangeal joint
IPK	intractable plantar keratosis
IS	interspace
iTCC	instant total contact cast
IU	international unit
IV	intravenous
IVIg	intravenous immunoglobulin
IVPB	intravenous piggyback
IVUS	intravenous ultrasound
JAMA	Journal of the American Medical Association
JAPMA	Journal of the American Podiatric Medical Association
JCAHO	Joint Commission on Accreditation of Healthcare Organizations
JNT	joint
JRRC	Joint Residency Review Committee
jt	joint
JVD	jugular venous distention
KA	ketoacidosis
KAFO	knee–ankle–foot orthosis
KAO	knee–ankle orthosis
KB	ketone bodies
KDA	known drug allergies
KFAO	knee–foot–ankle orthosis
KISS	keep it simple stupid
KJ	knee jerk
KOH	potassium hydroxide
KS	Kaposi sarcoma
KVO	keep vein open
KVp	kilovoltage
K-wire	Kirschner wire
L	left
LA	left atrium
	local anesthetic
LARD	length, angulation, rotation, displacement
LASA	Lisfranc articular set angle
LASER	Light Amplification by Stimulated Emission of Radiation
LAT	lateral
	left anterior thigh
LATAS	location, alignment, type, articular, stability
LCL	lateral collateral ligament
LCN	lidocaine
LCPD	Legg Calvé Perthes dz
LD	lactic dehydrogenase
LDH	lactic dehydrogenase
LDL	low-density lipoprotein
LE	lower extremity
	lupus erythematosus
LEA	lower extremity amputation

LEF	lower extremity fracture
LF	left foot
LH	luteinizing hormone
Lido	lidocaine
LL	left lateral
	left leg
	left lower
	long leg (brace or cast)
	lower leg
LLB	long leg brace
LLC	long leg cast
LLD	limb length discrepancy
LLE	left lower extremity
LLP	long leg plaster
LLQ	left lower quadrant
LLSB	left lower sternal border
LLWC	long leg walking cast
LLX	left lower extremity
LMH	Lesser Metatarsal Head Implant
LO	lateral oblique (x-ray)
LOC	local
	loss of consciousness
LOPS	loss of protective sensation
LC-DCP	limited contact dynamic compression plate
LR	lactated Ringer
LSB	left sternal border
LT	left
	light touch
LTT	lactose tolerance test
LUQ	left upper quadrant
LVN	Licensed Vocational Nurse
LX	lower extremity
M	male
	meter
	medial
	Monday
	mother
	muscle
mA	milliamperage
MAO	monoamine oxidase
MAC	monitored anesthesia care
	maximum allowable concentration
	minimum alveolar concentration
MAFO	molded ankle/foot orthosis
MBA	Maxwell–Brancheau arthroereisis
MC	metatarsocuneiform
	molluscum contagiosum
mcg	microgram (μm)
MCH	mean corpuscular hemoglobin

MCHC	mean corpuscular hemoglobin concentration
MCL	midclavicular line
MCV	mean corpuscular volume
MDC	medial dorsal cutaneous (nerve)
MDR	multidrug-resistant
MDRO	multidrug-resistant organism
MED	medication
	medial
MET	metatarsal
	metastasis
MFT	muscle function test
MHA-TP	microhemagglutination *Treponema pallidum*
MHW	medial heel wedge
MI	myocardial infarction
	mitral insufficiency
MIC	minimal inhibitory concentration
MIO	minimally invasive osteosynthesis
MIPO	minimally invasive plate osteosynthesis
MIS	minimally invasive surgery
MM	medial malleolus
	morbidity and mortality
	multiple myeloma
	malignant melanoma
MMP	matrix metalloproteinase
MMR	measles, mumps, and rubella
MO	medial oblique (x-ray)
MOA	mode of action
MOI	mechanism of injury
MPF	methylparaben free (an antifungal agent used as a preservative)
MPJ	metatarsophalangeal joint
MPV	metatarsus primus varus
MR	medical record
MRI	magnetic resonance imaging
MRSA	methicillin-resistant *Staphylococcus aureus*
MS	morphine sulfate
MSSA	multiple sclerosis
	methicillin-susceptible *Staphylococcus aureus*
MT	metatarsal
MTA	metatarsus adductus
MTJ	mid-tarsal joint
MTP	metatarsal phalangeal (joint)
MUA	manipulation under anesthesia
MVA	motor vehicle accident
MVC	motor vehicle collision
N	nerve
	normal
NA	not applicable
NAD	no apparent distress
NB	nail bed
	needle biopsy

NC	no change
	no complaints
NCV	nerve conduction velocity
NE	neurologic examination
NG	nitroglycerin
NGU	nongonococcal urethritis
NHD	normal hair distribution
NIDD	non–insulin-dependent diabetes
NIDDM	non–insulin-dependent diabetes mellitus
NINVS	noninvasive neurovascular studies
NK	not known
NKA	no known allergies
NKDA	no known drug allergies
NKFA	no known food allergies
NKMA	no known medication allergies
NL	normal
NLD	necrobiosis lipoidica diabeticorum
NMR	nuclear magnetic resonance (same as MRI)
NOACS	novel (or new) oral anticoagulants
non pal	not palpable
NOS	nitric oxide synthase
	no organisms seen
	not otherwise specified
NPH	neutral protamine Hagedorn (an intermediate-acting insulin), no previous Hx
NPO	nothing by mouth ("nil per os")
NPUAP	National Pressure Ulcer Advisory Panel
NR	no refills
	no response
NS	normal saline (0.9% NaCl)
NSAID	nonsteroidal anti-inflammatory drug
NSC	nonservice-connected
NSCD	nonservice-connected disability
NSR	normal sinus rhythm
NSS	normal saline solution
NSU	nonspecific urethritis
NTG	nitroglycerin
N&V	nausea and vomiting
NVS	neurovascular status
NWB	non–weight bearing
O	objective findings
OA	osteoarthritis
OACs	oral anticoagulants
OCD	osteochondritis dissecans
OCT	optical coherence tomography
OD	overdose
	right eye (oculus dexter)
OGTT	oral glucose tolerance test
OKC	open kinetic chain
OM	osteomyelitis

OMAHI	operations, medicines, allergies, hospitalizations, illnesses
OOC	out of cast
OOP	out of plaster
OPIM	other potentially infectious materials
OPS	outpatient surgery
OR	operating room
ORIF	open reduction internal fixation
OS	left eye
OSHA	Occupational Safety and Health Act
OT	occupational therapist
OTC	over-the-counter
OU	both eyes
$\bar{p}$	after
P&A	phenol and alcohol (matrixectomy)
PAB	pronation-abduction
PACU	postanesthesia care unit
PAROM	passive assistance range of motion
PASA	proximal articular set angle
PB	paraffin bath
PBN	polymyxin B sulfate, bacitracin, and neomycin
PC	after meals ("post cibum")
	packed cells
	present complaint
PCA	patient-controlled analgesia
PCC	poison control center
PCD	Phlegmasia cerulea dolens
PCN	penicillin
PCP	*Pneumocystis carinii* pneumonia
	primary care physician
P_{CO_2}	partial pressure of carbon dioxide
PCV	packed cell volume
PDR	Physician's Desk Reference
PDS	polydioxanone suture
PDU	pulsed Doppler ultrasonography
PE	physical examination
	pulmonary embolism
PEARL	pupils equal accommodation, reactive to light
PEARLA	pupils equal and react to light and accommodation
PER	pronation-external rotation
PERLA	pupils equally reactive to light and accommodation
PERRLA	pupils equal, round, and react to light and accommodation
PET	positive emission tomography
PFSH	past family and social history
PG	prostaglandin
PGA	polyglycolic acid
pH	hydrogen concentration
PH	personal history
PICC	peripherally inserted central catheter
PID	pelvic inflammatory disease
PIPJ	proximal interphalangeal joint
PITFL	posterior inferior tibiofibular ligament

PLLA	poly-L-lactic acid
PLT	platelet
PMH	past medical history
PMI	point of maximum impulse
PMMA	polymethylmethacrylate
PMN	polymorphonuclear leukocytes
PMR	posteromedial release (for clubfoot)
	Podiatric Medicine Residency
	Physical Medicine and Rehabilitation
PMS	premenstrual syndrome
PN	progress note
PNA	partial nail ablation
PO	by mouth ("per os")
PONV	postoperative nausea and vomiting
POR	podiatric orthopedic residency
PP	pedal pulse
PPAC	Podiatric Political Action Committee
	Practicing Physicians Advisory Council
PPBS	postprandial blood sugar
PPD	porokeratosis plantaris discreta
PPE	personal protective equipment
PPO	preferred provider organization
PPP	pedal pulses present
	piezogenic pedal papules
	Pseudomonas, Proteus, Providencia
PR	per rectum
PRBC	packed red blood cells
PRICE	protection, rest, ice, compression, and elevation
PRN	pro re nata (as needed)
PROM	passive range of motion
PRIB	Peacock, Reverdin, Isham, Bosch (a minimally invasive bunionectomy)
PSA	prostate-specific antigen
PSH	past surgical history
PSR	podiatric surgical residency
PSST	pressure sore status tool
pt	patient
PT	physical therapy
	prothrombin time
	posterior tibial (pulse)
PTA	percutaneous transluminal angioplasty
	physical therapy assistant
	posttraumatic amnesia
	prior to admission
PTF	posterior talofibular (ligament)
PTFE	polytetrafluoroethylene (artificial veins are made of this material)
PTH	parathyroid hormone
PTR	patella tendon reflex
PTT	partial thromboplastin time
PTTD	posterior tibial tendon dysfunction

PVD	peripheral vascular disease
PVNS	pigmented villonodular synovitis
PW	puncture wound
PWB	partial weight bearing
PWS	port wine stain
Px	physical examination
	prognosis
PYP	technetium Tc 99 m pyrophosphate kit
PZI	protamine zinc insulin (a long-acting insulin)
q	every
QAM	every morning
qd	every day
q4h	every 4 hours
qh	every hour
qhs	every night
qid	four times a day ("quarter in die")
qod	every other day
qpm	every night
QS	every shift
R	right
	respirations
RA	rheumatoid arthritis
RAD	radiation absorbed dose
RBC	red blood cell
RCW	removable cast walkers
RDW	red (cell) distribution width
RES	resection
	Resident
REM	rapid eye movement
	Roentgen equivalent man
RF	rheumatoid factor
Rh	Rhesus factor in blood
RICE	rest, ice, compression, and elevation
RIG	rabies immune globin
RLE	right lower extremity
RLQ	right lower quadrant
R/O	rule out
ROM	range of motion
ROS	review of symptoms
RPR	rapid plasma regain (test for syphilis)
	rotating podiatric residency
RR	recovery room
R&R	rate and rhythm
	recession and resection
RRR	regular rhythm and rate
RSB	right sternal border
RSD	reflex sympathetic dystrophy
RSTL	relaxed skin tension lines
RT	right
RTA	road traffic accident

RTC	return to clinic
RTx	radiation treatment
RUQ	right upper quadrant
RVU	relative value units
Rx	drug
	medication
	pharmacy
	prescription
	radiotherapy
RXN	reaction
S	subjective findings
s̄	without
SA	*Staphylococcus aureus*
SACH	solid ankle cushion heel
SAD	supination-adduction
SAS	San Antonio Shoes (commercially available extra depth shoes)
SATU	surgical Achilles tendon unit
SBE	subacute bacterial endocarditis
SBR	strict bed rest
SC	service connected
SDS	same day surgery
SER	supination-external rotation
SGA	small gestational age
SGOT	serum glutamic oxaloacetic transaminase
SGPT	serum glutamic pyruvic transaminase
SH	social history
	surgical history
SHIP	Sgarlato Hammertoe Implant Prosthesis
SIDS	sudden infant death syndrome
Sig.	let it be labeled ("signa")
SIS	small intestinal submucosa
SKAO	supracondylar knee–ankle orthosis
SLB	short leg brace
SLC	short leg cast
SLCC	short leg cylinder cast
SLE	systemic lupus erythematosus
SLNWBC	short leg non–weight-bearing cast
SLS	short leg splint
SLWC	short leg walking cast
SMA	sequence multiple analyzer (see CHEM)
SNF	skilled nursing facility
SNS	sterile normal saline
SNT	Suppan nail technique
SOA	swelling of ankle
SOAP	subjective, objective, assessment, and plan
SOB	shortness of breath
S/P	status post
SPG	scrotopenogram
S-PIN	Steinmann pin
SPVPFT	subpapillary venous plexus filling time

SQ	subcutaneous
SR	sedimentation rate
SS	super strength
SS#	social security number
S&S	signs and symptoms
SSD	silver sulfadiazine (Silvadene)
SSN	Social Security Number
SSSI	skin and skin structure infection
SSTI	skin and soft-tissue infection
STAT	immediately ("statim")
STATT	split tibialis anterior tendon transfer
STD	sexually transmitted diseases
STG	split-thickness graft
STJ	subtalar joint
SubQ	subcutaneous
SVS WIfI	Society for Vascular Surgery Wound, Ischemia, and foot Infection classification system
SWHT	Sussman Wound Healing Tool
Sx	signs
	surgery
	symptoms
T	temperature
T3	triiodothyronine
T4	thyroxine
TAC	triamcinolone cream
TAL	tendon Achilles lengthening
TAR	total ankle replacement
TATT	tibialis anterior tendon transfer
T-berg	Trendelenburg
TBW	tension-band wiring
T&C	type and cross
TCC	total contact cast
TCOM	transcutaneous oxygen monitor
TCP	transcutaneous pacing
$TcPco_2$	transcutaneous carbon dioxide
$TcPO_2$	transcutaneous oxygen
	tenotomy and capsulotomy
Td	tetanus and diphtheria toxoid
TENS	transcutaneous electrical nerve stimulation
TEV	talipes equinovarus
TF	to follow
TIA	transient ischemic attack
TIBC	total iron-binding capacity
tid	three times a day ("ter in die")
TIME	Tissue, Infection, Moisture, Edge
TLS	tiny little sucker (drain)
TMA	transmetatarsal amputation
TMC	triamcinolone
TMP-SMX	trimethoprim–sulfamethoxazole
TMT	tarsometatarsal

T&N	tingling and numbness
TNM	tumor, nodes, and metastasis
TOB	tobacco
TOC	treatment of choice
TP	thrombophlebitis
	total protein
TROM	total range of motion
TSA	type-specific antibody
TSH	thyroid-stimulating hormone
TSP	total serum protein
TTT	total tourniquet time
	turgor, texture, temperature
TURB	transurethral resection of bladder
TURP	transurethral resection of prostate
Tx	treatment
T&X	type and cross
UA	urinalysis
UGPF	ultrasound-guided plantar fasciotomy
Ung	unguentum (ointment)
USSC	United States Surgical Corporation
UTI	urinary tract infection
VA	Veterans Administration
VAN	vein, artery, and nerve
V&D	vomiting and diarrhea
VDRL	Venereal Disease Research Laboratory (test for syphilis)
VISA	vancomycin intermediate-resistant *Staphylococcus aureus*
VLDL	very low-density lipoprotein
VO	verbal orders
VRE	vancomycin-resistant *enterococci*
VREF	vancomycin-resistant *Enterococcus faecium*
VRSA	vancomycin-resistant *Staphylococcus aureus*
VS	vital signs
VSEF	vancomycin-susceptible *Enterococcus faecium*
VV	varicose veins
WA	with assistance
WB	weight bearing
	whole blood
WBC	white blood cell
WBTT	weight bearing to tolerance
WD	wet dressing
WDWN	well developed and well nourished
3-WEA	wetting, emulsifying, antiseptic (solution for softening calluses)
WHO	World Health Organization
WIfI	Wound, Ischemia, and foot Infection classification system
WNL	within normal limits
W-T-D	wet to dry
WWAC	walk with aid of cane
$\bar{x}$	except
XIP	x-ray in plaster
XOP	x-ray out of plaster

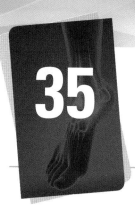

35   GLOSSARY

Adactyly Congenital absence of a digit.

Albright syndrome A polyostotic fibrous dysplasia with an associated endocrine abnormality. Clinical signs include café au lait spots and precocious puberty.

Allodynia Pain produced by a non-noxious stimulus.

Amniotic bands (Streeter bands) A partial or complete ring-like constriction around one of the limbs of the fetus during development caused by early rupture of the amnion, with the chorion remaining intact.

Anatomic neck Thinnest part of the metatarsal where the shaft meets the head, located proximal to the surgical head.

Anesthesia Loss of sensation.

Antistaphylococcal penicillins A group of penicillins also called penicillinase-resistant penicillins active against G(+), especially staph. This group includes cloxacillin, dicloxacillin, methicillin, nafcillin, and oxacillin.

Atelectasis Incomplete expansion of the lungs, collapse of alveoli. This is the number one reason for post-op fever.

Athetosis Repetitive, involuntary, slow, sinuous, writhing movements, especially severe in the hands.

Arthrocentesis Aspiration of a joint.

Axonotmesis Injury to an axon that results in Wallerian degeneration. The nerve can regenerate over time.

Bassett lesion A lesion on the anterior dorsal lateral aspect of the articular cartilage of the talus caused by rubbing from a hypertrophic anterior inferior tibiofibular ligament (<u>Bassett ligament</u>).

Bell palsy Sudden paralysis on one side of the face. Named after the physician who first described it. In the majority of patients, there is a preceding condition such as stress, fatigue, or a common cold. The disorder involves the 7th cranial nerve and the facial muscles it supplies. Patients usually recover completely within several months.

Bifurcate ligament A "Y" shaped ligament that originates on the anterior dorsal calcaneus. One arm of the inserts on the navicular and the other to the cuboid.

Blair fusion An ankle fusion salvage procedure used when the talar body is missing or cannot be salvaged. Consists of an anterior sliding tibial graft into the head of the talus.

BMI (body mass index) BMI is used as a screening tool to determine body fat percentage to indicate whether a person is underweight, overweight, or obese. Also referred to as Quetelet index.

BMI	Classification
<18.5	Underweight
18.5–24.9	Normal weight
25.0–29.9	Overweight
30.0–34.9	Class I obesity
35.0–39.9	Class II obesity
≥40.0	Class III obesity

BMI = pounds/inches^2 × 703
BMI + kilograms/meters^2

Bovie Electrocautery.

Brodie abscess A foci of bone destruction caused by osteomyelitis filled with pus or connective tissue.

Capsulorrhaphy Suturing of a joint capsule.

Carcinoma A malignant tumor arising from epidermis or visceral organ cells and tends to give rise to metastases.

Causalgia A burning pain due to a specific peripheral nerve.

Cervical ligament A very strong ligament that originates on the anterior superior surface of the calcaneus and inserts into the neck of the talus. This ligament helps resist inversion at the subtalar joint.

Charcot triad A symptom of MS consisting of nystagmus, intention tremor, scanning speech (syllables are separated by pauses).

Cheyne–stokes respirations Repeating cycle of gradual increase in depth of breathing followed by gradual decrease in depth of breathing until apnea occurs. Seen in CNS disorders and uremia.

Chopart joint The midtarsal joint.

Chvostek sign A clinical test to diagnose increased blood calcium levels. A light tap on the facial nerve will cause the facial muscles to contract.

Cicatrix Scar.

Clavus A corn on the toe.

Clinodactyly Congenital curly toe.

Coleman block test Determines whether a rearfoot varus deformity is flexible or rigid. The patient is placed on a wooden block 1 inch thick such that the entire foot is standing on the block, except the medial forefoot. In a flexible rearfoot varus, the 1st metatarsal will plantarflex down to the ground and the rearfoot varus will evert into a corrected position. Differentiates between a structural varus and a varus created by a plantarflexed 1st ray.

Constitutional symptoms
Symptoms that are indicative
of disorders of the whole body.
Symptoms involving more than
one body system (i.e., fever,
chills, weight loss, excessive
sweating).

Crescent sign The early sign
of avascular necrosis, which
represents a subchondral fracture
through the insertion of the
individual trabeculae.

Crista A ridge in the plantar
articular surface of the 1st
metatarsal head that separates
the sesamoids.

Crowe sign Axillary freckling,
pathognomonic for von
Recklinghausen disease.

Cyma line A smooth "S"
configuration formed by the
talonavicular and calcaneocuboid
joints seen on a lateral x-ray.
In the ideal foot, the cyma line
is intact. With a pronated foot
the cyma, line is anteriorly
displaced, meaning that the
talonavicular joint is anterior
to the calcaneocuboid joint
and does not follow a nice "S"
shape. With a supinated foot, the
talonavicular joint is posteriorly
displaced.

Cytochrome P450 Cytochrome
P450 constitutes a family of
enzymes that metabolize a
variety of endogenous and
exogenous substances in the
liver, most notably drugs. The
450 comes from the fact that they
maximally absorb light at 450 nm
wavelength. The significance of
the enzyme comes from the fact
that many drugs may be largely
dependent on a single form of
P450 for their metabolism in the
liver. If the enzyme is actively
metabolizing a particular drug
and another drug is administered
that relies on the same for P450
for its metabolism, the drug may
reach toxic levels at relatively low
doses.

Dancer's fracture A 5th metatarsal
diaphyseal (shaft) fracture.

Desiccate To dry out.

Diastasis Dislocation or
separation of two normally
attached bones.

Dolor Pain, one of the classic signs
of inflammation.

Dosimeter A device used to
measure radiation exposure. May
be a small badge worn on medical
personnel to monitor exposure in
surgery.

Down syndrome (a.k.a. trisomy 21)
An autosomal abnormality with
mental retardation. Classic facial
features include an epicanthal
fold, thick lips, large tongue
with deep furrows, and a small
nose with a broad bridge.
Other features may include a
broad short neck, clinodactyly
of the 5th finger, syndactyly,
polydactyly, and a simian line
(a single transverse palmer
crease).

Dyspareunia Painful sexual
intercourse.

Dysphagia Difficulty swallowing.

Eburnation The final end product
of bone sclerosis and is sometimes used as a term that is
synonymous with bone sclerosis.

Ecchymosis Bruise.

Ectrodactyly "Lobster claw" foot.

Ehlers–Danlos syndrome Collagen
and elastic tissues are abnormal,

resulting in thin, easily stretched hyperelastic skin. Ligamentous laxity, resulting in flat feet, genu valgus, congenital hip dislocation, and scoliosis. Aortic aneurysm is common.

Endoneurium The interstitial connective tissue in a peripheral nerve, surrounds a single nerve fiber.

Enthesitis Inflammation of the entheses, the site where a tendon or ligament attaches to bone.

Enthesopathy Disorder involving the attachment of a ligament or tendon to bone.

Epineurium The sheath of a peripheral nerve.

ESBLs ESBLs stands are extended-spectrum β-lactamases. ESBLs are enzymes produced by some bacteria, most notably *E. coli* and *Klebsiella*, that make them more resistant to certain antibiotics.

Eschar Scab.

Fibrous dysplasia An abnormal bone growth where normal bone is replaced with fibrous bone tissue. Radiographically, it is often described as having a ground-glass appearance. Causes abnormal swelling and expansion of the bone.

Fistula Abnormal communication between two hollow, epithelialization organs or between a hollow organ and the exterior (skin).

Foley Bladder catheter.

Foot drop Failure to raise the foot during the swing phase of gait. Often results in a "slapping" gait. Causes may include CVA, trauma, CMT, polio, Friedreich ataxia, infection, spinal tumor/lesion, Guillain–Barré syndrome, Dejerine–Sottas syndrome.

Genu valgum Knock knees, often seen in obese female children.

Genu varum Bowleg, may be associated with rickets, abnormal Ca and Ph metabolism, or Blount disease.

Gigli saw A bone saw that consists of a flexible roughened wire used to cut through bone.

Gower sign A classic sign of pseudohypertrophic muscular dystrophy. Because of muscle weakness, patients raise themselves to the standing position by crawling up their legs.

Grey Baby Syndrome A type of circulatory collapse that can occur from high levels of the antibiotic chloramphenicol. It is a result of circulatory collapse characterized by ashy skin, abdominal distention, vomiting, flaccidity, and death

Hallux interphalangeus Also called hallux valgus interphalangeus. This is lateral deviation of the hallux caused by an increased hallux abductus interphalangeus angle. It looking like a bunion but does not involve the 1st metatarsophalangeal joint.

Hanging heel sign Used in the diagnosis of metatarsus adductus, the deformity persists as viewed plantarly when the foot is lifted by the toes.

Hawkins sign A subchondral radiolucent band in the proximal talus. This indicates bone resorption and revascularization following AVN.

Heloma durum Hard corn over the top of the toe.

Heloma molle Soft corn found between the toes.

Hematemesis Vomiting of blood.

Hematoma Accumulation of blood within the tissue, which clots to form a solid swelling.

Hemoptysis Coughing up blood.

Hoffa sign Seen in calcaneal fractures. The tuber fragment displaces superiorly, relaxing the triceps and decreasing its plantarflexory power.

Hoke tonsil The fat plug in the sinus tarsi that is removed during sinus tarsi surgery.

Homan sign Calf pain with forced dorsiflexion of the foot. Indicative of venous thrombosis.

Homocystinuria Clinically very similar to Marfan syndrome, except that the patients are mentally retarded and excrete large amounts of homocysteine in their urine.

Hubscher maneuver When the hallux is dorsiflexed during WB, the arch will rise due to the windlass mechanism if no osseous restrictions are present. Also called Jack test.

Hunting response A secondary vasodilation response that occurs after prolonged vasoconstriction due to cold application. The purpose of this response is to prevent tissue damage.

Hyperalgesia Excessive sensitiveness to pain.

Hyperesthesia Increased sensation.

Hyperpathia Abnormally exaggerated subjective response to pain.

Hypesthesia Hypoesthesia.

Hypoesthesia Decreased sensation.

Ichthyosis Abnormal cornification of the skin, resulting in dryness, roughness, and scaliness. Results from hypertrophy of the horny layer resulting from excessive production of keratin.

Icterus Jaundice.

Induration Abnormal hardening of a tissue or organ.

Islet of Langerhans A type of tissue found scattered throughout the pancreas, involved in glucose metabolism. The islet of Langerhans contains α, β, and δ cells. The β cells compose about 60% of all the cells and secrete insulin.

Jack test Another name for the Hubscher maneuver.

Jones compression dressing The Robert Jones dressing is a thick, well-padded dressing. The firm even distribution of pressure is used to prevent or treat edema.

Kelikian test Tests whether or not the MPJ is reducible. Push up on the plantar surface of the metatarsal head and see if the toe straightens out.

Kussmaul respiration Deep, rapid respiratory pattern seen in coma or diabetic ketoacidosis.

Kyphosis Excessive primary curvature of the thoracic spine (hunch back), associated with aging, especially in women.

Lachman test Tests ligament stability in the MPJ by attempting to pop the metatarsal head out of the joint. Greater than 2-mm displacement is a positive test.

Lasègue test Also called the straight leg raise. This tests for a herniated disk in the back. Patient lying supine knees straight. Patient raises each leg, pain is a positive test.

Lemont nerve Intermediate dorsal cutaneous nerve.

Levine sign Classic sign of angina or MI, clenching of the fist and placing the fist over the chest.

Lister corn Painful corn that develops in the lateral nail groove of the 5th toe from the varus rotation of the phalanx.

Lordosis Excessive secondary curvature of the lumbar spine (sway back), often seen during pregnancy.

Maceration A white soggy appearance that the skin takes on after tissue is soaked. The connective tissue fibers are dissolved so that the tissue components can be teased apart. Often noted between the toes.

Marfan syndrome An autosomal dominant primary collagen defect resulting in a very tall and slender person. Clinical symptoms include arachnodactyly, hyperextensibility, muscle myotonia, joint dislocation, severe pes planus, scoliosis, lens subluxation, genu recurvatum, and aortic dilation with aneurysm.

Master knot of Henry An area in the rearfoot where the tendons of the flexor hallucis longus and the flexor digitorum longus cross. There is a thick band of connective tissue covering the tendons at this point and binding them to the navicular.

Marjolin ulcer A squamous cell carcinoma that arises in a chronic sinus due to osteomyelitis.

McGill pain index A pain scale based on comparing different diseases against each other. For example, RSD/CRPS is rated higher than chronic back pain.

Melorheostosis A flowing hyperostosis resembling dripping candle wax seen on x-ray of long bones.

Mercurochrome A weak antibacterial agent. Not recommended because it tends to dry out the wound and has been associated with contact dermatitis and aplastic anemia.

Metatarsalgia General nonspecific term referring to pain located in the ball of the foot. DDx includes stress fx, synovitis, capsulitis, tendinitis, neuroma, bursitis, IPK, foreign body, DJD, arthritis, tumor, and infection.

Metatarsus primus varus Clinical appearance is similar to metatarsus adductus, but only the 1st metatarsal is adducted and the IM is increased to >15°.

Metatarsus varus Metatarsus adductus with a varus component (often confused with clubfoot).

Methylparaben An antifungal agent often used as a preservative in local anesthetics.

MIC (minimum inhibitory concentration) Found on a C&S lab report, the MIC is the lowest concentration of the antibiotic needed to treat the cultured organism. The lower this value, the less antibiotic was required to kill the organism and, therefore, the more appropriate the antibiotic is.

Morton foot Short 1st ray.

Mosaicplasty Transplantation of cartilage and bone by way of a plug to fill a defect caused by osteochondritis dissecans.

Multiple myeloma (plasma cell myeloma) A malignancy beginning in the plasma cells of the bone marrow. Plasma cells normally produce antibodies to help destroy germs and protect against infection. With myeloma, this function becomes impaired, and the body produces anomalous immunoglobulins (Bence Jones protein), which are ineffective against infections. Symptoms include skeletal pain (especially in the back and thorax), renal failure, and recurrent bacterial infections.

Myasthenia gravis An autoimmune disorder of neuromuscular transmission involving the production of autoantibodies directed against the nicotinic acetylcholine (ACh) receptors. Women are affected twice as much as men. Symptoms include fatigable weakness and ocular problems (ptosis, diplopia, drooping eyelids). There is also often dysphagia and breathing difficulty. Treatment involves anticholinesterase drugs and thymectomy.

Neuralgia Pain in a nerve or along the course of one or more nerve.

Neurapraxia Bruising of a nerve with resulting numbness. Numbness is reversible (Seddon classification).

Neurectomy Excision of part of a nerve.

Neurofibromatosis (von Recklinghausen dz) A familial condition characterized by nervous system, muscles, bones, and skin changes. Occurs in about 1 in 3,000 people. Clinically, two of the following must be present to establish the diagnosis:

1. Six or more café au lait spots >15 mm in diameter, or >5 mm in the prepubertal patient
2. Two neurofibromas of any type or one plexiform neurofibroma
3. Axillary or inguinal freckling
4. Optic glioma
5. Two or more Lisch nodules in the iris
6. Distinctive osseous lesions (such as pseudoarthrosis)
7. A first-degree relative with neurofibromatosis type 1

Neurolysis Freeing up of a nerve.

Neurorrhaphy Nerve repair, suturing of a cut nerve.

Neurotmesis Complete severance of the nerve that is irreversible.

Neutral triangle The neutral triangle is an area of sparse trabeculation in the calcaneus. This triangle lies just inferior to the anterior edge of the posterior talar articular facet.

No-touch technique A surgical technique where K-wires are driven into surrounding bone and bend outwardly to clear soft tissue from the operative site. There is no retraction of the soft tissues necessary, with the exception of the initial placement of the K-wires. This technique is used a lot with surgeries with a precarious soft tissue envelops, such as Pilon and calcaneal fracture. Note that Allgöwer–Donati stitches are also recommended with these areas of friable tissue.

Nosocomial Originating in a hospital. Also, called "hospital-acquired infection" (HAI).

Odynophagia Painful swallowing.

Orthotist A person skilled in orthotics and their application.

Orthotripsy A treatment for plantar fasciitis whereby sound waves cause injury to the tissue in the area, thereby causing them to heal themselves and reducing the inflammation that created the pain. One machine available is called the OssaTron.

Osteoblast A bone cell associated with bone production.

Osteoclast A bone cell associated with bone destruction.

Osteomalacia A condition marked by softening of the bones with pain, tenderness, muscular weakness, and loss of weight resulting from a deficiency of vitamin D and calcium.

Osteoporosis A decrease in bone mass.

Paget disease A focal disorder of bone metabolism in which all the elements of bone remodeling are increased, resulting in bony enlargement and deformities. The condition is often asymptomatic, although pain and stiffness may develop. Symptoms include an enlarged skull, bowing of the long bones, and pathologic fractures.

Pantalar fusion A triple arthrodesis plus an ankle fusion.

Parabens Parabens (i.e., methylparaben) are used as preservatives in various pharmaceutical preparations, such as wound care products and local anesthetics. Parabens have been shown to be sensitizing agents and may cause allergic reactions in some patients.

Paralysis Loss of function.

Paresis Slight or incomplete paralysis.

Paresthesia Abnormal sensation.

Pedorthist A person skilled in the design, manufacture, fit, and modification of shoes and related foot appliances.

Percutaneous Performed through the skin.

Perineurium Surrounds a bundle of nerve fibers (fascicle).

Peroneus quartus An accessory muscle that originates from the peroneus brevis muscle and inserts into the retrotrochlear eminence of the calcaneus. Origin and insertion vary widely. Prevalence also varies widely from 6% to 20%. It may cause chronic ankle pain, swelling, and instability. For symptomatic cases, excision of the treatment of choice.

Polymethylmethacrylate (PMMA) A polymeric self-curing acrylic cement used as a mechanical filler to hold implanted prosthesis in position. This bone cement helps disperse mechanical stresses over a wider area. In addition to fixating prosthetics, PMMA can also be mixed with powdered antibiotics and rolled into "beads" for infected bone. The antibiotic should be broad spectrum, low allergenic, heat stable, and have the ability to leech from the cement. Aminoglycosides, such as tobramycin and gentamicin, fill these criteria and are often used. Antibiotics are mixed at a concentration of at least 500 mg, but no >1,000 mg per packet of cement.

Popliteal trifurcation Where the popliteal vein splits into the anterior tibial vein, posterior tibial vein, and peroneal vein. Located posteroinferior to the knee.

Porta pedis Entrance to the vault of the foot, the abductor hallucis comprises the floor and the quadratus plantae makes up the roof.

Prosthetist The field of substituting artificial parts for missing body parts, such as adding fillers to shoes of patients with amputations.

Pseudoequinus In a cavus deformity, the ankle appears to have less dorsiflexion because heel-off occurs earlier in the gait cycle from the plantarflexed nature of the forefoot in a cavus foot.

Pseudohypertrophy An apparent increase in size of certain muscles without true hypertrophy, the apparent muscle bulk is actually fat deposits. May be seen in the calves in certain types of muscular dystrophy.

Pseudomembranous colitis A superinfection of *Clostridium difficile* usually caused by antibiotics, most notably chloramphenicol. Treatment is with oral metronidazole or oral vancomycin. Vancomycin is not orally absorbed, so it has few oral indications. Because *C. difficile* is infecting the gut, it is effective against this type of infection.

Pyrexia A fever, or febrile condition.

Radiculopathy Impingement of the sciatic nerve within the spinal canal.

Radiolucent Black areas on a radiograph.

Radiopaque White areas on a radiograph.

Resupination test Have patient stand on tiptoes and see if the medial longitudinal arch develops.

Reye syndrome CNS and hepatic complication of influenza infection. Usually occurs about 4 to 6 days after a viral infection, and although the exact pathophysiology is uncertain, there seems to be a relation to children given aspirin. Symptoms include nausea, vomiting, and altered mental status consistent with encephalopathy. Cerebral edema is usually the main cause of death.

Rickets A condition due to vitamin D deficiency, especially in children. Signs include disturbances in normal ossification such as bowing of the legs and trumpeting of the metaphysis and epiphysis.

Rinne test An auditory test to compare air conduction with bone conduction. A tuning fork handle is placed on the mastoid process; when the sound can no longer be heard, the tuning fork is placed in front of the ear. Normally, the patient will be able to hear the tuning fork when it is held in front of the ear; in a patient with a conductive hearing loss, they will not hear the tuning fork when it is held by the ear.

Romberg test Tests position sense or cerebellar function. Patient stands feet together, and the arms outstretched with palms up. The patient is tapped by the examiner with eyes open and closed. A positive test is loss of balance.

Rubor Redness, classic sign of inflammation.

Sarcoma A highly malignant tumor made up of mesenchymal-supportive tissue (muscle, bone, cartilage, and tendon).

Saucerization The process of making a shallow "saucer-like" depression in a bone and/or skin ulcer. It allows the wound to drain freely without the threat of abscess formation. It is also used when removing a spur to compensate for scaring or bony regrowth that may occur.

Schober test A 10 cm length is measured along the erect lower lumbar spine; the patient bends forward. This measurement should increase by at least 4 cm. This test is positive in ankylosing spondylitis.

Sclerotic An increase in the density of bone.

Scurvy A disease due to deficiency of vitamin C marked by anemia, spongy bleeding gums, and brawny induration of calf and leg muscles.

Silfverskiold test Tests for gastrocnemius. Passive dorsiflexion of the ankle is measured with the knee extended and then with the knee flexed. If this value increases, there is an equinus due to a tight gastroc because the gastroc crosses the knee joint and the soleus does not.

Sinus tarsi An anatomic tunnel between the sulcus calcanei (on the calcaneus) and the sulcus tali (on the talus). The sinus tarsi is larger laterally and located between the posterior and middle facet of the calcaneus. The artery of the tarsal canal enters medially, and the artery of the sinus tarsi enters laterally.

Sinus tarsi syndrome Subacute or chronic pain on the lateral aspect of the sinus tarsi often following an inversion injury. Pain is elicited on ROM of the STJ and palpation laterally at the entrance of the sinus tarsi. Treatment includes steroid injections into the sinus tarsi or surgery to remove the fat plug (Hoke tonsil) in the sinus tarsi.

Somogyi effect A rebound phenomenon occurring in diabetics who take too much insulin in the evening, resulting in hyperglycemia in the AM. When a patient is given too much insulin at night, the body responds by releasing epinephrine, ACTH, glucagon, and growth hormones, which stimulate lipolysis, gluconeogenesis, and glycogenolysis, which, in turn, result in a rebound hyperglycemia when the patient wakes up in the morning.

Sphygmomanometer A device consisting of a blood pressure cuff with a pressure gauge on it used to take blood pressure.

Splay foot A foot type having a 1st IM angle of >12°, and a 4th and 5th metatarsal angle of >8°.

Stenosis Narrowing of a passage or opening.

Sudeck atrophy Posttraumatic painful osteoporosis. Associated with CRPS/RSD.

Surgical neck Part of the metatarsal neck located in the metaphyseal bone distal to the anatomic neck.

Tarsal canal Same as the sinus tarsi.

Telangiectasia A vascular lesion formed by dilation of capillaries that result in irregular clusters of red lines that blanch when pressed.

Tetralogy of Fallot A condition with pulmonary stenosis or atresia, intraventricular septal defect, right ventricular hypertrophy, and dextroposition of the aorta. It is the most common cause of cyanotic congenital heart disease.

Thalamic fragment A fracture fragment in a calcaneal fracture that contains the posterior articular facet.

Thalassemia A hereditary group of hemolytic anemias marked by a decrease in production of hemoglobin.

Tinel sign Tingling that radiates distally along the course of the involved nerve with percussion of the tarsal tunnel.

Tomography Any imaging technique resulting in sections or sectioning through the body such as MRI or CT.

Trendelenburg position Patient positioned with head lower than feet.

Triplane fracture This fracture is basically a Salter–Harris IV fracture that changes from the sagittal plane to the transverse at the physis to the coronal plane proximally. A fracture occurs in the distal tibia of a child whose growth plate is still open.

Turgor Poor skin turgor is a sign of fluid loss or dehydration. It can be tested by pinching and holding the skin for several seconds and noting if it rebounds back, and how long it takes to rebound back to its original shape.

Turk test Used as part of the diagnosis for tarsal tunnel syndrome. Determines whether the nerve is entrapped/compressed due to varicosities. Test is positive if symptoms increase once a tourniquet is inflated above venous pressure but below arterial pressure proximal to the site of suspected entrapment. Pain increased because the venae comitantes become engorged and cause pressure on the tibial nerve.

Valleix sign Tingling that radiates proximally along the course of the involved nerve with percussion of the tarsal tunnel.

Vamp disease A condition in which the vamp of the shoe causes irritation most commonly at the dorsal base of the hallux, resulting in a painful lesion or callus to develop.

Vasa vasorum Venous system around a nerve.

Virchow node (signal node) A palpable left supraclavicular lymph node often associated with gastrointestinal neoplasm such as pancreatic or gastric carcinoma.

Virchow triad Three factors that are commonly associated with the formation on thrombi: stasis, blood vessel injury, and hypercoagulability.

Volkmann contracture Contracture of the toes as a result of ischemia from an untreated compartment syndrome.

Volkmann fracture (fragment) An avulsion fracture of the posterior malleoli.

Watershed area Refers to an area that has poor blood supply. Most notably the Achilles tendon at a point 2 to 6 cm proximal to the insertion.

Weber test An auditory test to compare bone conduction of the two ears. Place a tuning fork firmly against the center of the patient's forehead. Ask the patient if they hear the sound more in the right ear, the left ear, or in the middle of their head.

Wernicke–Korsakoff syndrome A neuropsychiatric disorder due to thiamine deficiency usually due to alcohol abuse. Combining the features of Wernicke encephalopathy (confusion, gait ataxia, eye movement problems) and Korsakoff syndrome (amnestic component).

Wet-to-dry Damp gauze dressing placed on wound and removed after the dressing dries, providing debridement of the wound upon removal of the gauze.

Wolff law Final bone morphology is determined by the forces acting on it. Bone develops the structure, lamellae, and trabeculae, most suited to resist the forces acting on it. Areas of increased force are thicker, and areas of decreased force are thinner.

Xeroform Wound dressing with 3% bismuth tribromophenate in a petroleum base.

INDEX

Murphy procedure, 473
Muscles
  abductor digiti minimi quinti, 23
  abductor hallucis, 22, 25
  dorsal interossei, 26–27
  extensor digitorum brevis, 22
  extensor digitorum longus, 20, 377
  extensor hallucis longus, 20
  flexor digiti minimi, 25–26
  flexor digitorum brevis, 23
  flexor digitorum longus, 21
  flexor hallucis brevis, 24–25
  flexor hallucis longus, 21–22, 377, 378
  gastrocnemius, 21, 377
  lumbricals, 24
  peroneus brevis, 20–21
  peroneus longus, 20
  peroneus longus and brevis, 378
  peroneus tertius, 20
  plantar interossei, 26
  plantaris, 21
  popliteus, 21
  quadratus plantae, 24
  soleus, 21, 377, 378
  tibialis anterior, 20, 377
  tibialis posterior, 21, 377, 378
Muscular dystrophies, 466–469
Myasthenia gravis, 585
Mycelex, 30
Mycifradin, 54
Mycobacterium bovis, 71
Mycobacterium leprae, 71
Mycobacterium tuberculosis, 71
Mycobacterium ulcerans, 71
Mycology
  cutaneous mycosis, 75
  dermatophytes, 75
  opportunistic fungi, 77
  subcutaneous mycosis, 76
  superficial mycosis, 75–76
  systemic mycosis, 76–77
Myelin, 94
Myeloma, 207
Myositis ossificans, 288–289
Myotomes, 97–98

N

Nafcillin, 51
Naftifine, 30
Naftin, 30
Nail bed, 14

Nail curette, 342
Nail, IM, 366
Nail length, 382
Nails
  anatomy, 273
  chemical matrixectomy, 275–276
  pathology, 273–275
  subungual exostosis, 279
  surgical matrixectomies, 276–279
Naloxone, 34
Naltrexone, 34
Naproxen, 37
National Pressure Ulcer Advisory Panel (NPUAP), 253
Natural penicillins, 51
Nebcin, 54
Nebupent, 54
Necrobiosis lipoidica diabeticorum, 241
Needle holder, 343
Needles, 349
Negative-pressure wound therapy (NPWT), 265–266, 333
Neisseria gonorrhoeae, 71
Neisseria meningitidis, 71
Neisseriaceae, 71
Nelaton line, 439
Neomycin, 54
Neosporin, 48
Nerve conduction velocity (NCV), 106–107
Nerve tissue origin, 290–291
Nerve to the abductor digiti quinti muscle, 282
Nerves, 2
  anatomy, 94–95
  anterior femoral cutaneous, 99
  Baxter's, 5
  blocks, nerve, 96–99
    ankle block, 96
    Bier block, 96–97
    digital block, 96
    hallux block, 96
    local infiltration, 96
    Mayo block, 96
    mini-Mayo block, 96
    popliteal block, 96
  common dorsal digital nerve, 5
  common peroneal, 5, 376
  common plantar digital, 5
  communicating branch, 5
  cranial, 2